AF608845

Consultation–Liaison Psychiatry

1990 and Beyond

Consultation–Liaison Psychiatry
1990 and Beyond

Edited by

Hoyle Leigh
University of California, San Francisco
Fresno, California

SPRINGER SCIENCE+BUSINESS MEDIA, LLC

Library of Congress Cataloging-in-Publication Data

Consultation-liaison psychiatry : 1990 and beyond / edited by Hoyle Leigh.
p. cm.
Includes updated presentations at a workshop held May 1992 in Washington, D.C.
Includes bibliographical references and index.
ISBN 978-0-306-44725-9 ISBN 978-1-4615-2588-2 (eBook)
DOI 10.1007/978-1-4615-2588-2
1. Consultation-liaison psychiatry. I. Leigh, Hoyle, 1942-
[DNLM: 1. Psychiatry--trends--congresses. 2. Referral and Consultation--utilization--congresses. 3. Referral and Consultation--trends--congresses. WM 64 C7577 1994]
RC455.2.C65C663 1994
616.89--dc20
DNLM/DLC
for Library of Congress 94-16824
CIP

Proceedings of a workshop on Changes in Consultation–Liaison Psychiatry, held May 1992, in Washingtion, D.C.

ISBN 978-0-306-44725-9

Originally published by Plenum Press, New York in 1994

FOR VINNIE AND ALEXANDER

PREFACE

The essential role of the psychiatrist as consultant and educator of primary care physicians is increasing in importance as the American health care system faces fundamental restructuring. In a recent workshop during the annual meeting of the American Psychiatric Association, a number of prominent consultation-liaison psychiatrists reviewed major developments in consultation-liaison psychiatry during the past decade and looked toward the future. This book is based on these presentations, but it is not simply a proceedings book. A number of additional experts have contributed important chapters, and all the chapters based on the presentations are expanded and updated. Thus, this book reviews the current state of consultation-liaison psychiatry and anticipates future challenges. It also informs the reader about the state-of-the-art knowledge and skills in consultation-liaison psychiatry as of 1994.

This book should be a valuable up-to-date overview/refresher for both consultation-liaison psychiatrists and general psychiatrists who wish to update and formulate his/her consultant role. It should be especially valuable for psychiatric residents for whom the role as consultant to primary physicians assumes increasing importance, and for primary physicians and medical students who are interested in learning about commonly encountered complex biopsychosocial problems of their patients and integrating these dimensions in patient care.

I am grateful to Mary Safford and Eileen Bermingham of Plenum for their help with the preparation and production of this book. I am also thankful to Anita Shaw for her secretarial help.

Hoyle Leigh, M.D.
Fresno, California

CONTENTS

CONSULTATION-LIAISON PSYCHIATRY ON THE THRESHOLD OF A NEW CENTURY

Hoyle Leigh, M.D.

Professor and Vice Chairman
Department of Psychiatry
University of California, San Francisco
Director of Psychiatry, Fresno Division
Chief of Psychiatry, Fresno VA Medical Center
2615 East Clinton Avenue
Fresno, CA 93703

INTRODUCTION

At a workshop of the annual meeting of the American Psychiatric Association in 1980, the author and a number of his colleagues explored the values and assumptions then prevalent in consultation-liaison (CL) settings. The mood was generally upbeat, and most participants had great hopes for the biopsychosocial model potentially becoming a shared value among all physicians (Engel, 1977; Leigh, Feinstein & Reiser, 1980). The panelists described various forms of integrative biopsychosocial approaches in teaching medical students and other trainees. They also noted major changes impacting the CL psychiatrist in the 1970's due to changes in health care reimbursement system, and in medical ethics with the advent of newer medical technologies, such as hemodialysis, open heart surgery, organ transplants, and life support systems.

CHANGES IN THE 1980'S

The 1980's saw an escalation in changes in general hospital psychiatry practice, largely influenced by changing reimbursement patterns, advances in psychopharmacotherapy, and the widespread use of computer programs. With the advent of Diagnosis Related Grouping (DRG) and managed care, cost containment has become as important a mission of health care systems as is the provision of optimal care. The heady days of 1960's and 1970's when it seemed that an ideal health care system could be built on the biopsychosocial model, leading to comprehensive and technologically advanced care for all patients, are now but faint memories for many of us. There was enthusiasm for primary care in the 1970's as there is now, but with much more idealism and with far less concerns about cost containment. Consultation-liaison programs were considered notoriously cost ineffective then, following closely the heels of consultation-liaison

Consultation-Liaison Psychiatry: 1990 and Beyond
Edited by H. Leigh, Plenum Press, New York, 1994

psychiatry of the 1950's that emphasized proselytizing psychodynamic understanding of patients to nonpsychiatric physicians, even though the biopsychosocial model was far easier to understand, to operationalize, and was demonstrably more effective. Consultation-liaison psychiatry survived the 1980's, miraculous as it may seem for some. The reason it survived owes much to the contributors to this volume and those like them --- who have explored new areas and innovative techniques of consultation-liaison psychiatry. They range from developing adequate funding sources for CL psychiatry, dealing with difficult and challenging ethical and legal decisions, developing innovative techniques of psychotherapy, developing innovative curriculum in medical psychiatry, consultation-liaison with pediatric populations, and developing computerized CL programs that facilitate teaching, research, and remuneration for consultation work.

Strain, Gise, and Fulop discussed several alternative funding for CL in 1989, i.e., 1. high risk screening, renal transplant, geriatric units (Medicare), 2. salary stipends from collaborating disciplines, e.g., medicine, 3. consultation fees, 4. ambulatory CL clinics (Medicaid), and 5. grants from collaborative research. Koran and the Stanford group recently proposed the utilization of psychiatric comorbidity in enhancing revenues by moving patients from lower-paying to higher-paying DRG's. They calculated that in 1989, such strategy would have resulted in screening 142 Medicare patients (2.2% of Medicare admissions) and discovering 25 patients with comorbid psychiatric conditions, generating $51,800 in incremental hospital revenue. They suggested negotiating with the hospital administration for added funding of the CL service from this revenue. In this volume, Strain et al. discuss in depth these and other issues related to the funding of consultation-liaison psychiatry.

Ethical and legal issues have become increasingly important in consultation-liaison psychiatry over the past two decades. Some of the traditional ethical issues with which consultation-liaison psychiatrists used to deal have now become moot because of a change in the way medicine is practiced - e.g., whether or not to tell a cancer patient that he has cancer that used to agonize so many physicians (Leigh, 1973) - failure to disclose a diagnosis to a patient would be unthinkable now! The advent of sophisticated life support systems has made it possible to prolong the life of a seriously ill patient indefinitely, regardless of the quality of life. Many patients, on the other hand, opt not to receive life-prolonging measures, and, in fact, choose to die, bringing many health care professionals' values into conflict. These value conflicts are found among and between patients, physicians, nursing staff, and the society in general. Tong and Van Dyke provide in their chapter a comprehensive discussion concerning such changes in ethical and legal climate and attendant issues.

Few medical syndromes are as important, complex, and mysterious as the chronic pain syndrome. Chronic pain is, perhaps, the paradigmatic biopsychosocial syndrome, the evaluation and treatment of which requires a close collaboration of the primary physician and the psychiatrist. Streltzer and Eliashof provide an insightful discussion of chronic pain utilizing vivid case illustrations. Streltzer then discusses the intricate relationship between chronic pain and narcotic addiction, and provides useful guidelines in treating addicted patients with chronic pain.

Chemical dependence has reached epidemic proportions in the 1980s and 1990s, and the addiction psychiatry has attained "added qualification" status by the American Board of Psychiatry and Neurology. Griffith provides an extensive overview of the phenomena of chemical dependences and their treatments, and the role of the consultation-liaison psychiatrist in addiction psychiatry.

Organic Mental Syndromes, dementia and delirium, continue to be the most common syndromes for which psychiatric consultation is sought. With the increase in the number of the elderly population, the recognition and treatment of patients with dementia is becoming an ever important task for physicians. Robert Hanowell reviews important recent developsments in understanding and treating the dementia syndrome. It is of note that Hanowell is a senior resident at the University of California, San Francisco-Fresno program, and has written this chapter as a resident project, which is a requirement of that training program. Preparing trainees to a lifetime of self-learning through critical reviews of literature and synthetic thinking is an important part of an innovative curriculum of UCSF-Fresno Psychiatry Program. Ahles provides a detailed description of this residency training program which emphasizes medical psychiatry as taught in a consultation-liaison setting.

Consultation-liaison psychiatry has been lagging in the development of newer techniques and skills in comparison to some other areas of psychiatry, such as neuropsychiatry and psychopharmacology. Nevertheless, better conceptualization and description of effective techniques used in consultation psychiatry, exemplified by the chapter by Eisendrath in this volume, are receiving deserved attention. If few newer techniques have arisen in CL psychiatry, the same cannot be said of "behavioral medicine", unfortunately and unjustly often associated with the discipline of psychology. The practitioners of behavioral medicine have brought forth into the field of medicine such newer techniques as biofeedback, relaxation training, guided imagery, autogenic training, etc. In many medical centers, there are two separate mental health systems, psychiatric consultation-liaison service, and the "behavioral medicine practitioners", that operate in parallel and, often, without much communication between them. The former is usually a part of the psychiatry department, and the latter are often employees of the specific nonpsychiatric departments or services, such as cardiology and pediatrics. These parallel services often duplicate work, are confusing to the consultees.

The multiaxial approach of the American Psychiatric Association's Diagnostic and Statistical Manual (DSM) III and III-R have helped reduce the psychiatric versus medical dichotomy in understanding patients' behavioral and physiologic dimensions. Leigh proposes that a new diagnostic category should be included in a future DSM that recognizes the importance of physical conditions that affect psychiatric conditions through mechanisms other than direct chemical effect to the brain as in organic mental syndromes.

On a more developmental vein, Fox reviews the field of pediatric consultation-liaison and the challenges for the future. Streltzer provides an insightful account of the development of a consultation-liaison service in Hawaii, against the backdrop of national trends.

Teaching is an integral and pre-eminent part of consultation-liaison psychiatry. In many institutions, the CL service is the only educational site that actually integrates the biopsychosocial dimensions of the patient in daily practice. It is no wonder, then, that many CL psychiatrists participate actively in the education of both medical students and psychiatric and nonpsychiatric residents. Two of the contributors to this volume, Leigh and Streltzer, are also residency training directors of their respective institutions, and all the contributors are active in medical student teaching.

During the past decade, computers have become an indispensable tool for most physicians. CL services are probably in the forefront of psychiatry in utilizing computers for various functions. An overview of computers in psychiatry is provided by Powsner, followed by two chapters by Leigh, and by Hammer and Strain, respectively, describing their specific computerized databases.

How have the consultation-liaison psychiatrists fared during the past decade? Of the original five panelists in the 1980 workshop, two have left academia but are still practicing CL psychiatry as a part of their private practice, two out of the three who still remain in academia have now taken up administrative positions while continuing teaching in CL services, and one is still actively heading up a CL service. One sees a similar trend throughout consultation-liaison psychiatry --- there is considerable mobility, but, on the whole, CL psychiatrists tend to continue to teach and practice CL psychiatry in their new settings.

Challenges for the 1990's and Beyond: Consultation-Liaison Psychiatry in the 21st Century

The challenges for consultation-liaison psychiatry for the nineties and beyond lie in the successful resolution of the following seeming paradoxes: the need for comprehensive care vs. cost containment; the need for intense education of all psychiatrists in CL vs. the thrust for subspeciality status for CL; the assimilation of advances in neuropharmacopsychiatry vs. the maintenance of the biopsychosocial model; the need for integration with behavioral medicine vs. the need to maintain physician identity for CL.

The educational role of the CL psychiatrist seems to be firmly established, and through him/her, physicians of the future will be at least exposed to the notion of comprehensive, biopsychosocial care. I have heretofore opposed subspecialty status for CL psychiatry, mainly because I felt that CL training should be a requirement of any general psychiatrist. It seems clear, however, that, for a number of political and administrative reasons, the thrust for its subspecialty status is gaining momentum. The challenge, then, would be the differentiation between what part of CL psychiatry is essential for general psychiatrists, and what specialized knowledge and techniques within CL psychiatry should be considered to be unique to the members of the subspecialty.

Modern consultation-liaison psychiatrists are, perhaps, at the vanguard of those who advocate re-medicalization and maintenance of the physician role for psychiatrists. What is, then, the relationship between CL psychiatrists and the non-medical practitioners of "behavioral medicine" who are often consulted on the same patient as the CL psychiatrist? I believe that all the mental health workers who work with patients with medical/surgical diseases must accept the challenge of working together, synergistically, rather than working in parallel, causing unnecessary duplication and waste. One model of such working together would be to work toward an integrated mental health team, consisting of the psychiatrist, psychologist, social worker, nurse practitioner, etc. I had developed one such prototype at Yale New Haven Hospital (Leigh, 1987), in which the CL psychiatrist functions as the diagnostician and co-ordinator of the team. Once a three dimensional diagnosis has been made at a team conference with input from all the disciplines involved, a three dimensional treatment plan is devised, and the plans are implemented either in tandem or in sequence. For example, a course of relaxation training followed by explorative psychotherapy, while the patient receives an antidepressant medication. At the conclusion of the relaxation training, the patient and spouse would be evaluated for possible couples therapy.

With the increasing importance managed care systems will play nationally, an important task for the CL psychiatrist is to define its role within the managed care system.

All too often, the psychiatrist in managed care systems tends to be simply a dispenser of drugs to patients who are not even seen by the psychiatrist. I believe that CL psychiatrists can and should play a major role in managed care systems as the physician co-ordinator, diagnostician, and evaluator of treatment modalities of the mental health workers.

Together with the new health care proposals, consultation-liaison psychiatry faces an exciting but uncertain future. Much will depend on the evolution of the national health care system, which, in turn, depends on what we health care givers, and the people, choose it to be. Idealism is still the mainstay of CL psychiatry --- for comprehensive, integrative, non-reductionistic, biopsychosocial care of all patients. Future will tell whether this idealism will help rekindle the excitement of treating the whole person.

REFERENCES

Engel GL: The need for a new medical model: A challenge to biomedicine. Science, 1977, 196:129-136

Koran IM: Funding consultation-liaison psychiatry via Medicare screening. Gen Hosp Psychiatry, 1992, 14:7-14

Leigh H, Feinstein AR, Reiser MF: The patient evaluation grid: A systematic approach to comprehensive care. Gen Hosp Psychiatry, 1980, 2:3-9

Leigh H, Reiser MF: The Patient: Biological, Psychological, and Social Dimensions of Medical Practice, 3rd Edition, 1992, Plenum Publishing Co, New York

Leigh H: Multidisciplinary teams in consultation-liaison psychiatry: the Yale model. Psychotherapy and Psychosomatics 48:83-89, 1987

Leigh H: Psychiatric Liaison on a Neoplastic In-Patient Service. International Journal of Psychiatry in Medicine. 4:147-154, 1973.

Loebel JP, Borson S, Hyde T et al.: Relationship between requests for psychiatric consultation and psychiatric diagnoses in long-term care facilities Am J Psychiatry 1991; 148:898-903

Saravay SM, Steinberg MD, Weinschel B et al.: Psychological comorbidity and length of stay in the general hospital Am J Psychiatry 1991; 148:324-329

Strain JJ, Fulop G, Hammer JS: A new tool for consultation-liaison funding: Modified DRG's to reflect psychiatric comorbidity Gen Hosp Psychiatry, 1992, 14:119-23

Strain JJ, Gize LH, Fulop G: Consultation-liaison psychiatry. Possibilities for the 1990's. Gen Hosp Psychiatry, 1989, 11:235-40

Weiner MF, Sadler J, Fenton BJ, Fitzpatrick MC, Crowder JD, Goodkin K: A very modest proposal for 1990's C/L psychiatry Gen Hosp Psychiatry, 1989, 11:231-4

LEGAL AND ETHICAL CHANGES IN CONSULTATION PSYCHIATRY

Lowell Tong, M.D. and Craig Van Dyke, M.D.

Psychiatry Service
San Francisco Veterans Affairs Medical Center and
Department of Psychiatry
University of California, San Francisco
4150 Clement Street
San Francisco, CA 94121

INTRODUCTION

To illustrate how legal and ethical issues have changed over the past decade for the psychiatric consultant, we thought it would be instructive to compare how consultations on equivalent patients were handled in 1980 and 1990.

1980

Consultation Request: The patient is a 42 year old single, white male who was admitted for multiple medical problems. He wants to go on pass and is refusing bronchoscopy.

Psychiatric Evaluation:

Patient is a 42 year old single, white male who is admitted for evaluation of lymphadenopathy and a three month history of weight loss, lethargy, fever, chills, headache, cough and dyspnea. No prior medical illnesses.

The patient smokes two packs of cigarettes per day and consumes 12 beers per day when he binges. The patient states his last drink was two weeks prior to admission. He has no other history of psychiatric illness. The patient may be a homosexual.

The patient states that he is not eager to have bronchoscopy but would be willing to have the procedure after he is granted a weekend pass. His plans for this weekend are quite vague. He claims to have family and friends but will not give their names or telephone numbers.

Consultation-Liaison Psychiatry: 1990 and Beyond
Edited by H. Leigh, Plenum Press, New York, 1994

On mental status examination the patient is oriented times three, makes three mistakes on serial 7's and can remember Presidents Carter and Ford but is unable to recall Nixon. He appears depressed and states he feels so miserable at times that he wishes he were dead. He denies any suicidal ideation but says he might kill himself if he gets much sicker. Denies auditory or visual hallucinations. No evidence of tremulousness.

<u>Impression:</u>

(1) Alcoholism

(2) Personality disorder with mild depressive features

(3) No evidence of delirium tremens or other organic brain syndrome.

<u>Plan:</u>

(1) Multivitamins with thiamine

(2) Would not grant patient pass and would urge him to undergo bronchoscopy. Risk is that he will drink on pass.

(3) If patient insists on leaving, would recommend that he sign out against medical advice.

No other considerations occurred to consultant.

<u>1990</u>

<u>Consultation Request</u>: The patient is a 42 year old white, gay male with acquired immunodeficiency syndrome (AIDS), who is admitted for pneumocystis pneumonia. Patient wants to go on pass and refuses antibiotic therapy.

<u>Psychiatric Evaluation</u>:

Patient is a 42 year old white, gay male with a three month history of weight loss, lethargy, fever, chills, headache, cough and dyspnea. No medical illnesses prior to AIDS diagnosis two years ago.

The patient smokes two packs per day and drinks excessively under stress. He has attended Alcoholics Anonymous meetings sporadically in the past. He states his last drink was two weeks prior to admission. He does not use intravenous (IV) drugs and has no other history of psychiatric illness.

The patient states that he is not willing to take antibiotic therapy but would be willing to do so if granted a weekend pass. He accepts IV hydration but declines IV and oral antibiotics for unclear reasons. The patient *does* understand that he is suffering from AIDS but *does not* appear to fully appreciate that he has pneumocystis pneumonia, and that the severity of his condition requires immediate antibiotic treatment. His plans for this weekend are quite vague. He claims to have a lover, family and friends but cannot give their full names and telephone numbers.

The Neurocognitive Screening Exam (Kiernan et al., 1987) was administered and showed the patient to be alert and fully oriented, to have intact repetition, naming, and calculation abilities, but mild impairments in attention span and comprehension, and moderate impairments in constructions, memory and judgment.

The patient appears depressed and states that he feels quite miserable. He states that if he gets to the point of not being able to care for himself that he will commit suicide. At present he does not feel close to this point and denies current suicidality. He has contacted the Hemlock Society and states that his lover is fully supportive of his intentions. He denies auditory or visual hallucinations. No evidence of tremulousness.

The medical record contains a valid completed durable power of attorney for health care; the patient has named his lover as his proxy.

<u>Impression</u>:

(1) AIDS with pneumocystis pneumonia

(2) Cognitive deficits secondary to medical condition:
- (a) AIDS dementia
- (b) Central Nervous System (CNS) infection
- (c) CNS neoplasm
- (d) Alcohol abuse
- (e) Delirium tremens - doubtful

(3) Depression but difficult to evaluate in context of cognitive deficits.

(4) Patient is not able to understand the full nature of his medical condition or need for IV antibiotic treatment. Any procedures requiring informed consent should be discussed with his lover.

<u>Plan:</u>

(1) Patient should not be granted a pass. If he attempts to leave, his lover should be contacted.

(2) Primary physician should contact his lover to discuss patient's current medical condition and plans for treatment and clarification of durable power of attorney and patient's wishes about medical care. The lover may be able to convey to the patient the importance of IV antibiotics better than we can.

(3) CNS Evaluation
- (a) X-ray computed tomography or magnetic resonance imaging of head
- (b) Lumbar puncture
- (c) Neurology consultation

(4) Thiamine and multivitamins

Other considerations that occurred to the psychiatric consultant but were not addressed in the initial consultation note because of insufficient information were:

(1) Should this patient be committed for grave disability or suicidal ideation?

(2) Should the patient be observed frequently for risk of elopement or wandering off?

(3) Is the patient's suicidal ideation based on a depressive illness, irrational fears, or on a more rational "quality of life" basis?

(4) What is the patient's relationship with his lover and family of origin? Does the patient's family know about his human immunodeficiency virus (HIV) status, and how should we handle this issue given issues of confidentiality about AIDS and alcohol abuse?

(5) How closely should the patient's advance directive be followed?

(6) Does the patient's impaired mental state meet criteria for mandatory reporting to the Department of Motor Vehicles?

As can be seen from this example the same basic case results in a very different process in 1990 than it did in 1980. The medical and psychiatric diagnoses are quite different as are the suggestions for diagnostic workup and treatment. In addition, legal and ethical aspects of the case are much more prominent with the emphasis on respecting the patient's prior directives about his wishes for treatment under these circumstances. The patient's sexual orientation is an important part of the psychosocial picture, and his lover has a critical role in clinical and legal matters. A valid durable power of attorney for health care must be respected. The patient's confidentiality and autonomy as well as the profession's obligations to commit or report are weighed. Suicidality is assessed in a context broadened by contemporary health problems such as AIDS.

Moreover, this case illustrates that psychiatry has become "remedicalized" over the last decade, and that psychiatric consultation on medical/surgical patients is a prime example of this. As the clinical scope of the contemporary psychiatric consultant has expanded over the last decade, so has the expectation of expertise in legal and ethical areas grown. This has to do partly with the larger clinical scope, but also derives from changes in legal guidelines and changes in cultural attitudes about the roles and rights of patients.

Psychiatric consultants play a unique role in modern medical practice. The consultant needs to be well-informed about current medical and surgical practice, and like the primary caregiver, must be well versed in the wide array of ethical issues involved in caring for patients. It is the psychiatric consultant, however, who has the special expertise in assessing psychiatric issues such as cognition, depression, and suicidality in the medical patient.

In this chapter, changes in the legal and ethical issues facing the contemporary psychiatry consultant are addressed. By and large, California laws, court rulings and community standards shall be used as the basis for discussion of such changes. The principles discussed, however, are useful for consultation practice across the United States.

This chapter is not intended for use as legal advice, but rather to stimulate thinking about legal and ethical changes. Readers should be familiar with their own relevant local and state laws and should consult their own ethics committee and/or local legal counsel for advice on any specific case.

PATIENTS RIGHTS VERSUS STATE INTEREST

Over the last decade, the patient's right of self-determination has become an important principle in redefining relationships amongst patient, physician and other parts of the health care system. Examples of this are the rise of patient confidentiality laws, informed consent laws for medical treatment, advance directives for health care, the growing public and legal debate on rational suicide and physician-assisted death for the terminally ill and the ongoing national debate on abortion.

During this period, there has also been a rise in the state interest of protecting society against danger posed by certain patient conditions.

Examples of this are new or redefined laws mandating physicians or medical facilities to report to the state those patients who have disorders of impaired consciousness, who are abusive or a danger to others or who have certain communicable diseases.

MEDICAL /PSYCHIATRIC LAWS

California has three sets of laws related to issues of involuntary detention, competency, and surrogate consent for mentally impaired patients that the psychiatric consultant is likely to encounter. The first set is the Lanterman-Petris-Short Act of the California Health and Institutions Code which deals with psychiatric commitments. This Act defines criteria for the involuntary detention for psychiatric observation and treatment of patients who, 1) because of a mental disorder, 2) are gravely disabled or a danger to self or others, and 3) are unwilling and unable to consent to voluntary psychiatric treatment.

The second set of laws, in the California Civil Code, allows a *competent* individual to design a durable power of attorney for health care matters, and to assign this specified power to any second person whom the competent individual chooses. When the original individual becomes incompetent, the designated second person becomes the surrogate consentor for medical treatment as outlined by the first individual. The court is not involved in constructing durable powers of attorney, although witnesses are required. Often a durable power of attorney includes the patient's specific wishes or guiding principles regarding future health care such as life support and donating organs. This is sometimes called a "living will."

The third set of laws, in the California Probate Code, defines legal parameters for *incompetent* individuals who are not capable of making informed decisions about their medical care and who had not previously established a durable power of attorney. When a physician's assessment is that a patient is probably incompetent, the case can be referred to the courts. These probate laws allow *the judicial system* (State Superior Court) to evaluate and pronounce a patient incompetent, and then to consent to or refuse medical treatments on behalf of that incompetent patient. The courts may also give another individual the powers of surrogate consent for the incompetent patient's ongoing medical affairs.

There is a fourth and new legal area (not currently covered by California state laws) which is receiving national attention (Menikoff et al., 1992). This is the concept of statutory surrogate laws, in which there is a default list of surrogate consentors (e.g., guardian, family, friends) who are given the power of surrogate consent when a patient is found *by a physician* to be incapable of making rational medical decisions. The recently passed Illinois version applies to those patients who lack decision making capacity and who previously have not executed an advance directive for health care. Additionally, the patient must have a terminal condition, permanent unconsciousness or an incurable or irreversible condition. This type of law differs from California Probate laws in that the judicial system is not involved, instead it relies on the physician's clinical assessment of the patient's mental capacity.

In three of the four legal areas outlined above, physicians are required to make a clinical assessment of a patient's ability or inability to make decisions. In many cases this means that a psychiatric consultant will be asked to render a second clinical opinion on whether a patient is capable of consenting to voluntary treatment. It is entirely appropriate for the psychiatric consultant to render this opinion and to document the clinical assessment as an ability to give informed consent.

The psychiatric consultant should avoid rendering a judgment on *competency per se,* since it is the duty of the judicial system to make this legal determination. The way we handle this is in careful documentation. For instance we would use a phrase like, "This patient lacks the capacity to make reasoned decisions about the medical and surgical care of her gangrenous foot, because she cannot comprehend basic medical information given repeatedly." We would not use a phrase like, "This patient is incompetent to make medical decisions."

Laws such as those described above make an artificial distinction between mental/psychiatric disorders and medical ones. This causes problems for the psychiatric consultant who is often faced with a clinical dilemma in which the patient has psychiatric symptoms as part of a serious medical condition. For example, these laws may be quite helpful and clear for the psychiatry emergency room staff evaluating an acutely disorganized, wandering schizophrenic, or for a surgical team handling a comatose patient who needs an amputation. However, as will be described in the next section, these laws are less helpful to the medical team and psychiatric consultant in dealing with the previously described demented AIDS patient who has now developed septicemia, hallucinations and delusions and who wants to leave the hospital to escape imagined demons.

INVOLUNTARY PSYCHIATRIC COMMITMENT ON A MEDICAL WARD

Involuntary psychiatric holds are sometimes used on medical wards, when several conditions are met. These are: 1) The patient must have a mental disorder, 2) the patient must be incapable or unwilling to accept voluntary psychiatric assessment and treatment, 3) the patient must be a danger to self or others or gravely disabled (i.e., unable to provide for food, clothing or shelter), 4) the patient's medical condition warrants admission to or staying on a medical ward instead of a psychiatry ward, and 5) there is an overriding practical, ethical or legal need to instigate a psychiatric hold.

This last condition is most important; just because a psychiatric hold is *possible* does not mean that it should necessarily be used. Negotiating with the patient, compromising, diffusing a situation or helping the primary medical team consider a less optimal but still medically acceptable alternative should always be tried first. The involuntary psychiatric hold should be used as a last resort. This is the core of being an effective psychiatric consultant: knowing the law, knowing the patient, knowing the primary physicians and then negotiating a plan which still conforms to acceptable medical and ethical standards of care, yet respects the patient's self-determination and preserves the patient's best interest.

When a psychiatric hold must be used on a medical ward, it is important to remind all clinicians that the hold allows for psychiatric observation and treatment of the patient, but it does not obviate the need for standard informed consent for any non-psychiatric treatment.

In a California court ruling (Riese v. St. Mary's Hospital, 1987), it was found that psychiatric commitment laws do not eliminate the need for informed consent for psychotropic medications even for patients on an involuntary psychiatric hold. In other words, certain patients may be sufficiently disturbed to warrant an involuntary psychiatric hold, yet remain competent to refuse psychotropic medications. On a practical basis, it is common in California for both a probable cause hearing for the commitment and a *Riese* competency hearing to be convened simultaneously, so that the legal system can determine the patient's status for remaining on a hold and the patient's ability to accept or refuse psychotropic medications.

The psychiatric consultant is likely to be involved in probable cause hearings on a medical or surgical ward. Members of the psychiatric division of the judicial system (i.e., judge, as well as public defender or patient's advocate) are usually less knowledgeable and therefore more uncomfortable about making decisions on a medical/surgical patient. Therefore, to ensure fair judicial treatment of the patient, it is important for the psychiatric consultant to be objective and informative about both psychiatric and non-psychiatric conditions of the patient. Having the primary care physician available to explain the patient's medical condition and risks of discharge can be helpful.

Several times in recent years we have had to take the inconsistent positions of making both a strong case for commitment and then presenting the case for letting the patient go. These situations were the result of an uncertain judge and an anxious patient advocate not wanting to consider releasing patients who looked medically precarious because of multiple intravenous lines and medical monitoring devices.

Because the boundaries of "psychiatric" versus "medical" are artificial but still are part of laws, they are subject to varying interpretations. If the originally described demented AIDS patient, now septic, is insistent on actually leaving the hospital because of paranoid delusions and hallucinations, it would be reasonable to consider instituting an involuntary psychiatric hold to keep the patient on the medical ward while his lover is contacted. The psychiatric diagnosis would be delirium secondary to septicemia. The hold would allow only for involuntary psychiatric assessment and treatment and would not allow for involuntary non-psychiatric "medical" treatment.

Diagnostic lumbar punctures, blood cultures and empirical antibiotic therapy are standard "medical" interventions. They could also be thought of as "psychiatric" interventions, since they would be part of the evaluation and treatment of the delirium. If the now restrained, delirious AIDS patient specifically refused to have any needles or antibiotics, compromise would be the first order of business. Perhaps the patient's fears could be understood and pacified. Perhaps the patient would accept intramuscular or oral antibiotics. Perhaps one person could be found whom the patient trusted to start the IV line. Perhaps the patient would allow treatment after a cigarette.

If no compromise were possible, there are two directions which the clinician could take. The first would be to consider these procedures "psychiatric" and to institute an involuntary psychiatric hold. The second would be to consider the procedures non-psychiatric, and to determine whether the patient was capable of making reasoned and informed decisions about them. If truly capable, the patient's wishes would, of course, be respected. If the patient were not capable, then the clinician would refer to the patient's advance directive for guidance or obtain surrogate consent. In any event, the level of patient cooperation required for the treatment to be technically possible and safe would need to be considered. Both directions have their own unique merits, and it is up to the psychiatric consultant to decide which one is more appropriate under the specific circumstances. Seeking legal counsel should also be considered strongly whenever the psychiatric consultant is in such a professional dilemma.

The decision about which direction to take highlights the professional role of the psychiatric consultant. Waffling or referring everything to the courts is neither practical nor helpful. Legal advice can be helpful but does not substitute for professional clinical judgment. Being a useful contemporary consultant requires knowledge of community and local medical facility standards, an understanding of the scope, intent and limitations of relevant local laws, and professional judgment to make a decision about "medical" versus "psychiatric" boundaries.

RESTRAINING PATIENTS FOR MEDICAL REASONS

Not every patient who is restrained on a medical ward needs to be on an involuntary psychiatry hold. For instance, a confused and obtunded patient in the intensive care unit may be restrained either to prevent falling out of bed or pulling out IV catheters and nasogastric tubes. This patient may be delirious, but a psychiatric consult would not necessarily be called, since it may be standard practice on that unit to use soft wrist restraints at the discretion of the nursing staff and the primary medical team. Another example would be a severely demented patient with Alzheimer's disease admitted for an ophthalmologic procedure. This patient may be at great risk for wandering or falling and may be placed in a room with restricted exit or seated in a chair with a front table attached firmly in place. In both cases, the patients are being restrained without any specific legal hold. An important factor in these cases, however, is that the patient is neither expressing a desire to leave, nor making any attempt to do so. There is neither consent nor refusal. Family members should be kept appraised of the situation, but no specific consent is needed.

It would be a different matter if such patients were actively refusing their treatment or making attempts to leave the hospital. The first step would be to understand why the patient wants to leave and try to reach a compromise. A change in roommates, dietary alternatives, supervised cigarette smoking, fresh air strolls, comfortable clothing, a favorite nurse or doctor, mementos from home, and telephone access are just part of the list to consider in such negotiations.

If no compromises can be reached, then it would be imperative to make the clinical assessment whether patients were capable of understanding their medical conditions, treatments proposed, alternatives and probable outcomes. If they were capable and could make a reasoned decision, that decision, even if unwise, should be respected by the clinician. If they were not capable of making a reasoned decision, then two general approaches are possible.

The first approach would be to determine if an involuntary psychiatry hold were applicable. If so, it would still have to be remembered that an involuntary psychiatry hold does not allow for involuntary non-psychiatric medical intervention.

The second approach would utilize surrogate consent laws, which in California fall under the Probate Code. This allows for the State Superior Court to review a case and determine whether a patient should stay in the hospital for medical treatment. If the court finds the patient incompetent to consent to or refuse medical treatment, then the court may consent or refuse on behalf of the incompetent patient for a specific medical intervention. The court may also appoint a Probate conservator who is given the authority to consent or refuse on behalf of the incompetent patient.

CONFIDENTIALITY

A patient's medical information is confidential and cannot be released without permission. In most situations, consent is implied and primary clinicians often discuss the patient's medical condition with family and medical staff without any written consent. However, where inquiries are made by outside agencies, a written consent for release of this information is required.

There are certain conditions (e.g., HIV status, AIDS, and alcohol or drug abuse), where specific written permission is required for release of this information. Such information is highly sensitive and in most situations a signed release for general medical information is not sufficient. It is incumbent on the primary clinician to obtain specific consent. In the Veterans Affairs medical system, sickle cell anemia also enjoys this special confidentiality status. It is also of note that these special confidentiality requirements exist even after the patient's death. Since the laws on confidentiality vary greatly from state to state, it is incumbent on the reader to be aware of the particular state laws and the standard of practice in the community.

MANDATORY REPORTING OBLIGATIONS

There are several situations in which the primary clinician is required to report situations to state agencies. The reader is again urged to be familiar with local laws and standards of practice. Suspected or obvious child abuse is a mandatory reporting obligation so that children may be protected. Examples of child abuse include physical injury, sexual abuse, and neglect. It is important to emphasize that in many states the clinician is obligated to report this information even if it is based on suspicion or secondhand reports.

Many states have a similar reporting obligation for elder abuse. However, quite frequently elder abuse has to be reported in the context of actually seeing evidence of abuse or neglect in the elderly patient. Suspicion or secondhand reports of elder abuse may be reported, but may place the clinician at increased risk of breaching confidentiality.

Certain states have laws requiring that patients who suffer from epilepsy be reported to the State Health Department. These situations are reviewed by the Department of Motor Vehicles (DMV) to see whether an individual's driver's license should be suspended. Since driving is such an important aspect of the social and business life of most Americans, the DMV may take other factors such as response to treatment into consideration when deciding whether to suspend an epileptic patient's license (Krumholz et al., 1991). Certain states including California are now extending this principle to other conditions where there are lapses in consciousness. In California dementia and delirium are considered such conditions, so the primary clinician may need to report these patients to the State Health Department. It is also prudent for primary physicians to discuss with patients any condition that might impair driving skills and to document such discussion in the medical record.

There is an obvious conflict between a patient's right to confidentiality and the mandatory reporting obligations that physicians have for the good of society. This may occasionally place clinicians in awkward situations where decisions need to be made about how and when to break confidentiality and what should be revealed.

One guiding principle is to release the minimal amount of information that is necessary to meet the reporting obligation. For example in a situation where a drug abusing patient is abusing a child, it would be incumbent on the primary clinician to report the child abuse. Therefore reporting the patient's name and address, identification of the child and the nature of the abuse would satisfy the mandatory reporting requirement. However, it may be prudent for the clinician to withhold the information about drug abuse because of the particular strict confidentiality in regards to reporting that information. The other guiding principle is to consult others - fellow psychiatrist, legal counsel - when faced with awkward or complicated mandatory reporting situations.

Related to mandatory reporting obligations is the issue of breaking confidentiality in order to warn about a patient's intent to harm another. Varying from state to state, these are often called *Tarasoff* laws after a landmark case (Tarasoff v. Board of Regents of University of California, 1976) in which it was determined that the clinician should have forewarned the victim about the patient's stated intention to harm the potential victim. In California, there is now a Civil Code law which removes monetary liability from a psychotherapist who makes reasonable efforts to communicate a serious threat of physical violence to the potential victim and a law enforcement agency. It should be noted that failing to report such a serious threat is not a crime in California, but could be grounds for liability.

Standards for *Tarasoff* reporting obligations differ from those for psychiatric commitment for danger to others. In California the duty to warn does not require the patient to have a mental disorder, nor does it require the threat to be imminent. Because California commitment laws require a higher standard, the threatening patient may need to be reported but may not qualify for psychiatric commitment.

COMPETENCY

Adult patients are assumed to be competent and able to make decisions about their medical care unless there is evidence of impaired cognition or psychiatric disorders that compromise their ability to make reasoned decisions. While only the courts may declare such patients incompetent, in practice psychiatric consultants are often called upon to make judgments about whether patients can make an informed decision about their medical care. To be competent, a patient must be able to understand the basic nature of the relevant medical condition, its prognosis and planned course of treatment. The patient must also be able to understand the risk involved in the planned care as well as the benefits and risks associated with alternative forms of treatment. Moreover, a patient must be able to contemplate and choose amongst these alternatives. Whenever there is doubt, patients should be presumed to be competent and their preferences for treatment respected (Buchanan and Brock, 1989; Lo and Steinbrook, 1991; President's Commission for the Study of Ethical Problems in Medicine and Biomedical and Behavioral Research, 1983).

Competent patients are capable of giving informed consent for a certain medical intervention and are therefore capable of refusing that same medical intervention. Patients with full mental capacity are not required to make wise decisions, only reasoned ones. Occasionally deciding between an unwise decision and an uninformed decision may be very difficult. This is especially true when cultural differences exist. For example, certain cultures may lack a tradition of western medicine and be extremely resistant to surgery and other invasive procedures. Culturally determined notions about how the body works may differ markedly from our concepts and may sound irrational if not judged in the cultural context. Family members may be particularly crucial in understanding these situations.

In assessing competency, we find it helpful to have the primary clinician inform the patient of the medical condition, its prognosis and treatment as well as the risk and benefits of alternative treatments. This explanation is delivered in our presence so that we have a common set of information with the patient. We then ask patients to describe what was learned from the clinician and to inform us of their decision about treatment. It is in this context that we make our assessment of the patient's ability to give an informed consent and whether cognitive deficits or psychological factors are compromising that ability.

We also conduct a thorough cognitive status examination and psychiatric interview prior to evaluating the patient's response to the primary clinician (Jacobs et al., 1977; Folstein et al., 1975; Kiernan et al., 1987). It is of note that patients may have significant cognitive impairment, yet be able to render a competent decision about their medical care. For example, a patient with long term memory deficits may be perfectly capable of understanding at a particular moment the primary clinician's explanation of the medical condition and planned course of treatment and to render an informed judgment about medical care. However, a day or two later this same patient may have only the most rudimentary recall of the medical condition and planned course of treatment. In these patients, it is reassuring to the staff to give these explanations on several occasions and to have the patient render the same decision about treatment. The important point is that the patient must be able to understand the information at the moment of deciding about the medical care.

Another practical issue is that performing certain invasive procedures may be clinically risky for patients who are incompetent and unable to cooperate fully in their medical care. For example, a patient who has been deemed incompetent by the court system or for whom the family would like a certain invasive procedure to be carried out may be unable or unwilling to cooperate and therefore at greater clinical risk. Placing an arterial-venous shunt for hemodialysis in an uncooperative, demented patient may lead to acute medical complications that are worse than the chronic renal failure.

Finally, it is important to remember that incompetent patients may become competent in response to treatment. If a patient is found to lack ability to make reasoned medical decisions, the consultant should assess the likelihood of the patient regaining the ability. For instance, an acutely delirious patient may be expected to regain premorbid cognitive capacity in a matter of days while a patient with multiple infarct dementia would not be expected to improve cognitively. This information is an important piece of the clinical assessment of competency, and should be conveyed to the primary physician to optimize appropriate treatment planning.

ADVANCE DIRECTIVES

Ten to twenty years ago maximum efforts were employed, even in futile situations, to prolong the life of individuals. This was done routinely in comatose or incompetent patients under the principle of doing what was believed to be in the best interest of the patient which was almost always equated with maximum prolongation of life. Over time greater emphasis has been placed on respectful consideration of prior wishes of an incompetent patient about the extent to which invasive procedures and life support efforts should be utilized in prolonging life (President's Commission for the Study of Ethical Problems in Medicine and Biomedical and Behavioral Research, 1983; Council on Ethical and Judicial Affairs, American Medical Association, 1991).

On December 1, 1991 Congress put into effect the Patient-Self Determination Act (US Congress, 1990). This Act requires hospitals, hospices, nursing homes, and managed care organizations to advise patients of their rights to execute an advance directive about their medical care should they become incompetent to decide. The Act is tied to Medicare and Medicaid reimbursement and requires health care organizations to document whether patients have an advance directive. The same organizations are charged with developing policies and procedures for complying with advance directives or for informing patients of their rights to refuse or select treatment under state laws.

Advance directives take the form of verbal communications, written directives, living wills, and durable powers of attorney for health care. Each of these have advantages and disadvantages. For example, verbal communications are quite common with many people discussing with family members their preferences for care should they become seriously disabled or terminally ill. Many prefer palliative care and indicate that they would not like to live in a vegetative state. The court system, however, views such oral communication as less trustworthy than written documents (Cruzan v. Harmon, 1988; In re O'Connor, 1988). A living will attempts to put such guiding principles in writing, but it may be very difficult for a clinician to follow in practice because of the difficulty in anticipating various clinical circumstances at the time the living will is prepared. The durable power of attorney is gaining increasing popularity, because it places medical decisions for an incompetent patient in the hands of a specific concerned individual. However, there are difficulties with this approach as well.

Despite the growing awareness and the importance of advance directives, fewer than 20% of Americans have completed these (La Puma et al., 1991). While many reasons have been cited, one of the most important for the psychiatric consultant is discomfort on the part of the primary physician in discussing these issues with the patient. Physicians frequently feel that discussing death and dying with patients may demoralize them or otherwise adversely affect their care (Kohn and Menon, 1988). The psychiatric consultant has a growing role in facilitating discussions between primary physicians and their patients to overcome psychological barriers to such communication.

Another role for the psychiatric consultant is in assessing competency to complete an advance directive. Ideally, advance directives should be completed well before patients become seriously ill, at a time when patients are mentally competent and not experiencing the anguish associated with a life threatening illness. In practice, however, it is quite common for advance directives to be completed when patients are hospitalized for a serious medical illness and their cognitive capacity or emotional status may already be altered. Additional factors such as limited education, delirium, dementia, and major mental illness may influence patients' abilities to understand and validly execute an advance directive. Janofsky and colleagues (1992) have even developed a competency assessment instrument to help in making this judgment. This is an early effort in helping make this decision more objective and further efforts along these lines can be anticipated as we head into the next century.

Once an advance directive is completed there are several other roles for the psychiatric consultant. The most obvious is in helping decide that the patient's condition has reached the point where the advance directive must be put into effect. In the vast majority of cases this decision is reached by the primary physician after discussion with the patient's family and no psychiatric consultation is required. However, when there is disagreement or the mental status of the patient is difficult to assess, the psychiatric consultant may be called. Facilitating communication within the family or between family and primary physician is an appropriate role for the psychiatrist. Family members often disagree with one another and may have little awareness of the patient's actual desires. There is even recent evidence that patients vary considerably in how strictly they want their advance directives implemented (Sehgal et al., 1992). This places a greater burden on the primary physician to have in-depth discussions with patients about how strictly they desire their advance directives to be followed and what modifying factors should be considered.

There are also situations where proxies have projected their values onto the patient or have deliberately misrepresented or distorted a patient's wishes because of financial issues, a planned divorce, or the desire to be relieved of an emotional burden. The psychiatric consultant has a proper role in helping assess and resolve such situations. Consultation with an ethics committee and legal counsel is also appropriate.

One issue that is likely to increase in the next decade is the conflict of interest that health care providers have in controlling health care costs. Poorly educated, non-English speaking, and elderly patients without family support may be particularly vulnerable to pressure to limit their health care under the guise of maximizing their quality of life. Utilizing advance directives in order to decrease health care cost is totally inappropriate. However, safeguards to prevent this are beyond the role of the psychiatric consultant and belong more properly in the realm of government, the legal system, and health care providers who need to develop policies to address these issues.

We are obviously just at the beginning of the era when patients' knowledge and information about their own health care is increasing. Patients now read about their medications in their own copy of guidebooks such as the *Physician's Desk Reference*, watch video tapes of their pending operation, or participate in support groups with other patients with a similar condition. It is reasonable to anticipate that over the next ten years a much greater proportion of patients will have advance directives and their knowledge and instructions about how to care for them should they be unable to make their wishes known will be spelled out in much greater detail.

Another major trend for the near future is the increasing ability of medicine to diagnose and treat patients but at ever greater cost. With health care costs in the United States now reaching $1 trillion per annum, there will be major efforts by the government and the health care system to limit treatment. The balance between patient autonomy and society's need to provide the best care for everyone within a limited budget is the major issue ahead. The psychiatric consultant clearly has a role to play in seeing that new health care policy and laws are applied humanely and appropriately to a given patient whose cognitive, behavioral, or emotional status may be compromised.

FUTURE ISSUES

Euthanasia, Assisted Suicide, Rational Suicide

Since 1988 there have been an increasing number of medical journal articles, media revelations, and political and legal efforts addressing the topic of assisted suicide (Angell, 1988; Benrubi, 1992; Brody, 1992; Conwell and Caine, 1991; Hendin and Klerman, 1993; Miles, 1991; Quill, 1991; Quill et al., 1992; Singer and Siegler, 1990; Wanzer et al., 1989). This current debate about physician-assisted death of terminally ill patients is a very lively one that is likely to eventuate in some form of legalization or decriminalization in at least parts of the United States. The purpose of this section is not to provide a definitive review of the debate, which is a very complicated matter. Rather, it is to outline the most important aspects of the debate. Psychiatric consultants need to be part of the ongoing debate, since it is likely that they will be involved in the assessment of the mental status of at least some of the patients wishing that their lives be terminated.

Definitions of terms used in this debate vary, each with its own peculiar emotional derivation or response. *Euthanasia* itself is one of the most controversial terms, not often used in its most literal meaning, the "quiet" or "good" death. It often refers to the physician's act of purposely terminating the life of a patient with incurable or painful disease to prevent further suffering. Some make the distinction that the active intervention of a clinician injecting a single lethal dose of morphine is euthanasia, while the provision of narcotic prescriptions and information about lethal doses with the awareness of the patient's intention to end life is *assisted suicide*. Others propose that the use of morphine titrated to control severe pain in a terminally ill patient, when the "side effect" is respiratory cessation, is neither euthanasia nor assisted suicide but instead is medically-indicated analgesia.

Another controversial term is *rational suicide*. Some propose that rational suicide is an oxymoron; suicide and a rational mental state cannot co-exist. Others propose that if a terminally ill patient does not have a severe or treatable mental illness such as major depression, and if the patient is fully informed of the diagnosis, prognosis and treatment alternatives, then the patient may decide to commit suicide on a rational basis.

Whether legalized assisted suicide becomes commonplace, psychiatric consultants need to know how to make assessments of the role that psychiatric disorders play in a patient with suicidal ideation. If the availability of assisted suicide for terminally ill patients does become more common, it is quite probable that there will be a demand for psychiatric consultation requests for second opinions. The biggest challenge for the psychiatric consultant is to decide where on the spectrum of sadness to major depression a patient's mood state lies, and determining whether that mood distorts decision making to such an extent as to represent an impairment.

In addition to mood or other mental disorders like anxiety, other factors may cause a terminally ill patient to consider suicide. Uncontrolled pain, fear of pain, and the desire to take control over a hopeless situation are common factors. Often, physicians inadequately assess pain and underutilize analgesic treatment. The psychiatric consultant can play a very useful role in addressing this, both in specific clinical cases as well as by educating other physicians. For example, around the clock instead of "as needed" analgesia can provide a steady state of medication, and can help avoid patient-nurse conflict. We have also found that patient-controlled analgesia units delivering IV narcotics can be very effective for pain management in large part due to patient satisfaction with having control over dosing.

A setting where we have had occasion to evaluate suicidal patients is the hemodialysis clinic. From time to time a patient considers stopping dialysis with the full knowledge of the fatal outcome. One example was a patient with years of worsening debility who vowed to stay on dialysis until his granddaughter graduated from college. After the graduation, following full discussion with his family and the dialysis staff, the patient decided to stop dialysis. The nephrologist requested a psychiatric consultation even though no one believed that the patient was depressed or had any other psychiatric disorder. The renal staff just "wanted to be sure." On exam the patient had no evidence of psychopathology. He stated that he had considered stopping dialysis for years because of his serious physical deterioration, but had wanted to see his granddaughter through school since he was paying for her tuition. His wife and children did not want him to die, but respected his wishes. We concluded that there were no grounds for psychiatric intervention, because his decision was a fully informed one, and not the result of a mental disorder. The patient stopped dialysis and died at home. This was clearly a case of suicide, which required a passive act of staying home instead of an overdose or other active means of death. Some have argued that stopping cardiopulmonary life support or medical treatment like dialysis is ethically and legally the same as active suicide by overdose or suffocation.

The Hemlock Society has stimulated much of the public and legal debate on rational suicide and physician-assisted death of terminally ill patients (Humphry, 1991). The important but still unanswered question of the prevalence of treatable mental disorders in the whole population of terminally ill patients who might consider suicide is at the crux of much of the debate. The concern of the Hemlock Society and others is that analyses of this issue are always biased towards those patients who are preselected for psychiatric evaluations, and therefore the results are not applicable to all terminally ill patients. The Society believes strongly that terminally ill patients should not be assumed to have a mental disorder. However, the Society believes that if a terminally ill patient does have a mental disorder, that patient should not be assisted with suicide.

There are many concerns about the possibilities for abuse if physician-assisted suicide becomes legalized (Hendin and Klerman, 1993). Possible abuses include coercion of the elderly or frail to end their lives, inadequate attention to depression and other potentially reversible mental conditions and hastening death in the name of saving on health care expenditures.

Abortion

Psychiatrists are likely to have a prominent role in abortions if access to abortions becomes more restricted in the U.S. (Annas, 1992; Appelbaum,

1992). This is because there will probably always be clauses allowing abortions when there is danger to the health or life of the mother. Prior to the 1973 U.S. Supreme Court ruling in Roe v. Wade (1973), severe impairment to the mother's mental health became recognized as a legitimate exception to strict abortion laws. Psychiatric consultations were sought when mental anguish or suicidality was presented as the health risk for the mother.

Just as before Roe v. Wade, if there now come to pass more restrictive abortion laws, psychiatrists could be thrust into the role of gatekeepers of the narrowed access to abortion. Psychiatrists would be in the position of certifying danger to the mother's mental health in the absence of much objective data from scientific studies and the medical literature. Some psychiatrists may choose to not be involved in such consultations, while others may choose to be self-appointed social guardians of access to abortion, either keeping it open or closed. Obviously, individual psychiatrists as well as organized psychiatry will have to contend with their own moral, ethical and social reactions.

Contagious/infectious diseases

With the outbreak of drug-resistant tuberculosis, and certainly with the current HIV epidemic, there is the question of restricting patients' freedom for public health reasons. Psychiatrists may be consulted to assess the ability of a patient to follow appropriate infection control precautions, as part of determining whether involuntary confinement for public health concerns is appropriate.

Multiculturalism

Changing U.S. demographics will require the psychiatric consultant to be familiar with different populations of patients. An increase in a particular ethnic or cultural group may be the result of changed immigration laws, birthrate or interstate moves.

Each ethnic or cultural group has its unique social, health care and language issues. Familiarity with these is essential for the psychiatric consultant to be effective. For some patient populations, experience with using an interpreter may also be useful, since family members may not be available, and if they are present they may not be the most objective translators.

For example, familiarity with Vietnamese attitudes towards doctors, symptoms, medications and mental health, combined with knowledge of what to ask about life in Vietnam and immigration experience allowed us to make an appropriate intervention in an elderly Vietnamese woman. This woman presented with multiple physical complaints and had undergone an extensive medical evaluation including several invasive procedures. Her symptoms were so debilitating that the primary physician was debating between another round of medical procedures or withholding all active medical support. We were able to make the diagnosis of depression with multiple physical symptoms and to treat her accordingly.

Gay and Lesbian Patients

We are at a time when many patients are able to discuss their sexual orientation more freely. The effective psychiatric consultant must be able and willing to elicit relevant social and medical information without assuming that a patient, even if married, is heterosexual. The consultant needs to be aware of a gay, lesbian or bisexual patient's lover, spouse or other self-defined family system, as well as have knowledge of contemporary gay and bisexual health care and legal issues. Moreover, the consultant should be mindful of where a patient is along the continuum of the "coming out" process.

For example, it turned out that the main reason for suicidality in a middle-aged AIDS patient who had lost all of his two dozen friends to AIDS, was the terrifying prospect of having the social worker tell the next of kin, his elderly father, that the patient had AIDS and needed parental assistance. Through support and role-play practice, the patient made the telephone call himself revealing his sexual orientation, health status, and need for help. His father was quite gracious and generous, and the patient's level of suicidality decreased markedly.

In most hospitals and communities a gay lover or other unmarried partner is not recognized as legal next of kin. If there are no advance directives, an incompetent patient's blood relative's wishes are given more weight than those of a gay lover. A durable power of attorney for health care is a legal mechanism by which gay patients can assign a lover or any other specific person a full say if the patient becomes incapable of making reasoned decisions. This is most relevant for the gay patient with a serious illness where competency is expected to become impaired, although any gay couple should be educated about this. A durable power of attorney for health care can be very useful when there is unfamiliarity, disagreement or animosity between the lover and blood relatives of the patient.

In addition to ensuring that a gay patient is knowledgeable about durable powers of attorney, the psychiatric consultant can play an important role with other family matters. Sometimes blood relatives meet gay friends and the lover for the first time in the hospital during a gay patient's acute medical illness. The consultant can be instrumental in facilitating introductions, optimizing the chance for amicable relations, and developing a mechanism for opinions and wishes to be heard from all family members.

CONCLUSION

In this chapter we have discussed the changing legal and ethical issues that psychiatric consultants have faced over the last decade. We expect the pace and scope of such changes to quicken in the next decade, breaking new ground along the way. For example, our nation faces the dual challenge of providing health coverage to 37 million uninsured Americans at the same time it is trying to reduce the total health care budget. Since allocation of finite resources is central to such changes, important clinical dilemmas are inevitable. Another example is the impact that advances in neuroscience will have on society's understanding of and attitudes towards mental dysfunction.

New laws and ethical standards will follow new knowledge. A last example is the area of genetic manipulation which is now in the realm of high technology pioneers, but which may soon enter the clinical world. While policy, legal aspects, and ethics of such examples go far beyond the purview of the consultation psychiatrist, we will always have a role in applying them at the bedside.

ACKNOWLEDGMENT

We are indebted to Mrs. Gloria Patel for her editorial assistance.

REFERENCES

Acute Pain Management Guideline Panel, "Acute Pain Management: Operative or Medical Procedures and Trauma - Clinical Practice Guideline," 1992, AHCPR Pub. No. 92-0032, Rockville, MD: Agency for Health Care Policy and Research Public Service, U.S. Department of Health and Human Services.

Angell, M., 1988, Euthanasia, New England Journal of Medicine, 319:1348.

Annas, G.J., 1991, The health care proxy and the living will, New England Journal of Medicine, 324:1210.

Annas, G.J., 1992, The supreme court, liberty and abortion, New England Journal of Medicine, 327:651.

Appelbaum, P.S., 1992, Psychiatrists and access to abortion, Hospital and Community Psychiatry, 43:967.

Benrubi, G.I., 1992, Euthanasia-the need for procedural safeguards, New England Journal of Medicine, 326:197.

Brody, H., 1992, Assisted death - A compassionate response to a medical failure, New England Journal of Medicine, 327:1384.

Buchanan, A.E., and Brock, D.W., 1989, "Deciding for others," Cambridge University Press, Cambridge, Mass.

Conwell, Y., and Caine, E.D., 1991, Rational suicide and the right to die: Reality and myth, New England Journal of Medicine, 325:1100.

Council on Ethical and Judicial Affairs, American Medical Association, 1991, Guidelines for the appropriate use of do-not-resuscitate orders, Journal of American Medical Association, 265:1868.

Cruzan v. Harmon, 760SW2d 408 (Mo 1988).

Folstein, M.F., Folstein, S.E., and McHugh, P.R, 1975, Mini-mental state, Journal of Psychiatry Research, 12:189.

Hendin, H., and Klerman, G., 1993, Physician-assisted suicide: The dangers of legalization, American Journal of Psychiatry, 150:143.

Humphry, D., "Final Exit," 1991, The Hemlock Society, Eugene, Oregon.

In re O'Connor, 72 NY2d 517, 531 NE2d 607, 534 NYS2d 886 (1988).

Jacobs, J.W., Bernard, M.R., Delgado, A., and Strain, J.J., 1977, Screening for organic mental syndromes in the medically ill, Annals of Internal Medicine, 86:40.

Janofsky, J.S., McCarthy, R.J., and Folstein, M.F., 1992, The Hopkins competency assessment test: A brief method for evaluating patients' capacity to give informed consent, Hospital and Community Psychiatry, 43:132.

Kiernan, R.J., Mueller, J., Langston, J.W., and Van Dyke, C., 1987, The neurobehavioral cognitive screening examination: A brief but quantitative approach to cognitive assessment, Annals of Internal Medicine, 107:481.

Kohn, M., and Menon, G., 1988, Life prolongation: Views of elderly outpatients and health care professionals, Journal of American Geriatrics Society, 36:840.

Krumholz, A., Fisher, R.S., Lesser, R.P., and Hauser, W. A., 1991, Driving and epilepsy, A review and reappraisal, Journal of American Medical Association, 265:622.

La Puma, J., Orentlicher, D., and Moss, R.J., 1991, Advance directives on admission: Clinical implications and analysis of the patient self-determination act of 1990, Journal of American Medical Association, 266:402.

Lo, B., and Steinbrook, R., 1991, Beyond the Cruzan case: The U.S. Supreme Court and medical practice, Annals of Internal Medicine. 114:895.

Menikoff, J.A., Sachs, G.A., and Siegler, M., 1992, Beyond advance directives - Health surrogate laws, New England Journal of Medicine, 327: 1165.

Miles, S.H., 1991, The case of Helga Wanglie - A new kind of "right to die" case, New England Journal of Medicine, 325:511.

President's Commission for the Study of Ethical Problems in Medicine and Biomedical and Behavioral Research, 1983, Deciding to forego life-sustaining treatment, Washington, DC.

Quill, T.E., 1991, A case of individualized decision making, New England Journal of Medicine, 324:691.

Quill, T.E., Cassel, C.K., and Meir, D.E., 1992, Care of the hopelessly ill, Proposed clinical criteria for physician-assisted suicide, New England Journal of Medicine, 327:1380.

Riese v. St. Mary's Hospital & Medical Center, 243 Cal. Rptr., 241 (Cal. App. 1 Dist. 1987).

Roe v. Wade, 410 U.S. 113, 1973.

Sehgal, A., Galbraith, A., Chesney, M., Schoenfeld, P., Charles, G., and Lo, B., 1992, How strictly do dialysis patients want their advance directives followed?, Journal of American Medical Association, 267:59.

Singer, P.A., and Siegler, M., 1990, Euthanasia - A critique, New England Journal of Medicine, 322:1881.

Tarasoff v. Board Regents of the University of California, 131 Cal. Rptr. 14, 1976.

The Medical Letter on Drugs and Therapeutics, 1993, Drugs for pain, The Medical Letter, Inc., New Rochelle, NY, 35:1.

US Congress, Omnibus Budget Reconciliation Act of 1990, Pub L No.101-508.

Wanzer, S.H., Federman, D.D., Adelstein, S.J., Casel C.K., Cassem, E.H., Cranford, R.E., Hook, E.W., Lo, B., Moertel, C.G., Safar, P., Stone, A., and van Eys, J., 1989, The physician's responsibility towards hopelessly ill patients, A second look, New England Journal of Medicine, 320:844.

CHRONIC PAIN

Jon Streltzer, M.D. and Byron Eliashof, M.D.

Department of Psychiatry
Univeristy of Hawaii at Manoa
John A. Burns School of Medicine
1356 Lusitana Street
Honolulu, HI 96813

INTRODUCTION

The American Medical Association's Guides to the Evaluation of Permanent Impairment, third edition (revised), states that $60 to $100 billion are spent annually in the United States on chronic pain representing about one-fourth of the annual health care budget[1]. It estimates that 80 million individuals suffer from chronic recurring headaches and 30 million suffer from chronic lower back pain. The AMA Guides further states that chronic pain can become a pathological disorder in its own right which they call a chronic pain syndrome. This is characterized by pain perception and pain behavior which are both grossly disproportionate to any underlying noxious stimulus.

The AMA Guides states that chronic pain patients have certain typical characteristics. This includes dramatizing their pain and suffering, becoming dependent on drugs, alcohol and visits to their physicians. They receive repetitive diagnostic studies and sometimes unfortunate surgical procedures which provide no benefit but result in further pain and disability. Eventually they are referred to psychiatrists where they are typically told that they have no mental illness and that if they did not have their pain they would be fine.

The AMA Guides further states that psychogenic pain refers to somatoform pain disorder. This is a psychiatric disorder which, enigmatically, "differs from the chronic pain syndrome, which cannot be considered a mental disorder." Thus the official American Medical Association position seems to be that chronic pain is an immensely common and significant problem but that psychogenic pain or somatoform pain disorder is a different condition which tends to be only understood by psychiatrists.

Consistent with this view is the fact that there is an immense literature which has developed relevant to chronic pain. Only rarely does this literature refer to somatoform pain disorder however.

Consultation-Liaison Psychiatry: 1990 and Beyond
Edited by H. Leigh, Plenum Press, New York, 1994

Where does the field of psychiatry stand with regard to the relationship of mental disorders to chronic pain? Prior to 1980, pain did not have its own category in the American Psychiatric Association's Diagnostic & Statistical Manual. Pain which had no apparent organic basis and which was conceptualized as having primarily psychological roots was conceived in essentially the same manner that Freud had originally proposed 100 years ago.

In the case of Elizabeth Von R., Freud described a young woman who suffered from chronic pain which influenced her ability to walk and caused her substantial disability[(2)]. Freud initially used neurological treatments which were in vogue in that day, physical therapy and electrical stimulation to the affected areas. There are notable similarities to present day treatment which would typically include physical therapy and possibly the use of a TENS unit. The patient improved only slightly and eventually Freud began delving into her psychosocial history ultimately discovering psychological conflicts that seem to explain the development and the maintenance of the physical symptoms. Elizabeth had suffered the role of sick nurse to her invalid father until he died. This greatly limited her social activities and her desire to develop a life of her own went unfulfilled. She felt obligated to her father and was quite guilty about the slightest feelings of desire to engage in social activities rather than attend to her father. When she comforted him his legs would rest on areas of her thighs which eventually developed the pains. In addition, she became quite jealous of her sister and fell in love with her brother-in-law. When her sister died she repressed her unacceptable wishes for her brother-in-law and her symptoms became quite severe. Analysis of this patient ultimately led to a cure. Freud termed this a case of "conversion hysteria" in which powerful conflicting psychological affects were converted into somatic symptoms. This case and similar ones led Freud to appreciate the power of the mind and symptom formation and led to his profound influence on psychodynamic theory.

In the twentieth century, psychiatric views of chronic pain remained essentially the same as that originally proposed by Freud. Prior to 1980, a case of chronic pain could have been diagnosed as hysterical neurosis, conversion type, if the pain was considered to have been caused by psychological conflicts which were "transformed" into a complaint of pain.

In 1980, DSM-III was published[(3)]. This document was revolutionary in psychiatric nosology because it refused to infer a psychodynamic etiology to psychiatric conditions and it defined specific criteria which had to be met in order to confer a given diagnosis.

An exception was made, however, in the case of conversion disorder. Traditional views were so powerful in this condition that psychodynamic criteria were included. One had to judge that there was a psychological etiology to the symptoms. The etiology could be related to psychological conflict in the Freudian sense or it could be related to newer concepts of secondary gain. DSM-III also created a new category "psychogenic pain disorder" which was almost identical to conversion disorder except that the primary symptom was "severe and prolonged pain." Other criteria demanded that the pain complaints be "grossly in excess" of whatever physical pathology might be present and that psychological factors had to be part of the etiology. Specifically, the pain had to either result from psychological conflict or provide additional support from the environment or enable the patient to avoid some noxious activity.

The objectivity of DSM-III criteria led to an explosion of research that greatly enhanced our knowledge in many areas of pathology. This has not been equally the case in the area of somatoform disorders however. This is of concern to consultation liason psychiatrists since the somatoform disorders represent an area of psychopathology most likely to be seen in medical patients for whom psychiatric consultations is requested. The somatoform disorders are relatively rare in other subspecialties within psychiatry and other psychiatrists have relatively little interests in them. Of the somatorm disorders in DSM-III, somatization disorder had the most well defined criteria and thus had the most research performed in the 1980s[4,5]. The condition turns out to be quite rare as presently defined and as a result the knowledge of the disorder has not really been enhanced in recent years[4]. With DSM-IV[6], the criteria are broadened in order to attempt to make the disorder more inclusive.

In contrast to somatization disorder, psychogenic pain disorder was hardly studied at all. It was observed however that many patients with chronic pain who did not have an adequate organic explanation for the pain did not fulfill DSM III criteria for psychogenic pain disorder[7, p.424]. There was no obvious psychological conflict which was being solved by the pain disorder, and furthermore issues of secondary gain were not always very clear. The symptoms of pain only seemed to cause distress to the patient. It often appeared that no positive benefit accrued to the patient because of the pain nor did it always allow avoidance of noxious activity. While the DSM III criteria did seem to be present for many pain patients, for many others, they did not. Furthermore, the criteria are almost entirely subjective on the part of the evaluating psychiatrist. The old thrust of the scientific objectification of psychopathology in the 1980s was to specify diagnostic criteria which were highly reliable, reproducable, and atheoretical.

Because of observations that many cases of chronic pain which did not have a significant organic basis also did not have clear evidence of psychological factors in the etiology, in 1987, DSM-III-R changed the condition to "somatoform pain disorder (SPD)"[7]. Psychological factors were no longer required to make the diagnosis. Criterion A was also changed in that "severe and prolonged pain" was no longer required but merely preoccupation with pain. A specific timeframe was designated, six months minimum. The critical criterion for making the diagnosis became the judgment that the pain or the associated impairment was "grossly in excess" of what the physical findings would predict . These criteria for SPD are strikingly close to the definition of chronic pain syndrome as described in the AMA Guides. While the new diagnostic criteria eliminated the problem of using subjective psychological constructs. A definition of SPD presumes that medical findings are objective. In fact, as consultation liason psychiatrists are well aware of, medical diagnosis are often as subjective as any psychiatric diagnosis and frequently even more so. DSM-III-R leaves out the question of how the objectivity of the medical condition is determined.

Structured interviews were developed to test the reliability of DSM-III diagnoses as well as for utilization in psychiatric studies[8]. Somatoform pain disorder did not lend itself to these structured interviews and thus would be left out of epidemiological studies. The disorder cannot be diagnosed by interviewing the patient alone. Medical records were evaluations that other physicians required. Thus while the consultation-liason psychiatrist could frequently suspect the prsence of a somatoform pain disorder based on interview alone (and most likely would be correct), "objective" studies of the disorder could not be done. Furthermore, the sooner that one were to objectify the diagnosis by demanding, say, that a certain number of tests be negative or a certain number of other physicians failed to find an objective medical condition that would explain the pain, they would still be at a loss as to how to measure reliability of the other physicians' diagnoses. For no disorder is there any clear correlation between the amount of pain perceived and the amount of objective pathology. Cancer patients, for instance, with widespread mestastases sometimes reported little to no pain. Furthermore, supposedly objective findings such as abnormalities of the spine found on CAT scans or MRI turn out to be interpreted in widely varying manners by different practitioners and in fact the clinical significance of these objective abnormalitites is often unknown since they occur in high proportion in the general population[9,10].

ILLUSTRATIVE CASES

Case Report: Mr. L. was a 54 year old divorced man whose chief complaint was chronic low back pain. Medical records revealed that when first evaluated by an orthopedic physician for a work-related injury, he already had an attorney and was wearing a TENS unit all day long. The orthopedic surgeon obtained a history from the patient that he had fallen down at work injuring his right elbow and his low back rendering him unable to work. Older records however revealed that the orthopedic surgeon's initial history was in error. The patient had originally complained that while driving a piece of heavy equipment at a construction site, he ran over a rock which jarred him, causing him to hit his elbow and causing low back pain. The low back pain was an exacerbation of back pain which had been present for a year or two previously and was also associated with a prior work related injury and workers' compensation. After the current injury, the patient continued to work for a week or two and then stopped, indicating that the pain made him unable to continue working. The patient later revealed however, that he was also about to be fired. After stopping work, the patient traveled to another state where he reported that an orthopedic surgeon told him that he needed surgery on his low back.

Physical examination was essentially normal. X-rays revealed degenerated L4-5 and L5-S1 disk spaces. The surgeon recommended avoiding surgery and prescribed intensive physical therapy and exercise. In physical therapy, the patient complained of excruciating low back pain and also elbow pain. He was unimproved after four weeks. The patient was then evaluated by a neurosurgeon who obtained the history that the patient had a prior back injury for which he received workers' compensation. That injury occurred when the patient was moving a ladder while employed as a resident manager of an apartment complex. Physical examination revealed a stooped posture and muscle spasm in the left back. It was felt that the patient should only do "light work" and physical therapy was recommended.

A month later the patient was evaluated by a second orthopedic physician. The patient reported using his TENS unit 24 hours per day although the neurosurgeon had obtained a history that the patient was not using it. The patient's complaints had not improved and the pain had spread to his left side from its original location on the right side. The patient complained that the previous examination by the neurosurgeon had caused him so much discomfort that he had to remain in bed the next two days. The patient indicated that he was trying to keep active and was involved with ballroom dancing every night which made him feel better. Other activities were limited because of the pain. Physical exam revealed an "over reactive" patient. X-rays were interpreted as showing old degenerative disk disease. The diagnosis was "chronic pain syndrome." The patient was referred to physical therapy and to a psychologist. It was felt the patient could return to full duty work.

Further physical therapy resulted in no benefit and the impression by the physical therapist that the patient's attitude was poor. The patient was seen by a psychologist who believed that the patient's pain was in great part psychological. Biofeedback measurements of muscular tension however indicated very high levels and it was felt that biofeedback might be helpful. Follow-up visits indicated that the patient was responding well to biofeedback with regard to his levels of muscular tension but that the patient was reluctant to admit improvements. During this period of time the patient returned to the other state and again received a letter from an orthopedic surgeon recommending surgery.

Psychiatric evaluation occurred one and a half years after the injury. The patient complained that he was getting worse. He stated that he had "two herniated disks, bone spurs, arthritis of some form, nerve root compression, and a non-stable joint." The back pain was described as pinching, stabbing, and aching. Upon further discussion, the patient defined the pain as being of two types, the first type is a "lightning pain" which was a stabbing pain occurring suddenly and unpredictably. It would occur when his back was "unstable" and more likely to occur if he achieved too much relaxation. By holding his muscles tense, he was usually able to lessen the frequency of this kind of pain. The pain would typically be on the right side of his lower back but sometimes it would be on the left side. After the "lightning pain" comes the "fire." This was a pain caused by muscle spasms and was present all the time. He particularly got this pain if he relaxed too much, allowing his "loose joint" to become too unstable. Anti-inflamatory medication could control the pain and the TENS machine helped a great deal. Lying down would make the back pain worse. Sleeping was the worst because his body would become so relaxed it was vulnerable to the severe pain. If he noticed his body getting too relaxed, he would try to "jerk" himself out of it with a quick movement. Sometimes that way he could avoid severe back pain.

The patient indicated that his only medication for pain was an anti-inflamatory drug which was helpful but had significant side effects including sleepiness, impotence, and memory loss.

The patient also complained of difficulties developing in his legs. He would get pains in various parts of either leg and also numbness from time to time. He was also developing neck pain. This was due to kinking his neck in his sleep as a result of his back pain. The elbow pain was mild as long as he did not use it.

The patient's current activities consisted of going to doctors' appointments and physical therapy with his girlfriend who was also on disability and had similar appointments. He would go dancing at night and during the day would ride his motorcycle which was much more comfortable than riding in a car. He did not have financial concerns since his workers' compensation payments were substantially more than his monthly expenses.

The past history was remarkable for the contrast between the patient's high regard for his own abilities and talents his failure in almost everything that he did. In high school, Mr. L. stated that he was a class officer and an outstanding athlete. He was the captain of several sports teams and held records in a number of track events that stood for many years. Despite being president of his class, he got bored and dropped out of high school before graduating, running away from home to seek a warmer climate. He married a wealthy girl but suffered abuse from his in-laws who were drug and alcohol abusers. This caused him to leave the family and he lost contact with his only daughter.

Mr. L. was then drafted into the army but somehow managed to get into the navy and then was able to obtain an honorable medical discharge by hounding the doctors about a bad knee due to a football injury.

Mr. L. then intended to go to dental school but instead did a variety of things and ended up in Puerto Rico where he became an extremely successful businessman owning six retail stores, a night club and a restaurant. He married a Puerto Rican woman who turned out to be a "white witch." Unfortunately his wife became possessed by a "black witch" and a spell was put on his property. Ultimately they got divorced and Mr. L. lost everything.

Mr. L. then moved back to his home state to help his mother with her financial affairs since she had inherited a great deal from his father. Although he was very helpful to his mother, his siblings were all jealous and dishonest and they ended up obtaining a restraining order requiring Mr. L. to stay away from his mother.

Then Mr. L. moved to another state. He opened up a mail box rental business and a gift store. He was making a lot of money for the government because of all the gifts that were being mailed. He was doing so much business that he became the fifth largest "postal entity" in the state including all the regular post offices. The people in charge of the post office department however changed a contract which resulted in him losing money. Because of this dishonesty on the part of the postal officials, he had to sell his business.

Mr. L. then went through a series of three different jobs, working as a resident manager in apartment complexes. He was fired from each job. In each case, Mr. L. explained that he disagreed with the dishonest practices of the Boards of Directors. Doing one of these jobs, he claimed a back injury resulting from the moving of a ladder and received workers' compensation for it. Finally he obtained his most recent job operating heavy equipment at a construction site. Shortly after obtaining this job, he had his current injury and had not returned to work during the ensuing one and a half years.

Mr. L. expected that if he could get surgery for his back, he would be cured. After that he thought that he would like to get a job running a corporation. He felt it would not be difficult to get such a job. He noted that there are more jobs available at the top because people do not want to do those kinds of jobs.

Mental status examination revealed a sharply dressed man who gave the appearance of an executive much more than a construction worker. He carried a brief case in which he had medical records related to his case. He spoke freely and spontaneously. He appeared physically comfortable throughout the four hour interview. He showed no evidence of anxiety or depression. Affect was of normal range and appropriate to the conversation. He smiled frequently. He was not angry, hostile or guarded. Thought processes were logical, coherent and goal directed. There was some unusual ideation. He spoke at great length about his physical problems. He tended to describe them in terms of medical or pseudo-medical diagnoses rather than actual symptoms and complaints. His descriptions and belief about his bodily functions were often unusual and inconsistent. (Compression makes his back worse, but relaxing also makes it worse and tensing the muscles makes it better. Traction makes it better but lying down makes it worse. He has a loose joint that needs to be held in place. Anti-inflamatory drugs decrease his hearing, make him sleepy, make him impotent, and permanently affect his memory.) There were unusual ideas in other areas. (His belief in possession and the occult in Puerto Rico.) His descriptions of himself and others were typically in a very one dimensional fashion. With regard to himself, he is extremely talented, honest and capable. He is also mistreated and misunderstood. With regard to others, they tend to be dishonest, unreliable, untrustworthy and unappreciative. Attention, concentration and memory were intact. He could easily repeat six numbers forward and five numbers backward. Serial sevens were performed correctly. Presidents were named correctly back to Kennedy. Similarities and proverbs were interpreted correctly with the proper level of abstraction. He was pleasant and cooperative throughout the interview.

DSM-III-R diagnosis was as follows:

Axis I: Somatoform and pain disorder
Axis II: Narcissistic personality disorder
Axis III: Back pain and leg pain
Axis IV: 2-Mild (unstable residence and occupation)
Axis V: Current 66; past year 66

Two orthopedic surgeons and one neurosurgeon all concluded that the patient had minimal if any organic basis that would explain severe persistent complaints of pain and on-going disability. A letter from a surgeon in another state indicated that surgery was recommended on the low back. While the preponderance of medical evidence seemed to support the diagnosis of somatoform pain disorder, the psychiatric history of medical and mental status revealed factors which very much supported such a diagnosis. The patient's pain complaints, when explored in depth, turned out to be somewhat unusual even bizarre. They involved multiple areas of the body and they were shifting in character. The patient's history of ballroom dancing and motorcycle riding as well as his lack of discomfort during the long interview were all inconsistent with his pain complaints. Furthermore, the multiple problems in all areas of his life further suggested that the pain complaints should not be taken at face value. Thus the diagnosis of somatoform pain disorder seemed warranted.

Mr. L.'s history was also consistent with a narcissistic personality disorder. For example, he described himself as an immensely capable man who could run several businesses at the same time, an artist, a designer, a manufacturer, and who was also extremely knowledgeable about many aspects of construction. Despite this, the history listed many business failures, bankruptcy, and being fired repeatedly. In every instance, however, Mr. L. blamed the problem entirely on others whom he considered to be dishonest or, in the case of his second wife, possessed by an evil witch. This pattern even included his own family members. All of his siblings were considered to be dishonest and had conspired against him. He described himself as the "white sheep" in the family. Likewise all of his doctors failed to understand his medical problems which were unique, with the sole exception of the surgeon from another state. All of this was quite consistent with narcissistic personality disorder.

Case Report: Ms. T, a 63 year old divorced woman claimed several injuries while working as a nurse at a chronic care facility. The patient complained of pain which was present more often than not. The pain could be anywhere and everywhere. It included her neck, shoulders, arms, hands, legs, back and chest. Her pains began two years previously shortly after she began work at a new job. She was feeling fine and in good health, but then injured her back while attempting to transfer a patient . This injury did not cause her to take any time off from work but over the next couple months she was frequently criticized in her job and she believed she was given unfair assignments which caused her to deteriorate physically. She was trying to protect her injured back while she did her job and this caused problems in multiple other areas of her body.

Then the patient was assigned to the Medical Records Department because her supervisors did not feel that her performance was satisfactory when involving patient care. This angered the nurse. In addition, she felt that it would not be safe for her to work in

Medical Records since she would have to pull open stuck file drawers and lift and push files. She refused to work and filed another workers' compensation claim. The employer responded by firing the patient. She went to the union to fight her dismissal. She pointed out that someone who has a workers' compensation claim pending cannot be fired. The union was able to salvage the patient's job. She was rehired but not allowed to work as a nurse. She again felt that the job she had involved filing papers which was too physically stressful. She filed another workers' compensation claim. The patient decided that all of this was literally stressful also so she filed another workers' compensation claim for mental stress.

Ms. T denied any significant past history of pain problems. She acknowledged that she did have a condition called fibromyalgia which had caused pains all over her body for a few months. That condition, however, was easily treated with medication and exercise and then completely disappeared. Her current pains were nothing like the fibromyalgia pain that she had previously.

In addition to the pains all over her body, Ms. T complained of carpal tunnel syndrome. She noted numbness and soreness in her wrists and hands which would occur once or twice per week. She also complained of headaches, dizziness, nausea, and trouble swallowing. All of her symptoms had only been present since her employment at the chronic care facility. Ms. T denied any kind of emotional problems. She noted that she had been angry a lot but felt that was a healthy response appropriate to all that had happened to her. In fact, her anger was helpful. She needed "to have an edge on " to keep herself alert in order to catch problems that might occur when battling for her various claims and grievances.

Ms. T. was the fifth of six children. She was quite reluctant to talk about her past and gave few details. She did report that she had found school to be quite boring and did not attend class very much. She managed to graduate from high school and enlisted in the marines. She married another marine but the relationship ended up in divorce. She refused to talk about the issues that led to the divorce. Ms. T had four children and five grandchildren. She was not close to her children at present. She had been treated for alcoholism in the past but she had been sober for twenty years. Ms. T gave a history of many previous jobs which helped her develop many skills. Particularly in working with people. She had been living with a boyfriend for seventeen years but that relationship ended after she began work at the chronic care facility. Ms. T blamed her problems at that facility for the break up with her boyfriend.

Ms. T was living alone in a condominium that she owned. On occasion, she would go out with friends but otherwise kept to herself. Ms. T expected to win all her claims and return to her work. She felt that she could continue working for a number of years. She was also writing a book.

Medical records revealed a long past history of problems with pain. She had been injured in an automobile accident twenty-five years previously. Following this she developed chronic pain in her back, leg and other areas of her body. Two years after the accident, she had low back surgery. Post operative course was stormy and the patient had difficulties getting along with the nurses. A psychiatric consultation was obtained. The psychiatric consultant noted that the patient had initially been well to do with an inheritance but had been unable to hold a job and had ended up on welfare after her divorce. The patient was felt to have prominent dependency needs.

Six months after the surgery a consulting neurosurgeon reported that the patient's children called him at 4:00 am and reported that the patient had been lying on the floor unable to get up. The patient was quite angry with her attorney who had implied that Ms. T had unnecessarily had her surgery in order to get money. The neurosurgeon noted that the patient had complaints of headaches, dizziness, problems with her vision, problems swallowing , neck pain, shoulder pain, elbow pain, pain in her hands, back pain, abdominal pain, hip pain, and leg pain. All these symptoms had been present following the automobile
accident.

The neurosurgeon did not see the patient for the next six years. She returned again having multiple complaints. A year later, after a physical theraphy program, the patient's complaints were alleviated. The year following that however, the patient's complaints had reutrned.

The patient had a motor vehicle accident eleven years previously and two more two years following that. These were associated with multiple painful symptoms in the neck, back, and extremities.

Over the next few years medical records revealed that the patient sufferred from various additional injuries and pain complaints. One physician characterized the patient as having a "universal pain syndrome".

During the year prior to her employment with the chronic care facility, Ms. T saw a new physician who diagnosed her multiple complaints as fibromyalgia. This physician diagnosed the patient's current complaints as "fibromyalgia aggravated by work". The patient was referred to a psychiatrist who diagnosed major depression. Two anti-depressant medications were prescribed to be taken simultaneously and the patient was placed in twice a week group therapy with other chronic pain patients. The patient admitted that she had not taken the medication which was prescribed. She had attended the groups and had felt supported. She reported that the group members would "confirm" each other. She felt no need to continue the group however because she was at a different level from the other patients. She actually had been trained to lead groups rather than participate in them.

Mental status examination revealed a moderately overweight woman who sat ratherly stiffly in the chair. Periodically she would stand during the interview. Her affect was intense. She would become angry frequently in an abrupt fashion and recover quickly. Frequently she would smile and even laugh. Often this was incongruous as she was talking about such things as being mistreated and other events which were disconcerting to her. At thimes she spoke freely and spontaneously and at great length. Generally this was when she discussed her perceived mistreatment at work and her grievances. At other times she was very defensive and responded only in the most brief and general terms. On a number of occasions she refused to answer questions or talk about certain areas of her history. It was a constant theme that she was treated unfairly, misunderstood, discriminated, and conspired against, and her many talents and skills were unappreciated. For examle, as a nursing student, she tutored her peers successfully to the point that they got A's. She did not het as good grades herself, however.

Thought processes were logical, coherent and goal directed. When asked to describe her symptoms, however, she frequently strayed from the subject ot describe events that had occurred at work. it was as if the presence of physical symptoms was the same as "stress" or unfair treatment at work. The presence of one was equivalent to the presence of the other. When asked to distinguish the characteristics of the pain in different locations, she was unable to do so and became quite angry at this type of interest in her symptoms.

There was no deficit in attention, concentration or memory. She was almost comabtive in her response to the interview. At times, she verged on being hostile. Her descriptions of interactiojns with physicians, co-workers and supervisors were often laced with sarcasm. While she had paranoid tendencies in that she expected the worst from everyone, there were no formed delusions. Insight was poor. She acknowledged no personal contribution at all to any of her difficulties. She expressed no interest in gaining any understanding of herself or her situation. she expressed no interest in treatment. She was not at all concerned about resolution of her symptoms. She was preoccupied with her litigation and gleeful at the prospect of winning. She had no questions for me at the end of the interview.

DSM-III-R diagnosis was as follows:

Axis I:	Somatoform Pain Disorder
Axis II:	Paranoid Personality Disorder with Narcissistic and Passive Aggressive Traits
Axis III:	Multiple Physical Complaints
Axis IV:	3-Moderate (job disatisfaction, trouble with boss, litigation)
Axis V:	Current - 54; past year 54

Somatorform Pain Disorder was diagnosed becaused Ms. T was markedly preoccupied with pain as her primary symptom. Her multiple areas of pain were described in a rather bizarre fashion and fit no physiological disorder. Physical examinations had revealed no significant objective findings to account for the patients complaints. Her multiple complaints of pain been present off and an for at least twenty five years and were attributed to different things at different times.

The diagnosis of Ms. T's characteristic tendency to interpret the actions of people as deliberately demeaning or threatening. She expected others to attempt to exploit her. She was extremely mistrustful and was quick to react with anger. She would bear grudges and was unforgiving. She was extremely reluctanct to confide in others for fear the information would be used against her. She did not appear to have a true sense of humor nor did she demonstrate soft or tender feelings. She appeared to avoid intimacy and she had an extreme need to be self sufficient. She would exaggerate her self-importance.

The above two cases seem to clearly represent psychiatric disturbances in which organic factors play a minimal part. Without extensive review of medical records and without the benefit of a lengthy psychiatric interview, a physician could reasonably have difficulty making the diagnosis of somatoform pain disorder. A physician seeking to find an organic diagnosis, could focus the questioning along certain lines. A patient sensing areas of the physician's interest might focus the complaints in those areas and be less forthcoming in other areas which would place the history in a larger context. Thus, the diagnosis of somatoform pain disorder may be missed and an organic diagnosis mistakenly accepted.

In the 1980s new diagnostic entities were developed to account for many conditions with chronic pain such as fibromyalgia, myofascial pain syndrome, and temporomandibular joint disease[11,12,13]. Some authors have gone so far as to claim that most chronic pain patients have myofascial pain disorders and almost none have somatoform pain disorders[14]. It has even been claimed that non-physiological findings are part of the myofascial syndrome[15]. The lack of studies of somatoform pain disorder have likely contributed to the absence of recognition of this condition.

In our studies of somatoform pain disorder, we have found that pain appears to be a common occurrence in patients claiming workers' compensation injuries or motor vehicle injuries who are referred for psychiatric evaluation. Most of these appear seem to have somatoform pain disorder.

Our study of 49 such cases who appear to have unequivocal somatoform pain disorder revealed a number of interesting associated findings[16]. Ninety-eight percent of the cases had chronic pain in more than one site. In eighty-one percent the pain had spread beyond the original site of injury. The average number of distinct sites of chronic pain was five. More than two-thirds of the cases complained of frequent severe headaches.

For three quarter of the subjects the pain prevented them from working. More than half of the subjects had a history of pain prior to the current injury.

About half of the patients used daily prescription narcotics for their pain. One third of the patients used benzodiazepines daily. A number of cases had past histories of alcohol abuse which stopped when daily intake of narcotic medications was begun.

Almost half of the sample had a comorbid depressive diagnosis. Either currently or at some time during the course of their painful illness. Only twelve percent qualified for a substance use disorder diagnosis. Many patients on high doses of narcotics did not qualify for such a diagnosis because they took the medications as prescribed.

There were a large number of specialized diagnostic tests which were negative or equivocal. For a few cases these tests were repeated several times. Surgery was attempted in one quarter of the sample without any positive results.

A rating scale was devised to access the influence of litigation. Positive scores were given if symptoms increased in association with legal or insurance issues or contact with attorneys, insurance adjusters, or consulting physicians, or if treatment interventions, or rehabilitation efforts were resisted. Using this scale, thirty-nine percent of the cases were judged as having a major influence of litigation or compensation on their symptoms and fourteen percent were rated as having a moderate influence. Litigation issues were judged to have no or minimal influence on forty-seven percent of the cases.

The treatment history was remarkable in that no treatment of any type helped the patient's condition. Eighty-four percent of the patients had physical therapy which not only failed to improve their complaints of pain, but often made them worse. Thirty-one percent of the patients had massage therapy. Frequently the patients enjoyed this therapy and indicated it gave them temporary relief. The patients overall condition was never effected by this therapy however. The same held true for chiropractic treatments which were received by forty-seven percent of the sample.

Thirty-three percent of the sample had tried transcutaneous electrical nerve stimulation (TENS) . Most patients stated that this was not effective. A few patients proudly wore their TENS units which represented proof of their painful disorder. They stated that it was slightly helpful but did not change their underlying condition. Typically, they would rate the pain as nine or ten on a ten point scale without the TENS unit and seven or eight with it.

Anti-depresssant medication was used with fifty-five percent of the sample. Most of these patients had received the equivalent of 150 mg imipramine or more for at least one month. Several patients had been tried on a number of different anti-depressant medications. Some of these patients had improvement of depressive symptoms coincident with this treatment. None of the patients had amelioration of their pain complaints by use of these medications.

Seventy-six percent of the patients had been referred for psychotherapy. Medical records revealed that only nineteen percent of the therapists had diagnosed a somatoform pain disorder or the equivalent. Fifty-five percent of the therapists accepted the pain complaints as medically appropriate and they supported the patient in coping with a chronic physical disability. Some of the therapists became advocates for the patients in their litigation or their compensation claims.

We conclude that somatoform pain disorder is a condition of major medical and econonmic consequence and is not uncommon in a population of injured workers. Pain tends to spread from the original site of injury and occurs in multiple areas of the body. It is notoriously unresponsive to all types of treatment and iatrogenic complications of medication dependence and surgery are common.

DSM-IV

In DSM-IV[6] Somatoform Pain Disorder changes its name and is divided into two conditions. The first is Pain Disorder Associated with Psychological Factors. The psychological factors are judged to have a major role in the onset, severity, exacerbation, or maintenance of the pain. The second diagnosis is Pain Disorder Associated with Both Psychological Factors and a General Medical Condition. In this case both psycological factors and a medical condition are judged to have important roles in the onset, severity, exacerbation, or maintenance of the pain. The disorders are judged to be chronic if the duration is more than six months.

Utilizing DSM-IV criteria we evaluated the cases of somatoform pain disorder in the above study. All cases fulfilled DSM criteria for a pain disorder. Two-thirds fulfilled criteria for Pain Disorder Associated with Psychological Factors and the other third fulfiled criteria for Pain Disorder Associated with Both Psychological Factors and a General Medical Condition. For eighty percent of the latter group the general medical condition was judged to be important only in the onset of the disorder.

We conclude that DSM-IV criteria for pain disorder may be broader and more inclusive than DSM-III-R. Cases which did not qualify for somatoform pain disorder in our study because of the presence of significant medical pathology might have qualified for the DSM-IV disorder of Pain Disorder Associated with Both Psychological Factors and a General Medical Condition. It remains to be seen whether the increases specificity of DSM-IV criteria will help to advance our understanding of pain disorders and make them easier to study.

REFERENCES

1. Guides to the Evaluation of Permanent Impairment, American Medical Association (Third edition, revised), Chicago, 1990

2. Freud S: Fraulein Elisabeth Von R. In: The Standard Edition of the Complete Psychological Works of Sigmund Freud. Volume II. Strachey J., ed. London: The Hogarth Press, 1962, 135-181

3. DSM-III Diagnostic and Statistical Manual of Mental Disorders, (Third edition), American Psychiatric Association, Washington, D.C., 1980

4. Escobar JI, Burnam MA, Karno M, Forsythe A, Golding JM: Somatization in the community. Arch Gen Psychiatry, 44:713-718, 1987

5. Smith GR, Monson RA, Ray DC: Psychiatric consultation in somatization disorder: A randomized controlled study. N Engl J Med 314(22):1407-1413, 1986

6. Task Force on DSM-IV, DSM-IV Draft Criteria, American Psychiatric Association, Washington, D.C., 1993

7. DSM-III-R Diagnostic and Statistical Manual of Mental Disorders (Third edition, revised), American Psychiatric Association, Washington, D.C., 1987

8. Spitzer RL, Williams JB, Gibbon, M: Structured Clinical Interviews for DSM-III-R, New York, N.Y.: New York State Psychiatric Institute, 1987

9. Wiesel SW, Tsourmas N, Feffer HL, Citrin CM, Patronas N: A study of computer-assisted tomography 1. The incidence of Postive CAT scans in an asymptomatic group of patients. Spine 9(6):549-551, 1984

10. Boden SD, Davis DO, Dina TS, Patronas NJ, Wiesel SW: Abnormal magnetic-resonance scans of the lumbar spine in asymptomatic subjects. The Journal of Bone and Joint Surgery 403-408, 1990

11. Boissevain MD, McCain GA: Toward an integrated understanding of fibromyalgia Syndrome. I. Medical and pathophysiological aspects. Pain 45:227-238, 1991

12. Rosomoff HL, Fishbain D, Goldberg M, Steele-Rosemoff R: Myofascial findings in patients with "chronic intractable benign pain" of the back and neck. Pain Management 114-118, 1990

13. Nelson DA: Thoracic outlet syndrome and dysfunction of the temporomandibular joint: Proved pathology or pseudosyndromes? Perspect Bio Med 33:567-576, 1990

14. Fishbain DA, Goldberg M, Steele R, Rosomoff H: DSM-III Diagnoses of Patients With Myofascial Pain Syndrome (Fibrositis). Arch Phys Med Rehabil 70:433-438, 1989

15. Fishbain DA, Goldberg M, Rosomoff RS, Rosomoff H: Chronic pain patients and the nonorganic physical sign of nondermatomal sensory abonormalities (NDSA). Psychosomatics 32:294-303, 1991

16. Streltzer J, Eliashof, B: Somatoform Pain Disorder in "Injured" Workers. Presentation at the 7th World Congress on Pain, Aug. 22-27, 1993, Paris, France

CHRONIC PAIN AND ADDICTION

Jon Streltzer, M.D.

Professor of Psychiatry
Univeristy of Hawaii at Manoa
John A. Burns School of Medicine
Department of Psychiatry
1356 Lusitana Street
Honolulu, HI 96813

INTRODUCTION

Is addiction a problem in chronic pain? There is a school of thought arguing that it is not. The arguments include the following: Thousands upon thousands of patients have been treated with narcotics for acute post-operative pain. It is very rare that any of them become addicts[1]. Therefore treatment of pain with narcotics does not lead to addiction. Even long term use of narcotics is appropriate because, miraculously, tolerance does not develop[2,3]. The proof is that many patients reach a plateau and stay there with regard to medication dose. If patients increase their dose, then it must be because their pain got worse. It has even been argued that narcotics are not pleasant and therefore no one would take more than absolutely necessary. However, the fact that pain patients reach a standard dose of narcotics does not prove that dependence is not a problem any more than the fact that heroin addicts or methadone maintenance patients reach stable doses implies that they do not have a dependency problem.

It has also been argued that if indeed a patient is dependent upon opiates for pain then the best treatment is to maintain them upon opiates[4]. The reasoning is that the patients do not get off these medications easily. They resist detoxification and they complain of more pain if their medication is decreased. This argument is similar to the arguments for methadone maintenance as opposed to therapeutic communities or other drug-free modalities for street narcotic addicts. Narcotic addicts who become incarcerated however are not maintained on methadone. No one would argue that they need methadone maintenance when they have no access to narcotics. Similarly to argue that medical addicts need to be maintained on opiates is to consider that their access to medication is always present. If, on the other hand, these patients do not have physicians prescribing the medications for them, they will not and cannot continue to take them. In this sense, their dependence is iatrogenic.

Consultation-Liaison Psychiatry: 1990 and Beyond
Edited by H. Leigh, Plenum Press, New York, 1994

An analogy of the situation can be seen with regard to tobacco. Smokers will complain of significant symptoms if tobacco is denied them. These symptoms disappear completely if they continue their smoking. Physicians no longer argue that for such people smoking is worthwhile and the benefits outweigh the drawbacks. At one time physicians did argue this way however.

The argument that addiction is a problem in chronic pain states that tolerance is a problem with narcotic medication. Because of tolerance the patient taking regular doses of narcotics over the long term will receive little analgesic benefit. Thus, maintenance narcotic medication does not help chronic pain but adds secondary complications of medication dependence[5,6,7].

This model suggests that narcotics may actually make the pain worse[8,9]. Toward the end of the duration of action of the medication the patient goes into a mini-withdrawal state. The patient interprets pain as increased pain and therefore seeks more medication. Patients who use narcotics regularly report that their pain is always with them and they end up taking their medication on a fairly regular schedule. If they are on high doses of medication, they wake up of the middle of the night to take a dose. One would expect a painful condition to be associated with good days and bad days and to require more medication on some days than others. For most chronic pain patients who use regular narcotics however, their intake tends to be consistent and more dependent upon supply than fluctuations of pain[10].

Animal studies support this viewpoint[11]. Animals with no prior history of substance abuse would readily become addicted to narcotics when they are supplied in an easily available form. The animals will consume the narcotics on a regular schedule and at some point reach a plateau with regard to their intake. If the narcotic supply is cut back or eliminated, the animals will initially greatly increase their drug seeking behavior. An analagous situation is found in chronic pain patients who initially complain of increased pain and seek more prescriptions when their dose is cut down.

In the 1980s there was wide spread recognition that acute pain tended to be under-treated in the medical community[12,13]. Coincident with this there has been an increassed acceptance of the possibility of treating chronic pain with narcotics. It is the authors contention that for most chronic pain patients this is not helpful. This is particularly true for patients with somatoform pain disorder but is also probably true for most cases with significant organic pathology. For many patients, pain can be markedly alleviated or even eliminated by weaning the patient off of narcotics[10]. For other patients the complaints of pain continue but the persons functioning greatly improves.

ILLUSTRATIVE CASES

Case Report: Mr. A, a 55 year old veterinarian was referred for evaluation of his chronic headaches. His wife had become quite concerned when he had passed out during dog surgery recently and thought it might be related to his headache medication. Mr. A stated that he suffered from daily headache since veterinary school. He used narcotic pain pills to treat the headaches and his medication requirements and frequency of headache had gradually increased over the years. He was currently using a variety of codeine, propoxyphene and oxycodone preparations. He did not have a fixed schedule for any of these medications but rather used them at various times and in varying combinations according to his sense of the quality of the headache and its severity. His first dose, however, was usually shortly after arising in the morning. He took more pain pills during the day and he always took a bedtime dose. In addition, most nights the headache woke him up and he had to take more medication in order to get back to sleep. Medications were prescribed by a phsycian friend on demand.

There was no significant past medical history aside from the headaches and there was no past psychiatric history. The man did no drink or smoke. Aside from his work, his only interests were watching news on TV and reading veterinary journals. He tended to be quite shy and withdrawn in contrast to his wife who was quite outgoing and managed all the household affairs. Mr. A. was minimally involved in the raising of his children. On mental status examination, he was not anxious or depressed, but was quite formal and intellectual. He was unable to talk at any length about any subject other than his work and he denied experiencing strong emotions such as anger or joy. Diagnostically he was thought to have a somatoform pain disorder, opiate dependence, and obsessive and schizoid personality traits.

He was asked to provide a diary of his headaches and also the medications that he took. He was happy to do this and provided a detailed typewritten sheet specifically documenting his experiences of the week. The diary revealed that the patient took 14 to 16 narcotic doses each 24 hour period where a dose was considered equivalent to 60 milligrams of codeine. The patient was told that his headaches were probably caused to a great extent by his dependence on medication and that it was recommended that he be detoxified from narcotics as the critical step in the management of his headaches. The patient was told that this could be done as an outpatient but it could also be done more rapidly and more easily as an inpatient. The patient stated he would like to do it as an inpatient because he thought he would have great difficulty following the protocol as an outpatient.

Arrangements were made for an elective admission. The patient was easily detoxified using methadone over a six day period. The patient was entirely compliant in the hospital and only complained of a headache when asked.

Upon discharge, the patient was given a small dose of an antidipressant medication to use as needed for headaches. The patient was initially followed weekly but as he did very well the visits were quickly spread out to the point where he was followed every six months for several years. Each visit followed a typical pattern. Mr. A. would come in smiling and act very cordial. Then he would state "Doctor, I still have headaches. Is there any medication you could give me that would help my headaches?" Mr. A. was then asked about his headaches and the medication that he was using and about what was going on in his personal life. Then a slight adjustment was made in the medication either changing the dose or switching to a new medication. The patient always appeared satisfied at the end of the interview.

One month after discharge from the hospital, Mr. A's wife was seen and she reported that her husband seemed like a new man. He was much more attentive and less forgetful. His personality had greatly improved and had returned to the way it once was, very reliable and predictable. He no longer had any difficulties doing surgery in his veterinary practice.

This patient was quite easy to treat. He never gave up his complaint of headaches but the headaches caused no difficulties whatsoever after he was withdrawn from narcotic analgesics. The patient had used narcotics for many years for his headaches. When he was younger, this did not seem to cause him significant disability. Over the years, however, the dose kept increasing until significant behavioral affects were finally recognized by his wife.

The following case is of a patient who had a history of intermittent alcohol and street drug abuse prior to his dependency on pain medications.

Case Report: Mr. D, a 35 year old construction worker, had a minor injury on the job causing him to complain of shoulder and neck pain. The patient received workers' compensation benefits and stayed out of work while he recovered. The orthopedic surgeon prescribed physical therapy and gave him pain medication, Percodan. Mr. D, an experienced street drug user, asked for a lot of medication. He then suddenly developed a massive GI bleed requiring hospitalization. One consultant felt that the cause might be the aspirin in Percodan which the patient was taking. Following this hospitalization, the orthopedic surgeon prescribed Percocet. Over the next two and a half years, Mr. D took this medication in steadily increasing doses and complained of constant pain which had spread to his low back. In addition to receiving narcotic pain medications, the orthopedic surgeon periodically gave cortisone injections into the shoulder area.

Finally the rehabilitation counselor suggested to Mr D that he see a psychiatrist interested in pain management when the patient had become almost nonfunctional and afraid to drive following a motor vehicle accident in which the patient almost fell asleep at the wheel. Mr. D was told that his pain medications were making his pain worse and that he needed to be admitted for detoxification. On the day of admission, Mr. D indicated that he had been so afraid of developing withdrawal symptoms in the hospital that he had stopped all the medications himself several days previously. He developed withdrawal symptoms which were now gone. Indeed in the hospital Mr. D required no narcotic medication. He had also been dependent on Valium taking 40 milligrams a day for two years. This medication was reduced to 30 mg and gradually tapered off over a four month period.

Off of narcotics, Mr. D's pain diminished markedly. After discharge, an agreement was made with the orthopedic surgeon that he would not prescribe narcotic medications. Mr. D remained drug free and resumed normal activities. He still complained of some pain but much milder than before.

This patient became cooperative when the psychiatrist took control of the pain medications and Mr. D knew that he would not be maintained on narcotics. He had insight in to his substance abuse problem and was able to improve when the proper controls were instituted.

The following case is of a patient who had significant physical pathology but for who pain medication greatly complicated his course.

Case Report: Mr. P, a 42 year old man, first injured his back 20 years previously when working as a painter. He was diagnosed as having a ruptured disk with sciatica. He improved gradually after surgery. He continued to use Darvocet off and on for about four years. The maximum dose was four pills per day. Then Mr. P obtained a new nonlaboring job as a hospital aide. His symptoms completely disappeared and he enjoyed this job for four years. He then slipped on a wet floor and fell, injuring his back and developing sciatica and a foot drop. Mr. P had excruciating pain and was immediately operated on. The neurological symptoms improved but pain continued and three months later Mr. P was operated on again. He patient improved somewhat. He was taking about six to seven Percodan per day and his surgeon was unhappy with this. A second opinion was obtained and the patient switched to the new surgeon. This surgeon indicated that the narcotic medications were part of the problem and needed to be reduced and eliminated. He repeated a myelogram, however, and felt that Mr. P still had a surgical lesion. Six months after the previous surgery, he reoperated. After that, Mr. P seemed to improve slowly. He was referred to a psychiatrist for possible depression and to help cope with his disability. Within a year he had returned to work part time. He was fearful that he would reinjure his back at work however. The psychiatrist initially felt that Mr. P needed his pain medications because of his definite organic disease. After a while however the psychiatrist came to believe that the intake of the pain medications was excessive and that Mr. P was addicted. The patient's pain meds were reduced when he went back to work and continued to be reduced until he was taking only two or three Darvocet per day. After this reduction, Mrs. P indicated that her husband seemed to do much better. He was more active and his old personality had returned. He was no longer so irritable.

The surgeon had been contemplating another operation for some time however because Mr. P's complaints had persisted so long. Another operation was performed three years after the injury and fourteen years after the initial surgery. The patient's low dose of pain medication and his improved functioning had only been present only for a month prior to the operation. This improvement was not factored into the decision to operate.

Following this last operation, Mr. P did much worse. His pain became more severe and had spread to include pain down the right leg as well as the left. Pain medication increased to an equivalent of about 10 narcotic pills per day. Six months after the operation, the surgeon was concerned about the level of narcotic intake and felt it was quite excessive. Mr. P was admitted to a rehabilitation facility for treatment of his chronic pain. He was to be detoxified from narcotics while receiving physical therapy. Mr. P seemed to do pretty well in the hospital and was doing well in physical therapy. However, Mr. P became concerned in the third week when the methadone dose became low. He signed out of the hospital and immediately resumed his regular medications. Mr. P was then referred to a physician who was considered to be a specialist in addiction medicine. This physician judged that the patient needed narcotics for his pain but that they should be limited to no more than seven narcotic tablets per day. Over the next few months, this physician gradually increased the prescriptions in response to the pain complaints until Mr. P was again taking about ten narcotic tablets per day. Care was then taken over by the patient's family doctor.

Mr. P also stopped seeing the psychiatrist. He was angry that the psychiatrist had supported the idea of surgery which the patient felt had made him much worse. At the time the patient stopped seeing him, the psychiatrist was also strongly indicating to the patient that he needed to reduce his pain medications.

Within the next five years, the patient was maintained on pain medications by his family doctor. The dose gradually increased until it was up to 20 - 23 narcotic tablets per day. The patient withdrew from social activities and for the most part was a recluse.

Mr. P was then referred to a "pain management specialist". This physician indicated he would treat the patient with anti-depressant medication and immediately begin weaning the patient from his narcotics until they were eliminated. He also placed the patient in group therapy with other chronic pain patients. In addition, the physician provided physical therapy on the same day as the group therapy. The physical therapy consisted of massage and heat.

The patient felt better with this treatment. He was no longer a recluse and attended therapy sessions three times per week. He made friends with some of the other group members and the patient found it helpful to talk with these people particularly about how to manage finances since they were all dependent upon disability payments. After that experience, the patient believed that his mood and attitude improved which he attributed in part to the antidipressant medication. The patient denied any change at all in his pain however. Physical therapy was enjoyable but within an hour after the massage his pain was the same as always. Mr. P strongly resisted the tapering of his narcotic medications. When he was given small prescriptions, he would run out and call in needing more. After six months of this new treatment, his narcotic intake had remained the same.

Although the patient had positive physical findings which included a diminished patellar reflex on the left and some mild weakness of the dorsiflexors of the left foot, he was able to ambulate without difficulty. He could easily get up and down from the chair and he was able to sit comfortably throughout an evaluation interview lasting almost four hours. He drove his car frequently. When interviewed, he was quite pleasant and cooperative, engaging and convivial. He was not depressed. He had a history of periodic moodiness and irritability with loss of temper followed by feelings of guilt for his outburst. Other interviewers noted that at times he presented with slurred speech. He expressed great fear that if he reduced his medications the pain would be intolerable. He had no interest in any kind of treatment other than the continuation of his pain medication.

The patient had no prior history of drug or alcohol abuse. There was a history of alcoholism in a brother and his father. He originally was treated with a narcotic pain medication for a bonafide medical condition known to be associated with acute pain. Treatment of acute pain with narcotics as well as treatment of postoperative pain with narcotics is thought to be very rarely associated with addiction problems. On the other hand, medication dependence is noted to be commonly associated with chronic pain.

Overall, during his ten year course of illness, Mr. P had treatment or consultation with ten physicians all of whom felt that he was dependent on his medication or recommended that the narcotic medication be eliminated.

TREATMENT OF CHRONIC PAIN IN THE ADDICTED PATIENT

If we accept the premise that maintenance narcotics are problematic in the chronic benign pain patient, then certain treatment approaches logically follow. We have found the following approach quite workable:

1. Explanation of the role of narcotics in maintaining pain

The patient must be informed of the diagnosis in a supportive and optimistic manner. One might say in effect to the patient "You have been suffering immensely from your painful disorder for a long time. You have been treated with numerous medications, physical therapy, TENS, surgery, etc. ... none of which have prevented your condition from continuing and even gradually worsening. Your activities have greatly diminished and your relationships are deteriorating. You need help. I am not surprised that your pain has failed to improve because you are taking medication that actually causes pain." The patient often becomes intensely interested. Then the phenomenon of tolerance is discussed pointing out that their pain medications do not last as long as they did when they were originally taken nor do they work as effectively. It may be pointed out to the patient that he is able to take narcotic medications and not become intoxicated or drowsy on doses that would have powerful effects on other people. It may be useful to suggest that the patient's body is resisting these medications. Some patients may be offered neurophysiological explanations that involve receptor sites and endorphins. It is useful to acknowledge that the medications seem to help since the patient feels better immediately after taking them, but that the medication wears off quickly causing the patient to feel significant pain. This occurs regularly as the patient's pain medication wears off; as a result the medication dose remains relatively constant from day to day which would be unlikely with mechnical pain or most types of pain. Many patients resist such explanations and insist that the pain medication is the only thing that helps. The greater the associated features of addiction, the more likely this response is to occur. Nevertheless, the rationale has been established for proceeding to detoxify the patient from their medications. Even if they do not agree, the physician is able to say that he is treating the pain, not treating drug addiction.

2. Detoxification

Detoxification can be done in a number of ways. It is easiest as an inpatient since there is complete control of the patient and behavior and activity levels can be monitored. As an inpatient, methadone can be used which provides the smoothest and simplest detoxification because it is long acting and reliably absorbed when administered orally. Twenty-four hour observation of the patient is also quite helpful in assessing pain behavior and the psychological component of the pain. Outpatient detoxification can be done readily using codeine. Clonidine can be used but it is less comfortable for the patient and generally takes longer. Codeine should be given on a fixed schedule usually three or four times per day. The dose must be reduced daily until it reaches 0 in seven to ten days. It may be necessary to give daily prescriptions. Extra narcotic medication is absolutely forbidden. If the patient takes his medications too early and runs out, then he may go through minor withdrawal symptoms. If the patient seeks other sources of narcotics, either from other doctors or illicitly, then no further prescriptions are given. In any case, the patient is no longer dependent upon legitimately prescribed narcotics by the primary career.

3. Treat pain independently of detoxification

The patient should be clearly told that the narcotics are not for the purpose of treating his pain. Other medications will be given. These medications can include acetaminophen, NSAIDS, small doses of antidepressants, small doses of major tranquilizers or small doses of antihistamines. For example, one might prescribe an anti-inflammatory drug on a regular basis and give 10 to 25 milligrams of amitriptyline or hydroxazine as needed for severe pain. The patient is cautioned not to take too much of this medication but he can take it every three hours if absolutely necessary. Pain complaints will initially increase (similar to animal behavior during detoxification). At that point the PRN medication should be changed or the dose adjusted slightly. It is critical that detoxification proceed through this period unchanged.

After detox, the NSAIDS typically are more effective for pain than the previous narcotic regimen. The antidepressants or major tranquilizers are often given up by the patient. Their on-going prescription does not become a critical issue.

4. Coordinate care and mobilize support

There must be agreement by all physicians involved in the care not to prescribe narcotics; otherwise the detoxification makes no sense. All caregivers must understand the rationale for the program and the goals. Ideally the patient's family is included.

Frequently the spouse considers the patient to be a drug addict. If the spouse understands that the purpose of detoxification is to improve the pain and that the pain meds are actually causing pain, the spouse stops being so critical of the patient. Support from the spouse in going through this process is immensely beneficial to the patient.

5. Provide psychological support

It is critical to spend time talking with the patient about his concerns. Patients become very anxious about losing medications that have been such a constant part of their lives for years. Listening to the various concerns and fears goes a long way to alleviate anxiety and change the patient's attitude about narcotic medications.

6. Promote healthy behaviors

To reinforce the idea that the treatment is for the patient's health and not punishment for being a drug addict, promoting other healthy behavior should become part of the treatment. Simple regular exercise should be prescribed in a manner that the patient can be successful at. For example, he might be prescribed to walk five minutes per day. Every few days that should be increased by one minute. In general the prescription should be within what the patient is able and willing to do and allow for improvement. This gives the patient the feeling of success and becoming more healthy. If the patient were a smoker, there should be strong encouragement to stop smoking. While this is unlikely to be successful most of the time, it reinforces the idea that the physician is truly interested in the patient's health. The physician may also want to discuss such areas as leisure activities and family activities indicating that all these areas are important for the patient's health and well being.

In conclusion, it must be clear in the physician's mind, that whatever the source of the patient's pain, maintenance narcotics are not helpful for treatment of the pain (in some instances they may be appropriate for other reasons). Other methods of treating pain will not result in the elimination of narcotic dependence. The narcotic medications must be eliminated first for other treatments to have any potential benefit.

REFERENCES

1. Porter J and Jick H: Addiction rare in patients treated with narcotics. N Engl J Med 302:123, 1980

2. France RD, Urban B, and Keefe F: Long term use of narcotic analgesics in chronic pain. Soc. Sci. Med. 19:1379-82, 1984

3. Portenoy RK, Foley KM: Chronic use of opioid analgesics in non-maglignant pain: Report of 38 cases. Pain 25:171-186, 1986

4. Tennant FS, Rawson RA: Outpatient treatment of prescription opioid dependence. Arch Intern Med 142:1845-1847, 1982

5. Barr Taylor C, Zlutnick SF, Curley MS, Flora J. The effects of detoxification, relaxation and brief supportive therapy on chronic pain. Pain 8:319-329, 1986

6. Mathew NT, Kurman R, Perez F. Drug induced refractory headache--clinical features and management. Headache 30:634-638, 1990

7. Arner S, Meyerson BA: Lack of analgesic effect of opiods on neuropathic and idiopathic forms of pain. Pain 33:11-23, 1988

8. Turner JA, Calsyn DA, Fordyce WE, Ready LB: Drug utilization patterns in chronic pain patients. Pain 12:357-363, 1982

9. Buckley FP, Sizemore WA, Charlton JE: Medication management in patients with chronic non-malignant pain. A review of the use of a drug withdrawal protocol. Pain 26:153-165, 1986

10. Streltzer J: Treatment of iatrogenic drug dependence in the general hospital. General Hospital Psychiatry 2:262-266, 1980

11. Gardner FL: Chapter 7, Brain reward mechanisms. In: Lowinsen JH, Ruiz P, Hillman RB, eds. Substance Abuse: A Comprehensive Textbook. 2nd ed. Baltimore: Williams & Wilkins, 1992:70-99

12. Marks RM, Sacher EJ: Undertreatment of medical inpatients with narcotic analgesics. Annals Int Med 78:173-181, 1973

13. Streltzer J, Wade TC: The influence of cultural group on the undertreatment of postoperative pain. Psychosomatic Medicine 43:397-403, 1981

PSYCHIATRIC CONSULTATION WITH CHEMICALLY DEPENDENT PATIENTS

Stephen R. Griffith, M.D.

Associate Clinical Professor of Psychiatry
Fresno Division
Department of Psychiatry
University of California, San Francisco
Fresno Veterans Affairs Medical Center
2615 E. Clinton Ave.
Fresno, California, 93703

INTRODUCTION

With the move towards psychiatric subspecialization occurring over the past few years, there has been rapid parallel developments in both the fields of consultation - liaison psychiatry and addiction psychiatry. Recently, the field of addiction psychiatry was approved for added qualifications certification status, and the first certification examination was administered March 1993. During the 1992-93 academic year, there were 46 active fellowships in addiction psychiatry, with a total of 170 trainees currently enrolled in programs (1).

Added qualifications status is currently under active review for the subspecialty area of consultation-liaison psychiatry, with a strong possibility of approval in the very near future. Although the wisdom of subspecialization has been seriously called into question, the process has been set in motion. Both areas of psychiatry can be expected to undergo rapid growth in terms of research and training program development as a consequence. It is inevitable, given the intimate involvement of both addiction and consultation -liaison psychiatrists with patients in the general medical setting, that the new specialists will share much common ground. Subspecialists in both addiction and consultation psychiatry will be involved with the chemically dependent medical patient, with access to an increasingly larger and more sophisticated knowledge base than has been available in the past. This future development is certainly encouraging, as substance abuse in the hospitalized medical patient still frequently goes unrecognized or is ignored by the treating physician.

It can be anticipated that some of the future addiction psychiatrists will assume an increased role in hospital consultation with chemically dependent and chronic pain patients. Indeed, there may be a substantial number of clinicians interested (and trained) in both addiction and consultation psychiatry. However, it is also clear that the numbers of these

Consultation-Liaison Psychiatry: 1990 and Beyond
Edited by H. Leigh, Plenum Press, New York, 1994

addiction subspecialists will be relatively small over the near future, and most will probably be located at major training institutions. At least for the immediate future, the consultation- liaison psychiatrist will continue to assume consultation responsibility for the majority of in-hospital psychiatric consults with substance abuse related issues.

Given the large numbers of chemically dependent individuals encountered in the general medical setting and the increasing recognition of patients with combined substance use and mental disorders, it seems essential that the consultation-liaison psychiatrist possess a reasonable level of experience and knowledge in the addictions. A detailed discussion of substance abuse training in a consultation-liaison fellowship is beyond the scope of this chapter. However, it would appear that at least a minimal degree of emphasis in addiction psychiatry is necessary during the C&L training experience.

The remainder of this chapter will address three general areas of the chemical dependence field which seem to be of most relevance to consultation-liaison psychiatry. In the first section, national epidemiological factors related to substance abuse will be examined. An appreciation of past, current and predicted trends in substance use and dependence is necessary for the physician to anticipate and recognize the complex multifactorial clinical and psychosocial issues related to the chemically dependent patient. The knowledge of changing drug usage patterns or perhaps an impending drug epidemic is critical to the adequate assessment of patients presenting with drug induced medical\psychiatric problems. The second section will address specifically some current and expected clinical issues related to the substance dependent medical\surgical patient. This section will not serve as a guide or handbook for dealing with clinical problems, but will focus on projected problem areas in the 90's and beyond. Finally, in the third section, some recent and possible future pharmacological treatment interventions for chemically dependent patients, will be reviewed. Some knowledge of the state of the art pharmacological treatment of addicted patients is essential for the appropriate management of these individuals in the medical setting.

The economic and political aspects of substance abuse policies, although of critical importance in this age of managed care, budget deficits, and resource cutbacks unfortunately cannot be satisfactorily addressed in this chapter. However, in terms of the consultation-liaison psychiatrist, these issues will most certainly affect the availability and quality of treatment referral sources.

EPIDEMIOLOGIC DATA

The epidemiological information related to substance use and dependence in the US comes from a number of sources. The measurement of the nature and extent of drug abuse is determined by large scale instruments such as the National Household survey and the University of Michigan survey of high school seniors (currently called the Monitoring the Future Study)(2). The national household survey has been conducted since the early 1970's, and currently the sample size is over 32,000. The Monitoring the Future survey has been conducted each year since 1975. There has been some criticism of this instrument inasmuch as it misses many students who drop out of school or have school related difficulties. (This of course is the population that is most likely to be involved in drug use) (3).

Another important source of information is the National Institute of Mental Health (NIMH) Epidemiological Catchment Area (ECA) program. This large survey involves five major catchment sites(Los Angeles, New Haven, Baltimore, St. Louis,and Durham-

Piedmont). Included in this project are interviews with individuals in homes, prisons, nursing homes, and other institutions.

A significant source of data is provided by the Drug Abuse Warning Network (DAWN) which provides valuable information in terms of " drug mentions" from selected hospital emergency rooms and medical examiners. Also included in the DAWN data are other agencies involved with medically ill or deceased drug abusers. This data is helpful in determining the adverse consequences of drug abuse.

The epidemiology of alcohol and drug abuse is in a continual state of flux. As of this writing, there are multiple changes taking place that will impact on the future incidence of substance usage. Factors such as economics, law enforcement policies, drug availability, drug preparations and route of administration, expense, as well as health issues and media exposure in our society all have significant effects on the incidence of substance abuse. This section will briefly review some epidemiological trends of the major substances of abuse. Because of the fluidity of substance use patterns, a review of current trends is by no means a necessarily accurate projection of future conditions. Also, substance abuse patterns demonstrate marked geographical variability throughout the country, such that drug use which is virtually epidemic in one section of the nation will not present major problems in another.

An example of the changing epidemiology of drug usage is the trend in cocaine usage over the past century. Cocaine was used extensively in the US as early as the 1880's and was considered a dangerous and highly addicting drug by some physician's at that time (4). Cocaine usage declined nationwide until the 1970's when the drug was "rediscovered", partly it seems as a result of increased controls over amphetamine use. The use of cocaine then rapidly spread throughout the country. At first it was largely administered intranasally, and because of its expense and the perception that it was a "safe" recreational drug, cocaine became very popular with the upper middle class.

In the 1980's, the relatively less expensive, more potent smokable crack cocaine made its appearance. The development of crack cocaine resulted in a cocaine epidemic among the unemployed inner city population. Since crack cocaine is pharmacologically more potent, there was a significant increase in medical as well as psychiatric complications associated with its use. According to data from the DAWN system , there was a five-fold increase in the number of emergency room visits by people using cocaine in 1988 compared to 1984. During the same period, there was a 28 fold increase in the number of visits by smokers of cocaine (5). The use of crack cocaine has also been increasingly associated with the spread of AIDS. This aspect will be addressed in more detail later in this section.

The problems with crack cocaine have occurred despite an overall decrease in the number of cocaine users in the US. According to the National Household Survey, 1990, there was a decline in cocaine users from 5.8 million in 1985 to 1.6 million in 1990 (5). The overall decreased usage appears to have at least partly come about as a consequence of media attention to the dangers of the drug.

These figures point to a paradox in the drug treatment field. Clearly, from a positive standpoint, there are many individuals who have responded to the frequent warnings regarding the potential harmful effects of cocaine. Yet at the same time, there has evolved a more heavily addicted population of cocaine abusers, who are developing much more severe physical and psychiatric complications. Galanter and al in a study at a major teaching hospital serving an inner city population, reported a prevalence of 38% cocaine abuse in patients admitted for general psychiatric treatment (6). Of this group, almost one third were given no other Axis I diagnosis other than cocaine abuse, indicating that the psychiatric problems resulting in admission were frequently drug induced. It was estimated that cocaine usage was responsible for as many as 20% of the total psychiatric admissions to that facility. Additionally, Galanter reported that among the cocaine users referred to a cocaine treatment program, there was a high incidence of polysubstance abuse particularly alcohol (72%), marijuana (33%), and heroin (24%). The group was more likely to be black and homeless. Of the 20% who were tested for HIV, over one-half were seropositive. In another survey by Levin et al (7), over half of an inner city general hospital referrals to a substance abuse consultation service (53%) reported a history of cocaine abuse. In view of the above cocaine data, it can be projected at least for the near future, that consultation -liaison psychiatrists, will be dealing with large numbers of cocaine abusers in medical\surgical services in the hospital. This is particularly true for institutions serving inner city populations. Many of these patients will have secondary psychiatric disorders. Because of the severe psychosocial problems and poor treatment motivation of many of these individuals, such consultation work will present a formidable challenge.

Amphetamine abuse began to be reported about the time these drugs first appeared on the licit market in the 1930's. The abuse of amphetamines peaked during the 1960's as a result of widespread diversion of these legally prescribed drugs. Usage subsequently declined following the implementation of much more strict government regulations regarding amphetamines in 1970 (8).

During the 1980's, there has been an apparent increase in amphetamine abuse, largely as a result of illicit production. There were 2,439 amphetamine mentions in the DAWN report in 1988 compared with 1,370 mentions in 1985 (9). Methamphetamine, the most popular and abused amphetamine, has been illegally manufactured by clandestine laboratories, particularly in California since the late 60's. The potential of a serious amphetamine problem developing in the Western US and elsewhere is evidenced by the frequent findings of portable methamphetamine labs found in California, mostly in rural, isolated locations in the state. "Ice", a relatively inexpensive, longacting and very potent smokable form of dextroamphetamine, has yet to make a significant impact in the mainland US, although it has been a major problem in Asia and Hawaii. However, it may just be a matter of time before this drug presents major problems, particularly in the Western US. As is the case with the cocaine epidemic, it seems that later generations tend to "forget" the problems associated with drugs used by earlier generations. It does not seem so long ago that the expression "speed kills" was widely acknowledged in our society.

Alcohol continues to be the most widely abused substance in our society, and despite some data demonstrating an overall decrease in US alcohol consumption, there is no convincing evidence that the prevalence of "problem drinking" and alcohol dependence is lessening. Approximately 10% of adult Americans currently are problem drinkers, and there does not appear to be any data suggesting a significant change from that figure in the near future. Alcohol related problems are even more frequently encountered in the hospital setting. Surveys have demonstrated a prevalence of alcoholism on the hospital medical surgical units to be in the range of 20%-29% (10). Particularly high numbers of patients with alcohol problems are found on medical services with gastrointestinal disorders (i.e. pancreatitis, liver disease, peptic ulcer), as well as in the hospital emergency departments. One investigator reported that about 40% of patients in one emergency room had consumed alcohol prior to being evaluated (11).

Table I shows data collected by Moore et al in which patients in a general hospital screening positive for alcohol abuse are reported. The results were recorded for each of the clinical departments. The figures indicate a large percentage of patients screening positive for alcohol problems, and significant rates found in all the major services (psychiatry, medicine, general surgery, and surgical specialties)(12).

TABLE I. Prevalence of Patients Screening Positive for Alcohol Abuse by clinical Department*

DEPARTMENT	PREVALENCE (%)
Psychiatry	30
Medicine	24
Neurology	19
Obstetrics	12
General Surgery	21
Surgical Specialties	28

* Modified from Moore RD, Bone LR, Geller G, et al: Prevalence, detection, and treatment of alcoholism in hospitalized patients. JAMA 261:403-407,1989,"Copyright 1989, American Medical Association.", with permission.

Despite the significant incidence of problem drinkers as well as other substance abusers in the hospital, there is generally a low rate of psychiatric consultation requests for evaluation. Reports from surveys by consultation-liaison psychiatric services indicate that a substantial number of this population is not referred for psychiatric assessment (13,14). The patients that are referred are often individuals with advanced alcohol problems and present management difficulties because of organic mental disorders. It has also been reported that once a patient with alcoholism or other drug problems is referred for consultation, psychiatrists tend to spend less time with the patient and there are fewer followup visits than with other referrals (14). The issue of psychiatric underconsultation for patients with alcohol or other drug problems is of paramount importance, and will be further addressed later in this chapter.

The prevalence of heroin use is difficult to accurately estimate because of obvious sampling problems with this particular population of substance abusers. However, there is some evidence that heroin use has been on the increase recently, particularly among males, African Americans, and residents of large metropolitan areas of the Northeast (2). This apparent trend seems likely to continue in the 90's and beyond. There has been reports suggesting an increase in the availability of a cheaper, more potent heroin known as" black tar" in some locations of the country. The increased accessibility of a more potent heroin associated with a reduced cost is reminiscent of the crack cocaine epidemic. The consultation-liaison psychiatrist can expect to be dealing with a substantial population of opiate addicted patients on the general medical-surgical services particularly in terms of the management of opiate withdrawal symptoms and recommendations for assistance with pain control in this difficult population.

In a recent survey by a substance abuse consultation service, Levin (7) reported that over 60% of the referrals involved polysubstance abuse issues (the use of two or more substances concurrently). Alcohol was the most frequently mentioned ever-abused substance with 68% of individuals reporting its use. Following were cocaine (53%), opiates (46%), and marijuana (22%). The current trend towards polysubstance use is indeed a challenge to professionals, who must deal with many individuals addicted to two or more substances simultaneously. Substance abusers tend to present with unreliable drug use histories, and with multiple substances involved, the consultant may be presented with very confusing medical and psychiatric picture.

On a more optimistic note, the University of Michigan survey of high school seniors has reported marked decreases in the use of illicit drugs and alcohol during the 80's (3). In 1990, the rate of illicit substance use among High school seniors was half the rate it was in 1979. In 1980, 72% of high school seniors reported that they had consumed alcohol in the past month. This figure was down to 57% in 1990. Marijuana use peaked in 1979 with 37% of the surveyed group reporting use in the previous month. This rate had dropped dramatically to 14% in 1990. Cocaine use has followed a similar pattern since 1985. Of some concern, however, was the increased reported usage of LSD and inhalants among high school seniors surveyed in 1992 (15). It would appear that the potential dangers of LSD so evident in the 1960's are not as well appreciated by the current youth generation. This so called "generational forgetting " is similar to the situation with cocaine and amphetamines.

A recent survey of 8th graders across the country revealed that in 1992, the surveyed group reported higher rates in their use of marijuana,cocaine including crack, LSD, stimulants, and inhalants than did 8th graders in 1991. This troubling finding may reflect a decreased perception of the potential dangers involved with drug usage, perhaps as a consequence of decreased media coverage during the early 90's (15).

Westermeyer (16) has recently speculated that substance abuse in the 90"s will remain at a high level because of anticipated drug favoring environmental factors. These considerations would include the relative decrease in the cost of drugs and alcohol, weakness in social controls and prohibitions against substance usage, and a lack of improvement in the socioeconomic status of many long -disenfranchised individuals in the nation. He indicated that mass media efforts to reduce alcohol and drug usage in the country had not had demonstrable effects on the drug use patterns among certain socioeconomic deprived ethnic and racial minorities. Westermeyer pointed out the increases in the number of "at risk" children, including those raised by a single parent, addicted parents, or those who have lost a parent in childhood.

Comorbity Data

Over the past decade, there has been a significant increase in interest in the psychiatric aspects of substance abuse. It has long been known that the alcoholic or drug abusing individual is at increased risk for mental disorders. (The alcoholic or opiate abuser was often reported to be depressed and/or anxious). However, until recently the specific associated psychiatric disorders could not be accurately assessed. With the implementation of DSM-III in 1980, a much greater degree of diagnostic clarity was possible. DSM -IIIR added even further clarity to the diagnosis and the upcoming DSM IV takes into account the latest research data, to enable more sophisticated diagnostic precision. In addition, the development of structured diagnostic instruments allowed for more objective data gathering and has resulted in more exactness and reliability in psychiatric diagnoses. With these innovations, it has became possible to more objectively identify the psychiatric condition of substance abusers. During the past decade, data related to psychiatric co-morbidity has rapidly accumulated.

It is clear, in terms of outcome, that psychiatric impairment in the substance abuser is an unfavorable prognostic indicator (17). With improvements in the pharmacological treatment of mental conditions also rapidly developing over recent years, treatment professionals are increasingly able to offer pharmacotherapies for the specific mental conditions found in substance abusers. Hence,there is a greater likelihood of an improved prognosis for the treatment of the addiction. (For example; the depressed patient with secondary alcoholism will often decrease the consumption of alcohol following successful treatment of the depression with antidepressants.)

A large database of comorbid alcohol and drug disorders and mental disorders has been accumulated by the extensive Epidemiologic Catchment Area (ECA) study of the NIMH. Data was gathered during 1981-1984 in multiple locations throughout the country, using the Diagnostic Interview Schedule (DIS). This study convincingly demonstrates the magnitude of the comorbidity between substance use disorders and mental disorders (18). Of those individuals with an alcohol disorder, 37% had a comorbid mental disorder. For those with a drug disorder (other than alcohol), a striking 53% were diagnosed with an associated mental disorder. (see Table IIA) The most commonly diagnosed comorbid conditions were the Axis-II antisocial Personality disorder, affective disorders, and anxiety disorders.

In the ECA study, there was also found a very high incidence of substance abuse disorders among individuals with severe mental disorders. About 29% of all persons with

TABLE IIA. Lifetime Prevalence of Various Mental Disorders Among Persons with Any Alcohol and Other Drug Diagnosis : Five Site ECA Combined Community and Institutional Sample Standardized to the US Population*

	ANY ALCOHOL	ANY OTHER DRUG
COMORBID DISORDER	%	%
ANY MENTAL	36.6	53.1
SCHIZOPHRENIA	3.8	6.8
ANY AFFECTIVE	13.4	26.4
ANTISOCIAL PERSONALITY	14.3	21.0
ALCOHOL ABUSE OR DEPENDENCE		47.3

* Modified from Regier DA, Farmer ME, Rae DS, et al: Comorbidity of mental disorders with alcohol and other drug abuse. JAMA 264: 2511-2518, 1990.

mental conditions have a lifetime diagnosis of a substance use disorder. The rates are particularly high for antisocial personality disorder (84%), schizophrenia (47%) and for bipolar disorder (56%). (see Table IIB) The association between mania and alcohol or drug use disorders is eight times the predicted "normal" value.

Ross et al (19) in a survey of 501 patients seeking treatment for alcohol and other drug problems, using the Diagnostic Interview Schedule (DIS),found that 78%of the sample had a DIS lifetime psychiatric disorder, and 65% had a current DIS mental disorder.In this survey, psychiatric impairment was correlated with the severity of the alcohol and drug problem. Polysubstance abusers (those who abused both alcohol and other drugs) were significantly more mentally impaired than patients who abused either alcohol or other drugs but not both. The great majority of lifetime diagnoses in this sample consisted of antisocial personality disorder, anxiety disorders(including phobias), psychosexual disorders, and affective disturbance. Many of the reported mental disorders may have been secondary to substance use.

TABLE IIB. Lifetime Prevalence of Alcohol and Other Drug Disorders Among Persons with Schizophrenia, Antisocial Personality, and Bipolar Disorders: Five Site ECA Combined Community and Institutional Sample Standardized to the US Population

	SCHIZOPHRENIA	ANTISOCIAL PERSONALITY	BIPOLAR
COMORBID DISORDER	%	%	%
ANY SUBSTANCE DEPENDENCE	47.0	83.6	56.1
ANY ALCOHOL DIAGNOSIS	33.7	73.6	43.6
ANY OTHER DRUG DIAGNOSIS	27.5	42.0	33.6

* Modified from Regier DA, Farmer ME, Rae DS et al: Comorbidity of mental disorders with alcohol and other drug abuse. JAMA 264: 2511-2518, 1990.

The comorbitity data is quite revealing. Whether an associated psychiatric disorder is secondary to a substance use disorder or represents a primary condition, there is a very high probability of a psychiatric impairment being found in substance users. Conversely, for those individuals with severe mental disorders especially schizophrenia or bipolar disorders, an associated substance abuse problem is quite likely. The implications of this data on future psychiatry consultation-liaison work is obvious. Patients seen for psychiatric consultation will need to be carefully screened for alcohol and drug usage, and many should be referred for further evaluation and treatment by chemical dependency programs. On the positive side, the identification of an associated comorbid condition presents an opportunity for the consultatant to initiate effective treatments for the patient.

HIV Data

Any review of future epidemiological factors in the substance abuse field must take into account the status of the HIV epidemic. As of this writing, there are no major breakthroughs in the treatment of this devastating enigmatic disease, despite years of painstaking research. There are some preliminary encouraging reports regarding the development of an AIDS vaccine, but as of now, a successful immunization still seems in the distant future.

Current data shows an increase over the past few years in the prevalence of HIV infection among substance abusers (20). Although the risk of HIV infection has been assumed to be overwhelmingly associated with intravenous drug abusers, increasingly there are reports of rapid spread of the infection in the non IV drug abusing population (21). This seems especially true of abusers of crack cocaine. Although accurate figures regarding this problem are not available, some clinicians in several locations of the country (i.e. Miami and New York) are reporting the majority of their HIV positive substance abusing clients are non IV users, and presumably contracting the virus through unsafe sexual practices.

Since the phenomenon of AIDS in non IV drug abusers is primarily associated with the use of crack cocaine, it would seem to be a consequence of cocaine induced hypersexuality and disinhibition. In many instances there is a an additional factor of prostitution and transactions that involve "sex for drugs". It appears that many substance abusers have responded to the wide media attention regarding the dangers of "dirty needles", but have not reacted to warnings about unsafe sexual practices. At this time, it appears that the AIDS epidemic among drug users will closely parallel developments with the crack cocaine problem.

Batki reported that 84% of HIV+ patients at a substance abuse treatment program were given a psychiatric diagnosis (22). Of these, 33% had a depressive disorder, 33% had an anxiety disorder, and 18% were diagnosed with organic mental disorders. Johannet and Muskin, in a survey of AIDS patients admitted to a general hospital, reported that psychiatric consultation was requested for 23% of the IV drug abusers. The drug abusing AIDS patients tended to be seen more frequently for behavior problems than the non drug using AIDS patients(23).

These figures would indicate that HIV+ substance abusers will probably generate large numbers of psychiatric consultation requests in the near future. This is particularly true in areas of the country with high HIV seropositive rates where a large percentage of the consultation load will involve AIDS patients.

CLINICAL ISSUES IN THE 90'S

The epidemiological data indicate that substance abuse issues will continue to be a significant factor in psychiatric consultation work in the foreseeable future. Because of the magnitude of the problem, the overall numbers will be large despite the relatively low rate of consultation requests for chemical dependence cases currently being reported in the literature.

Given the likely scenario of a large number of substance abuse related consultations, what will be the nature of the clinical work facing the psychiatrist? To begin with, and of most importance, the attitudes of both the consultant and the consultee towards chemically dependent patients must be examined. It seems clear that substance abusers are still often perceived as "undesirables" in the medical setting. Many physicians feel that these patients do not "deserve" or require more than a minimal degree of medical attention. These perceptions need to be examined, as there is no reason to expect significant changes in attitudes in the near future.

It would appear that negative perceptions about addiction exist as a consequence of several common factors.

1. There is a strong tendency of the alcohol or drug abuser to deny that there is a substance use problem. Denial is assumed to be a major defense mechanism in the phenomenology of addiction, perhaps a necessary condition. However, many treatment professionals have difficulty conceptualizing denial as a symptom, and tend to view the patient in denial as deliberately "lying" or at least being evasive about the condition. In addition, the patient is perceived as wanting to continue the addiction rather than seek treatment.(Indeed, on the surface, this may appear to be the case.) Consequently, the clinician's response is quite often anger, intolerance and avoidance of the individual rather than attempting to understand the meaning of the behavior. To be sure, experienced chemical dependence staff members frequently struggle with the same negative feelings towards denial, since addicted individuals will continually resist many aspects of treatment.

2. For a variety of reasons, there is frequently strong negative counter-transference feelings on the part of physicians and other treatment personnel towards the substance abuser. This would seem to be especially true in the case of the HIV+ substance abuser.(This particular situation is so emotionally laden and fraught with problems, that it will dealt with in more detail later in this chapter.) Negative reactions may be conscious or unconscious. The doctor may have a current or past problem with chemically dependence, and unable to objectively evaluate the patient. There may be a significant chemically dependent family member in the physician's life who has contributed to a pessimistic view towards addiction. The physician may simply be responding to very definite negative attributes on the part of the addicted patient, attributes which the majority of people would find offensive. There is unfortunately a frequent association between substance abuse and antisocial behavior, poor impulse control, poor treatment compliance, and defiant attitudes. Psychiatric consultants,(and this is to be emphasized), obviously are not immune to negative counter-transference responses. Indeed, in many cases, the primary difficulty might be between the psychiatrist consultant and the patient. This issue will be dealt with further in this section.

3. The prevalent feeling that alcoholism and drug addiction are "hopeless conditions", and not amenable to treatment. This common attitude largely reflects lack of education and experience in treatment of the addictions. It is often not appreciated that addiction is a "relapsing condition" and one or more relapses does not necessarily imply treatment failure. Unfortunately, patients presenting on the medical/surgical units of the hospital frequently have been refractory to multiple treatment efforts, and such patients may contaminate the physician's overall perception towards substance abusers. It is indeed in this writer's experience a rare medical or surgical attending who feels positive about the chances of a successful treatment outcome with a patient who has a history of frequent hospital admissions for complications of drug or alcohol abuse. Often the consultation

request is simply a strong demand to move the patient from a medical service to a psychiatric unit or chemical dependence program without any expectation of recovery.

4. Finally, there is a strong possibility that the physician may "miss" the diagnosis of a substance use disorder, and focus on the manifest clinical pathology while overlooking the basic cause. Such diagnostic problems are partly a result of the preceding factors, and partly a consequence of inadequate training in addiction medicine. The following case vignette illustrates the type of problems and consequences of negative attitudes that occur when a medical attending refers a chemically dependent patient for psychiatric consultation.

" The patient is a 65 year old divorced man admitted to the medical service for the treatment of medical complications of chronic alcoholism. He had been drinking heavily prior to the admission, and treatment was initiated for alcohol withdrawal as well as malnutrition, hypokalemia, and a severe peripheral neuropathy. This was one of several similar admissions for the patient over the past five years." A psychiatric consultation was requested when the patient began reporting auditory hallucinations on the third day of hospitalization.

The psychiatrist made a diagnosis of alcohol hallucinosis, and recommended the use of haloperidol in conjunction with the oxazepam being administered for withdrawal. The consultant felt that the patient required further medical stabilization prior to a referral to a chemical dependency program. The attending physician agreed with the use of haloperidol, but was not optimistic concerning a referral for chemical dependence treatment. He stated the patient had repeatedly been instructed not to drink following previous admissions, but had not chosen to quit. It was the attending doctor's opinion that the patient had no interest in alcohol treatment and he planned to discharge the man as soon as he was medically stable. The patient's hallucinations abated within several days, and the psychiatrist continued to recommend a treatment program. However, the consultant did not directly confront the patient regarding his addiction, nor did he request that an addiction counselor see the patient. The patient was subsequently discharged home without a direct link to a treatment program being established."

This case is a typical example of negative, pessimistic attitudes interfering with an appropriate referral for substance abuse treatment. The attending physician was irritated with the patient, and not interested in treating the man beyond medical stabilization. He did not feel there was any point in a chemical dependence referral as he didn't think the patient had any motivation to change his behavior. The psychiatric consultant's reluctance to directly confront the patient may have ben related to his own negative expectations or counter transference issues.

In order for an appropriate intervention to have take place, there must have been an attitude of positive expectations displayed. The psychiatric consultant needs to somehow impart to the physician as well as to the patient that he expects recovery to be a possibility (24). If a consultant is unable to convey that attitude, he should at least obtain the assistance of an experienced drug counselor who could.

The available data would suggest that the psychiatric consultant has often displayed a less that enthusiastic interest in the substance abusing patient. In the report by Burton et al (14), it was shown that consultation liaison psychiatrists on the service spent less time with addicted patients, and made fewer treatment recommendations with this group than with non substance using patients. In addition, the physicians when making assessments and referrals with substance abuse patients, seemed to have less ongoing involvement with these individuals than with the non chemically dependent patients.

These findings could indicate either a lack of interest in substance abuse issues on the part of the consultants, and/or an attitude of "therapeutic nihilism" towards chemically dependent patients. Negative expectations may well indicate a lack of training in addiction medicine, and in particular, inexperience in terms of active involvement in the longer term rehabilitation of chemically dependent people. Quite often, a training experience in chemical dependency is limited to the medical aspects of detoxification.

It would seem that at least a minimal exposure to the longer term recovery process of the chemically dependent patient would enhance the training programs for consultation liaison psychiatrists. The psychiatrist needs to experience firsthand the treatment process beyond detoxification, including involvement in twelve step groups, family treatment, and outpatient maintenance of the recovering addict to fully appreciate the recovery process. The physician must get a sense of the emotional, feeling aspects of recovery to realize that there is hope. Finally, the doctor must talk with and listen to recovering people in order to understand that successful longer term outcomes are possible. There needs to develop an empathetic appreciation that the truly addicted individual desperately wants recovery, and that his or her life is existentially miserable.

Much of the existing literature related to substance abuse and consultation psychiatry involves work with exclusively alcoholic patients. As noted earlier in the section on epidemiology, the consultation-liaison psychiatrist of the 90's and beyond is increasingly more likely to encounter individuals with polysubstance abuse patterns (including alcohol). The patients are more apt to be younger, male , and non-white, at least in the larger public inner city institutions. There will be a greater incidence of comorbid substance use and psychiatric conditions, and the patients will present more severe behavioral management problems.

Exclusively alcoholic patients, although by no means free from behavioral problems, tend to be less antisocial and impulsive, and at least superficially more compliant with treatment than the polysubstance abusers. Polysubstance abusers (particularly abusers of crack cocaine, and heroin are far more likely to have severe defects in personality function, associated with multiple social, legal and behavioral problems. (These individuals would tend to have very high ratings on the addiction severity scale as developed by McClellan et al (17). The following case report illustrates the severe pscho-social problems manifested by a polysubstance user. Such cases have become increasingly common, and should continue to present diagnostic and management problems for the consultant in the near future.

"A 28 year old single homeless unemployed African-American male was admitted to the medical service for evaluation and treatment of acute chest pain. On initial evaluation in the emergency room, he reported recent heavy smoking of crack cocaine in addition to consuming 12-15 beers per day. He was noted to have an elevated blood pressure as well as a tachycardia. An admission blood alcohol concentration was .124. A urine toxicological screen was positive for cocaine, marijuana, and phencyclidine. He seemed restless, mildly agitated, with mild impairment of concentration. There was no evidence of psychotic thinking or marked confusion. He was admitted to rule out an acute myocardial infarction. Several hours following his admission, the patient became markedly agitated, confused, and reported hearing voices of a threatening nature. A stat psychiatric consultation was requested. A review of the medical record showed a psychiatric hospitalization five years previously. At that time, the patient was given a diagnosis of paranoid schizophrenia. There was no mention in the previous admission of substance abuse. He was treated with haloperidol during that admission for one week and discharged. There was no indication that the patient had become involved in the outpatient followup that was scheduled."

This case illustrates the complex diagnostic and treatment aspects of a patient with polysubstance abuse and severe psychosocial impairments. From a diagnostic standpoint, the psychiatric consultant must ask whether this patient has a true Axis I diagnosis of schizophrenia or is experiencing a substance induced mental disorders. It is not immediately clear whether the psychotic behavior is a complication of cocaine, alcohol, or PCP. The consultant will have to make some decisions regarding pharmacotherapy both for the acute psychiatric signs as well as possible drug withdrawal. Most likely, the clinical picture represents a drug combination effect, and pharmacotherapy will not be specific for any particular substance induced disorder. Fortunately,if used judiciously, high potency neuroleptics and benzodiazepines can be used quite safely in most cases.

Of greater concern, however,is the management of the patient once the acute psychiatric and medical symptoms are stabilized. He is homeless, unemployed, and most likely without a sober support system. How can this individual be convinced to enter a drug treatment program.? What incentives does this person have to become drug free? In Galanter's recent series of hospitalized cocaine addicts, more than 50% were homeless and the majority were treatment dropouts. Because of the difficulty in engaging this type of patient into treatment, Galanter recommended the use of recovering peer addicts in initiating therapeutic interventions (6). In this particular institution, a peer leadership self-help model was introduced into the general hospital service. The use of professionally supervised recovering peer addicts may indeed be necessary to break through the enormous socioeconomic and transcultural barriers to developing a therapeutic relationship.

The HIV+ substance abuser has become a major focus of psychiatric consultation over the past decade, and this will certainly continue during the 90's and beyond. The following brief case vignette is typical.

"A 32 year old homeless Hispanic male IV abuser of cocaine and heroin was admitted to the hospital for treatment of an abscess of his left arm. The patient was told that he was HIV+ almost one year previously. He had no medical complications of AIDS at the time of the current hospitalization. A psychiatric consultation was requested when the patient was observed to be very depressed and expressing suicidal thoughts. There was no previous history of psychiatric treatment."

The HIV+ individual presents with overwhelming medical and psychosocial problems. The patient must cope with multiple losses and stressors including the facing of a terminal illness, loss of health, sexuality, and significant relationships. This particular patient also is homeless and without any meaningful support system. As noted in the section on epidemiology, there is a very high rate of psychiatric disorders associated with AIDS, particularly depression. Suicidal ideation is very common (25).

Because of the complex problems associated with the AIDS patient, Batki has suggested the need for different levels of intervention in managing the mental health needs of these individuals (22). The psychiatric approach may need to follow a "case management " model, as patients require frequent contacts and extensive networking with different agencies. Fortunately, some consultation services in high HIV seropositive regions of the country have established multidisciplinary teams for dealing with AIDS patients (25).

The psychiatrist must also be especially cognizant of negative perceptions in dealing with HIV+ individuals. The consultant must cope with feelings of helplessness in dealing with patients who are terminally ill. In addition, the physician may have strong negative countertransference feelings towards substance abusing AIDS patients. However, with the appropriate ancillary services available to assist in the overall care, the psychiatrist can assume a critical treatment role. The consultant is in a position to diagnose and manage acute psychiatric symptoms such as depression or organic mental disorders. The psychiatrist also can actively recommend and support the patient's involvement in a drug treatment program.

There are as yet no good controlled studies demonstrating that HIV+ patients who continue drug usage have a more rapid progression of the disease. Substance abuse treatment, however, is of utmost importance in order to prevent further spread of the condition. The patient in treatment, moreover, has increased access to other modes of psychosocial intervention. To continue drug use puts the HIV+ patient at a high risk for other infections including TB, hepatitis, pneumonia, and other sexually transmitted diseases (26).

Another relevant clinical issue involving the consultation psychiatrist in the 90's and beyond is the differentiation of primary psychiatric disorders from those that are secondary to substance use disorders. The often confusing relationship between depression and alcoholism has been examined and reviewed over the past decade. Schuckit found that the vast majority of depressed alcoholics were experiencing a secondary depression that would reverse with abstinence (27). A number of investigators have shown that depression secondary to alcoholism improves within two weeks of abstinence, and that treatment with antidepressant medication is not indicated in these situations (28,29,30). Some investigators have advocated waiting even longer than two weeks following drinking to initiate treatment (29).

It does seem clear that depression, in the great majority of alcoholics, resolves without the need for antidepressant medication following a period of abstinence. Unfortunately, there seems to have developed a tendency for some clinicians to assume that all depression is secondary to alcohol or drug use in a substance abusing individual. The clinician must be wary not to overreact to the chemically dependent individual, and withhold antidepressant treatment from an individual solely because the patient reports drinking associated with depression. It must be remembered that there are considerable numbers of primary depressives or bipolar patients who escalate their drinking during depressive episodes. Moreover,it doesn't seem reasonable to withhold pharmacotherapy from a severely depressed individual after a period of about two weeks has elapsed since the last drinking episode.

There is also an inclination for some clinicians to assume that any psychosis associated with the use of drugs especially cocaine and amphetamines is drug induced. Many schizophrenic patients are abusers of cocaine, and need treatment for both conditions. Because of the common association between substance abuse and psychopathology, a number of facilities have developed dual diagnosis units for the purpose of assessment and treatment of these problematic cases. The consulting psychiatrist needs to be aware of the often confusing relationship between mental disorders and substance abuse and use his or her best judgement in making treatment decisions.

One other clinical issue that should be briefly addressed is the management of the chronic and acute pain patient. Problems frequently occur with the use of opiates in the management of pain in the patient with a substance abuse history. It can be assumed that the consultant will at some time be asked to evaluate the use of opiates in the heroin addicted patient. It must be remembered that any individual on methadone maintenance will need to continue the present dose of methadone in addition to any other indicated analgesia. The heroin addicted patient not taking methadone will have a very high tolerance for opiate analgesia, and substantially larger than normal dosages will be necessary for the relief of acute pain. There is almost never an indication for opiate treatment in the substance abusing individual with non malignant, non acute pain.

The use of opiates for chronic non-malignant pain in any individual almost always presents a treatment dilemma. This is particularly true for the patient who has been maintained chronically on opiates for a questionable clinical indication. This type of patient often is found to have a history of past alcohol abuse if a careful assessment is made. Many patients maintained on chronic opiate treatment are addicted to prescription opiates, but unwilling to discontinue them. This writer is aware of a few suicide attempts by patients who have had opiate prescriptions abruptly discontinued by clinicians concerned over opioid abuse. The psychiatric consultant must deal with such cases carefully. There is frequently a co-existing depression or other mental disorder present as well as a possible history of alcohol or substance abuse. Some hospitals have ongoing pain programs, which would appear to be the treatment of choice for such individuals. The typical pain program offers a multidisciplinary, multi faceted approach to the pain patient which the individual clinician cannot possibly achieve.

PHARMACOLOGICAL TREATMENTS

There is currently active and exciting research into the neurochemistry of alcohol and drug addiction. With advances in the elucidation of brain mechanisms involved in the phenomenon of substance dependence, the development of effective pharmacotherapies should theoretically be possible. As of this writing, research into brain neurochemistry with animals has lead to the model of a dopamine mediated central brain reward system (31). It has been suggested that the major drugs of abuse, although involving disparate neural transmitter mechanisms, may all enhance the activity of this reward system which serves as a final common pathway for drug reinforcement. Drugs of different classes could act at different anatomical sites in this system. Cocaine, for example, may act directly on the dopamine mediated reward system, whereas benzodiazepines, would exert activity directly on GABA neurons, which then would input into the central location.

Obviously, the proposed system is overly simplistic, but it represents a great advance in thinking about the neurophysiology of addiction during the past decade. Using the theoretical model, pharmacological interference or attenuation of activity in the reward system could alter the addicted individual's perception of euphoria or craving associated with the reinforcement of drug usage. As of now, there are no therapeutic agents developed which have proven consistently efficacious in breaking the complex process of addiction. On the other hand, less ambitious pharmacotherapies have proven useful in the addiction field. Methadone maintenance, for example has proven to be effective as a substitution treatment for heroin and opiate addiction. The benzodiazepines are very effective as a substitute pharmacotherapy in the treatment of alcohol and sedative hypnotic withdrawal states.

The remainder of this section will focus on some current as well as possible future pharmacological interventions in the treatment of chemical dependence. In the pharmacotherapy of alcoholism, there has been some interesting preliminary work in the use of selective serotonin reuptake inhibitors. In earlier experiments with rats, it was shown that increased alcohol consumption was associated with decreased levels of brain serotonin (32). The use of serotonin reuptake inhibitors with these animals was shown to decrease alcohol consumption, presumably by increasing the level of brain serotonin. This effect has been demonstrated with a number of agents including zimelidine, norzimelidine, citaprolam, fluoxetine, and fluoxamine (33).

In work with human subjects, thus far the results have been considerably less dramatic than with animals. Several investigators, in small trials with non- depressed subjects have documented modest reductions in the craving and consumption of alcohol following treatment with fluoxetine, zimelidine and citaprolam (34).

No human studies to date have evaluated the use of serotonin uptake blockers in the longer term maintenance treatment of alcoholics. Larger, placebo controlled studies are needed to determine if these agent have any practical use in the treatment of alcoholism. The serotonin reuptake inhibitors may be found to have value in a relapse prevention stratagem for certain individuals. At this time, it would seem from an empirical standpoint that these drugs may be first choice considerations in the pharmacotherapy of the depressed alcoholic.

A brief mention should be made concerning the use of disulfiram (Antabuse). The drug has been utilized in the treatment of alcoholism for over 40 years, but it remains somewhat of a controversial therapeutic agent. In a review of disulfiram treatment, Wright and Moore concluded that disulfiram is effective in the short term reduction of alcohol consumption, but only if taken under supervision in the context of a comprehensive treatment program (35). There was no evidence from the available literature that unsupervised use of the drug is of any value. Generally, the prescribing of disulfiram to an alcoholic patient following a single consultation or interview without followup treatment arrangements is inappropriate. Disulfiram, of course has been associated with a number of serious side effects, and there are relative contraindications to its use including hepatic dysfunction, ischemic cardiovascular disease, history of psychoses, renal impairment, and diabetes mellitus.

Naltrexone is a longacting opioid antagonist which has been utilized for the treatment of opiate addiction. By effectively blocking the pharmacological effects of heroin for at least 24 hours, the daily oral use of naltrexone eliminates the euphoria as well as the analgesia associated with the injection of heroin. Many opiate addicts who have taken naltrexone also report a significant decrease in craving for opiates. It is not entirely clear whether this effect is a direct pharmacological property of naltrexone, or a behavioral consequence of the knowledge that the individual cannot obtain an opiate "high" while using the drug.

On a theoretical basis, naltrexone would appear to be an ideal pharmacological treatment for heroin addiction, given its almost complete opiate blocking characteristics, an effective oral preparation, and long half-life. However, its use has been limited by extremely poor acceptance by most heroin addicts. As of this time, the successful use of naltrexone in the treatment of opiate addicts is limited to a relatively few highly motivated individuals, who in general possess significant psychosocial and material assets. These individuals tend to have a great deal to lose by their continued opiate use. There also has been some reported success with the prescription of naltrexone to some heroin addicts who have recently been released from prison and take the drug as a condition of parole (36).

Naltrexone has been shown in animal studies as well as early human investigations to decrease alcohol consumption and craving (37). These findings suggest that alcohol consumption is influenced by activity at the opiate receptor site. In a study by Valpicelli et al, naltrexone was reported to decrease the craving for alcohol, and seemed particularly effective in decreasing the continued drinking by patients who had experienced at least one "slip" during followup (38). Valpicelli theorized that alcohol may increase "opiate system activity" which in turn stimulates further drinking by the individual. Naltrexone by blocking the opiate receptor, decreases this "priming effect" of the initial drink of alcohol and thereby decreases the impulse to continue drinking. This study was limited by its short length of time (only 3 months). Consequently, the longer term effects of naltrexone on alcohol consumption were not addressed.

O'Malley et al have recently reported in a double bind placebo controlled study, that the probability of relapse to drinking during the initial period of recovery can be decreased with a combination of naltrexone treatment and behavioral psychotherapy (39). The intriguing findings utilizing naltrexone in the treatment of alcoholism await further controlled investigations, particularly in terms of longer term outcome results.

On a theoretical basis, naltrexone could have beneficial effects on in the treatment of other drug addictions as a consequence of interference with the opiate input into the brain reward system. Naltrexone has not been shown to be effective with cocaine addiction to date. One report has in the literature has indeed described a potentiation of the stimulatory and euphoric cocaine effect by naloxone, a short acting opiate antagonist (40).

There continues to be much controversy concerning the clinical us of methadone in the treatment of opiate addiction. However, the accumulated data conclusively demonstrates that methadone treatment decreases the use of intravenous heroin, associated criminal behavior, and improves overall health status and employment (41). These indices of life improvement are particularly true if the daily methadone dosage used is at least 60 mg. The overall success of a methadone program has also been shown to be related to other program variables, such as the presence of individual psychotherapy, provision of medical treatment, and the quality of therapists, ect. (42)

Despite the proven efficacy of methadone maintenance, there remains considerable moral and ethical objections to its usage. It is the most stringently regulated form of medical treatment in the US today. Many physicians and other treatment personnel are not comfortable with the use of a pharmacologically addicting opiate as a long term treatment modality. For these individuals, the goal, however unrealistic, remains total abstinence.

The consultation-liaison psychiatrist, as previously mentioned will continue to be dealing with acute and chronic pain issues involving patients on methadone maintenance. In the management of pain these patients must be continued on the current dosage of methadone in addition to any additional required analgesia while in the hospital. Moreover, the discontinuation of methadone will result in a delayed but significant opiate withdrawal syndrome. It is remarkable how often this basic phenomenon is not appreciated by clinicians, and the opiate withdrawal symptoms are attributed to "drug seeking" behavior.

Levo-methadyl acetate (LAAM) is another synthetic opiate similar to methadone but having a longer half life. LAAM has been shown to be as effective as methadone in controlled studies in the treatment of heroin addiction (43). LAAM has some advantages over methadone. Because of the longer duration of action, the drug can be administered three times weekly, thus obviating the need for take home medication, and the concomitant problem of street diversion. LAAM is not currently available for clinical usage despite years of familiarity with its potential by clinicians in addiction medicine. LAAM, as is the case with methadone, might certainly be criticized as a pharmacotherapy that substitutes one addiction for another.

Buprenorphine, a partial mu-opiate agonist, offers another approach to the treatment of heroin addiction. Buprenorphine binds very strongly to the mu opiate receptor. It produce agonistic effects at the receptor, but the inherent mu agonist effects are less than maximal. As a consequence, Buprenorphine (a) produces subjective morphine-like effects; (b) produces only limited withdrawal signs and symptoms following abrupt discontinuation; and (c) blocks the euphoria produced by morphine (44). Because of these pharmacological properties, buprenorphine is more acceptable as a treatment modality to opiate addicts than naltrexone and may decrease illicit intravenous opiate use .(To date, the only consistently successful pharmacological interventions in the maintenance treatment of opiate addicts, involve drugs with significant intrinsic mu agonist activity.) Buprenorphine could prove to be successful as a agent for opiate detoxification as well as maintenance. There have also been reports suggesting that buprenorphine may be useful in the treatment of cocaine addicts (45).

Problems with buprenorphine include poor oral bioavailability. Currently, the sublingual route is primarily used. There are increasing reports of buprenorphine abuse appearing in the literature. A recent report from Europe seems to indicate that opiate abusers who have switched from IV heroin to IV buprenorphine, reported that the drug produced subjective effects very close to IV heroin (46). Widespread diversion and abuse of IV buprenorphine would obviously render this drug counterproductive in any treatment of opiate addiction.

The pharmacological treatment of cocaine and amphetamine addiction to date has been characterized by limited success. It has been theorized that chronic heavy cocaine and amphetamine usage lead to a dopamine postsynaptic supersensitivity secondary to a depletion of dopamine stores. This hypersensitive postsynaptic state has been postulated to cause the anhedonia so frequently associated with stimulant withdrawal. The tricyclic drugs have been utilized because of the pharmacological effect of downregulation of postsynaptic dopamine and B-adrenergic mediated receptors (47). There have been some reports of decreased cocaine craving and depression in studies using the tricyclic antidepressant desipramine (40). Other reports have indicated some improvement with other tricyclics as well as trazodone (40). In a recent double blind, placebo controlled 12 week study, Arndt et al were unable to demonstrate a decrease an cocaine usage in a group of methadone maintenance patients treated with desipramine (48).

Dopamine depletion secondary to chronic cocaine use has been reported to be causally related to the intense craving for the drug seen following discontinuation. The dopamine agonist drugs, bromocriptine and amantadine have been used in an attempt to treat cocaine craving by a pharmacological correction of the dopamine depletion (47). Both drugs have been reported to decrease initial cocaine craving in double blind studies.

Overall, the pharmacotherapeutic approach to cocaine addiction with both antidepressants and dopamine agonists has been disappointing. No agents have been found to be efficacious in the longer term maintenance treatment of cocaine addiction as of this writing. The psychiatric consultant, however, may find the use of amantadine or desipramine quite useful in individuals on medical services experiencing severe withdrawal craving or anhedonia.

A novel approach to the treatment of cocaine addiction involves the development of an antibody that binds specifically to cocaine, and hastens the degradation of the drug in the body. Recently, Landry et al reported the development of a catalytic monoclonal antibody capable of catalyzing the hydrolysis of the cocaine benzoyl ester group (49).

Although this work is in a very early stage of development, the possibility exists of the development of an immunization with an enzyme that could effectively block cocaine reinforcement .It may be feasible for an immunization of this type to remain effective for a prolonged period of time. The treatment of cocaine abuse as well as other addictions with monoclonal antibodies could well be the pharmacological approach of the future. Further developments in this work are anticipated.

A brief mention should be made in this section regarding the phenomenon of "protracted withdrawal". It has been long appreciated that the addicted person may experience a multitude of clinical symptoms long after the completion of the acute substance specific withdrawal state. These reported symptoms range from chronic depression and anxiety to abnormalities in sleep and other biological parameters and have collectively been referred to as "protracted withdrawal" (50). The various post-withdrawal clinical presentations have been felt by clinicians to contribute significantly to relapse.

In a recent review of protracted withdrawal, Satel et al, concluded that there was insufficient documentation in the literature to include this diagnostic entity in the upcoming DSM-IV (50). This group concluded that the current usage of the term lacked consistency and required more precise diagnostic clarity. Nevertheless, there seems to be sufficient evidence in the literature indicating that persistent abnormalities in physical and psychological functioning following acute withdrawal do occur. This is particularly true for alcohol and opiate addiction. The pharmacological treatment of protracted abstinence symptoms would appear to be of value in preventing relapse in certain individuals. At this time, such drug treatments must be individualized based on the presenting symptoms. Antidepressant treatment, for example, would seem appropriate for persistent depressive symptoms following acute withdrawal. Buspirone may be helpful in some cases as a non addicting approach to chronic anxiety states. The addiction field is in need of further investigations to specifically identify signs and symptoms of protracted withdrawal leading to the future development of pharmacological treatments.

CONCLUSIONS

Addiction psychiatry has recently attained added qualifications status, increasing the appeal of subspecialty training in chemical dependence. However, it would appear that the number of addiction psychiatrists working in the general hospital setting and performing inpatient consultations will be small in the forseeable future. Consultation-liaison psychiatrists, although by no means numerous, will continue to be dealing directly with the majority of substance abuse issues on the hospital medical units.

Current epidemiological trends suggest that alcohol and polysubstance dependence, particularly various combinations of cocaine, heroin, and alcohol, will continue to be a major problem in the US. Other substances which may be re-emerging as significant problems include amphetamines and hallucinogens. It can be expected that the consultation-liaison psychiatrist will be confronted with numerous substance abuse related clinical consultations in the hospital setting. It is also increasingly clear that there will be a high incidence of comorbid psychiatric and substance use disorders encountered. The consulting psychiatrist will need to be careful in the assessment of psychopathology with medical patients. A comprehensive drug use history as well as urine toxicological screens will be required in many cases. Even in situations where drug or alcohol use is obvious, treatment decisions with these disorders may be problematic.

Major clinical issues in the future will include; (1) dealing with continued negative attitudes towards chemically dependent patients; (2) management of polysubstance abusers with associated psychosocial impairment including homelessness; (3) opiate addicted chronic pain patients; and (4) working with HIV+ substance abusers. These clinical situations may be quite frustrating and demanding of the psychiatrist's clinical skills and patience. However, with the increased emphasis on addictions research and the development of new treatments for substance use disorders, consultants may find future work in this area rewarding as well as challenging.

Because of the magnitude of substance abuse in the hospital setting, it seems necessary that the consultation psychiatrist be exposed to some chemical dependence training during the fellowship. Not to be ignored in this training is at least a minimal experience with a substance abuse rehabilitation program.

REFERENCES

1. Postgraduate medical fellowships in alcoholism and drug abuse.
Prepared by Center for medical fellowships in alcoholism and drug abuse, 1993

2. Winick C: Epidemiology of alcohol and drug abuse, in Lowinson JH, Ruiz P, Millman RB et al (eds): Substance Abuse, A Comprehensive Textbook, 2nd ed. Baltimore, Williams and Wilkins, 1992

3. Dusenbury L, Khuri E, and Millman RB: Adolescent substance abuse: A sociodevelopmental perspective, in Lowinson JH, Ruiz P, and Millman, RB (eds): Substance Abuse, A Comprehensive Textbook, 2nd ed. Baltimore, Williams and Wilkins, 1992

4. Musto DF: Opium, cocaine, and marijuana in American History.
Scientific American, July, 1991, 40-47

5.Closser MH and Kosten TR. Alcohol and cocaine abuse: A comparison of epidemiology and clinical characteristics, in Galanter M (ed): Recent Developments in Alcoholism: Alcohol and Cocaine: Similarities and Differences. New York, Plenum Press, 1992

6.Galanter M, Egelko S, DeLeon G et al: Crack/cocaine abusers in the general hospitals. Assessment and initiation of care.
Am J of Psychiatry 149:6 810-815,1992

7. Levin FR, Weddington WW, Haertzen, CA, et al. A substance abuse consultation service: Characteristics of patients and pedagogical potential.
NIDA Research Monograph, 105: 291-292, 1991

8. Hall JN, Broderick PM: Community networks for response to abuse outbreaks of methamphetamine and its analogs, in Miller MA, Kozel NJ (eds):National Institute on Drug Abuse, Research Monograph Series: Methamphetamine Abuse, Epidemiologic Issues and Implications, 1991

9. Miller MA, Kozel NJ: Introduction and overview, in Miller MA, Kozel NJ (eds): National institute on Drug Abuse, Research Monograph Series: Methamphetamine Abuse, Epidemiologic Issues and Implications, 1991

10. Mitchell WD, Thompson TL, and Craig SR: Underconsultation and lack of follow-up for alcohol abusers in a university hospital.
Psychosomatics 27:431-437, 1986

11. Holt S, et al:Alcohol and the emergency service patient.
Br Med J 281(6241):638-640, 1980

12. Moore RD, Bone LR, Geller G, et al:Prevalence, detection, and treatment of alcoholism in hospitalized patients.
JAMA 261:403-407,1989

13.Dulit RA, Strain JJ, and Strain JJ: The problem of alcohol in the medical/surgical patient.
Gen Hosp Psychiatry 8:81-85, 1986

14. Burton RW, Lyons JS, Devens M et al: psychiatric consultations for psychoactive substance disorders in the general hospital.
Gen Hosp Psychiatry 13:83-87, 1991

15. Kaplan A: Illicit drug use rises among young teenagers, signals possible reversal in usage decline trend.
Psychiatric Times 10 (5):40.1993

16. Westermeyer J: Substance use disorders: Predictions for the 1990's.
Amer J Drug Alcohol Abuse 18 (1):1-11, 1992

17. McLellan AT, Luborsky L, Woody GE, at al:Predicting response to alcohol and drug abuse treatments- Role of psychiatric severity.
Arch Gen Psychiatry 40:620-625, 1983

18. Regier DA, Farmer ME, Rae DS, at al: Comorbidity of mental disorders with alcohol and other drug abuse. Results from the epidemiologic catchment area (ECA) study.
JAMA 264:2511-2518, 1990

19.Ross HE, Glaser FB, and Germanson T: The prevalence of psychiatric disorders in patients with alcohol and other drug problems.
Arch Gen Psychiatry 45: 1023-1031, 1988

20. Centers for Disease Control. HIV/AIDS surveillance report. Atlanta: Centers for Disease Control, Sept 1990

21.Klimas N: HIV infection and substance abuse. Substance abuse treatment in the 90's. VA Teleconference, 1993

22. Batki SL: Drug abuse, psychiatric disorders, and AIDS: Dual and triple diagnosis. West J Med 152: 547-552, 1990

23. Johannet C and Muskin PR: Mood and behavioral disturbances in hospitalized AIDS patients.
Psychosomatics 31: 55-59, 1990

24. Gill DJ: Alcoholism and the consultation-liaison psychiatrist.
Psychiatric Clinics of North America 10:129-139, 1987

25. Orr DA and Wallack JJ: Multidisciplinary approaches to consultation-liaison psychiatry: the C-L psychologist on an AIDS treatment team.
Psychosomatics 31:441-447, 1990

26. Karan LD: Primary care for AIDS and chemical dependence.
West J Med 152:538-542, 1990

27. Schuckit MA: Genetic and Clinical implications of alcoholism and affective disorders.
Am J Psychiatry 143:2 140-148, 1986

28. Dackis CA, Gold MS, Pottash ALC, at al: Evaluating depression in alcoholics.
Psychiatry Research 17:105-109, 1986

29. Brown SA and Schuckit MA: Changes in depression among abstinent alcoholics.
J of studies on Alcohol 49 (5): 412-417, 1988

30. Dorus W, Kennedy J, Gibbons RD, et al: Symptoms and diagnosis of depression in alcoholics.
Alcoholism: Clinical and Experimental Research 11 (2) 150-154, 1987

31. Gardner EL: Brain reward mechanisms, in Lowinson JH, Ruiz P, and Millman RB (eds): Substance Abuse, A Comprehensive Textbook, 2nd ed. Baltimore, Williams and Wilkins, 1992

32. Zabik JE: Use of serotonin-active drugs in alcohol preference studies, in Galanter M (ed): Recent Developments in Alcoholism, vol 7, New York, Plenum Press, 1989

33. Gorelick DA: Serotonin uptake blockers and the treatment of alcoholism, in Galanter M (ed):Recent Developments in Alcoholism, vol 7, New York, plenum Press, 1989

34. Naranjo CA, Sellers EM, Jullivan JT, et al: The serotonin uptake inhibitor, citalopram, attenuates ethanol intake.
Clin Pharmacol Ther 41: 266-274, 1987

35. Wright C and Moore RD: Disulfiram treatment of alcoholism.
Amer J of Med 88: 647-655, 1990

36. Brahen LS, Henderson RK, Capone T, et al:Naltrexone treatment in a jail work-release program.
J Clin Psychiatry 45:49-52, 1984

37. Volpicelli JR, Davis MA, Olgin JE: Naltrexone blocks the post-shock increases of ethanol consumption.
Life Sci 38: 841-847, 1986

38. Volpicelli JR, Alterman AI, Hayashida M, et al: Naltrexone in the treatment of alcohol dependence.
Arch Gen Psychiatry 49: 876-880, 1992

39. O'Malley SS, Jaffe AJ, Chang G, et al: Naltrexone and coping skills therapy for alcohol dependence: A controlled study.
Arch Gen Psychiatry 49:881-887, 1992

40. Taylor WA and Gold MS: Pharmacologic approaches to the treatment of cocaine dependence.
West J Med 152 (5): 573-577, 1990

41. Zweben JE and Payte JT: Methadone maintenance in the treatment of opiate dependence: A current perspective.
West J Med 152:(5) 588-599, 1990

42. Lowinson JH, Marion IJ, Joseph, H, et al: Methadone Maintenance, in Lowinson JH, Ruiz P, and Millman RB (eds): Substance Abuse, A Comprehensive Textbook, 2nd ed. Baltimore, Williams and Wilkins, 1992

43. Ling W and Wesson DR: Drugs of abuse-Opiates.
West J Med 152 (5): 565-572, 1990

44. Jasinski DR, Pevnick JS, and Griffith JD: Human pharmacology and abuse potential of the analgesic, buprenorphine.
Arch Gen Psychiatry 35:501-516, 1978

45. Kosten TR, Kleber HD, and Morgan C: Role of opioid antagonists in treating intravenous cocaine abuse.
Life Sci 44:887-892, 1989

46. Torrens M, San L, and Cami J: Buprenorphine versus heroin dependence:Comparison of Toxicologic and psychopathologic characteristics.
Amer J of Psychiatry 150 (5): 822-824, 1993

47. Hall WC, Talbert RL, and Ereshefsky L: Cocaine abuse and its treatment. Pharmacotherapy 10 (10): 47-65, 1990

48. Arndt IO, Dorozynsky L, Woody GE, at al: Desipramine treatment of cocaine dependence in methadone-maintained patients.
Arch Gen Psychiatry 49: 888-893, 1992

49. Landry DW, Zhao K, Yang GX, et al:Antibody-Catalyzed Degradation of cocaine. Science 259: 1899-1901, 1993

50. Satel SL, Kosten TR, Schuckit MA, at al: Should protracted withdrawal from drugs be included in DSM-IV?
Amer J of Psychiatry 150 (5): 695-704, 1993

THE DEMENTIA SYNDROME IN CONSULTATION PSYCHIATRY

Robert Hanowell, M.D.

Fresno Division
Department of Psychiatry
University of California, San Francisco
2615 East Clinton Avenue
Fresno, CA 93703

INTRODUCTION

Patients with dementia suffer from an acquired impairment of cognitive function. The consequences of dementing disorders are often nothing less than tragic. A large percentage of such patients suffer a downward spiralling course into cognitive oblivion despite the most diligent efforts of the medical profession. The demented patient is not the only one touched by the affliction, since the patient's family faces the burden of caring for a loved one whose quality of life has been all but obliterated. As such, treating the demented patient is probably one of the most frustrating tasks encountered by the psychiatric consultant. Nonetheless, timely intervention by the psychiatrist is often of great palliative value and can soften the blow to both the patient and the family. If this were not the case, there would be, perhaps, little point to this chapter.

PHENOMENOLOGY

Dementia has been accurately and succinctly defined by Cummings and Benson (1992) as being "an acquired persistent impairment of intellectual function with compromise in at least three of the following spheres of mental activity: language, memory, visuospatial skills, emotion or personality, and cognition (abstraction, calculation, judgement, executive function and so forth)." DSM III-R also provides criteria for diagnosing dementia, and these are shown in Table 1 (American Psychiatric Association, 1987). It should also be noted that such vague terms as *organic brain syndrome* and *senility* are not uncommonly used by physicians; however, these terms are imprecise and are best avoided entirely.

Consultation-Liaison Psychiatry: 1990 and Beyond
Edited by H. Leigh, Plenum Press, New York, 1994

Table 1. DSMIII-R Criteria for Dementia

A. Demonstrable evidence of impairment in short- and long-term memory. Impairment in short-term memory (inability to learn new information) may be indicated by inability to remember three objects after five minutes. Long-term memory impairment (inability to remember information that was known in the past) may be indicated by inability to remember past personal information (e.g., what happened yesterday, birthplace, occupation) or facts of common knowledge (e.g., past Presidents, well-known dates).

B. At least one of the following:

(1) impairment in abstract thinking, as indicated by inability to find similarities and differences between related words, difficulty in defining words and concepts, and other similar tasks
(2) impaired judgement, as indicated by inability to make reasonable plans to deal with interpersonal, family, and job-related problems and issues
(3) other disturbances of higher cortical function, such as aphasia (disorder of language), apraxia (inability to carry out motor activities despite intact comprehension and motor function), agnosia (failure to recognize or identify objects despite intact sensory function), and "constructional difficulty" (e.g., inability to copy three-dimensional figures, assemble blocks, or arrange sticks is specific designs)
(4) personality change, i.e., alteration or accentuation of premorbid traits.

C. The disturbance of A nd B significantly interferes with work or usual social activities or relationships with others.

D. Not occurring exclusively during the course of Delirium.

E. Either (1) or (2):

(1) there is evidence from the history, physical examination, or laboratory tests of a specific organic factor (or factors) judged to be etiologically related to the disturbance
(2) in the absence of such evidence, and etiologic organic factor can be presumed if the disturbance cannot be accounted for by any nonorganic mental disorder, e.g., Major Depression accounting for cognitive impairment.

Criteria for severity of Dementia:
Mild: Although work or social activities are significantly impaired, the capacity for independent living remains, with adequate personal hygiene and relatively intact judgment.
Moderate: Independent living is hazardous, and some degree of supervision is necessary.
Severe: Activities of daily living are so impaired that continual supervision is required, e.g., unable to maintain minimal personal hygiene; largely incoherent or mute.

From : American Psychiatric Association: Diagnostic and Statistical Manual of Mental Disorders, Third Edition, Revised. American Psychiatric Association, Washington, D.C., 1987. Used with permission.

Dementia is unfortunately a common phenomenon, and it is destined to become even more common as the number of elderly people continues to climb. The exact prevalence of dementia is somewhat unclear (Cummings and Benson, 1992). In a review of the topic, Ineichen (1987) noted that the prevalence of dementia in patients over sixty-five years old ranged from 2.5 to 24.6 percent. In a recent study of patients in the Framingham Study cohort, it was noted that the incidence of dementia increased with age. More specifically, the incidence rose from seven new cases per thousand at ages sixty-five to sixty-nine to 118 new cases per thousand at ages eighty-five to eighty-nine (Bachman, Wolf, Linn, et al, 1993).

The clinical course of dementia is highly dependent on the etiology of the dementia. A patient suffering from dementia resulting from head trauma may well have a static deficit, or may even show improvement in cognitive function with time. On the other hand, a patient with Alzheimer's disease will almost always have a progressive dementing course.

It is essential for the consulting psychiatrist to keep in mind that cognitive impairment per se may not always be the most problematic aspect of dementia. It is often the behavioral sequelae of dementia that are most disabling to the patient. Problematic behaviors are seen commonly, occurring in up to seventy percent of demented patients (Wragg and Jeste, 1988). Behaviors such as wandering, physical violence, and refusal of assistance with dressing, feeding, and toileting are obviously disruptive and sometimes life threatening. Indeed, the generation of a psychiatric consult often results from such problematic behaviors.

Demented patients commonly exhibit psychotic symptoms, although the existing literature is rather conflicted with respect to the exact prevalence of psychosis in these patients (Burns, 1992). It is certainly of note that behavioral problems may be, in some demented patients, a manifestation of psychosis (especially persectory delusions). Indeed, it has been suggested that the effectiveness of neuroleptics in treating such patients may result primarily from their antipsychotic properties (Leibovici and Tariot, 1988).

DIFFERENTIAL DIAGNOSIS

The psychiatric consultant must keep in mind that many patients with gross impairment of cortical function are not demented. This is not a trivial matter. Not only does the clinician do such patients a disservice by inappropriately labelling them as demented, but missing certain alternative diagnoses could potentially result in a fatal outcome.

Aphasia can sometimes be mistaken for dementia. Indeed, it can be nearly impossible to rule out a coexisting dementia in patients with certain types of aphasia because of the difficulties inherent in interviewing these patients. Patients with receptive aphasia are particularly difficult to assess. These patients exhibit fluent but often incomprehensible verbal output and have poor comprehension of the questions presented by the clinician. Patients with expressive aphasia, on the other hand, tend to have intact comprehension but limited verbal output. Such patients usually understand the questions presented to them but are unable to provide articulate responses (either verbal or written); they may communicate their responses with very brief phrases or single words expressed seemingly with great effort. With such patients, the psychiatrist may find it useful to conduct the mental status examination in a "yes-or-no" format, or a multiple choice format, in which the patient is allowed to choose the correct answer presented by the interviewer.

Amnestic disorders may sometimes be mistaken for dementia. These disorders would include psychogenic amnesia, transient global amnesia and Korsakoff's syndrome. The key to distinguishing these disorders from dementia lies in the fact that although patients afflicted with these disorders may have profound impairment of memory, other cognitive abilities are at least relatively spared. Psychogenic amnesia is an interesting disorder in which the patient develops profound amnesia, which is usually retrograde. this disorder often follows on the heels of a profound psychosocial stressor, and is, in fact, a fairly common type of dissociative disorder (Kaplan and Sadock, 1991). Transient global amnesia is an unusual illness which involves the sudden onset of amnesia. It is felt to result from ischemia of the temporal lobes, and indeed these patients may have temporal lobe spikes on EEG (Kaufman, 1990; Bannister, 1992). Korsakoff's syndrome is a well known amnestic disorder, usually resulting from chronic alcohol abuse. Such patients have pronounced memory deficits and may confabulate. Korsakoff's syndrome is characteristically seen in patients who have suffered one or more past episodes of Wernicke's encephalopathy, a syndrome of ophthalmoparesis, nystagmus, ataxia, and an acute confusional state. Many patients with Korsakoff's syndrome may also suffer from alcohol dementia (discussed later in this chapter) (Victor, Adams, Collins, 1989).

A number of functional psychiatric disorders can mimic dementia, including schizophrenia, factitious disorder and anxiety disorders; however, depression is the most frequent culprit (Kaufman, 1990). The term *pseudodementia* has been used to describe this phenomenon, although some have argued that this term is vague and misleading (Reifler, 1982). One clue that the patient may be suffering from pseudodementia is the presence of symptoms consistent with depression. Indeed, Reynolds and associates (1988) compared patients with depressive pseudodementia with patients with primary degenerative dementia and found a significantly greater number of pseudodemented patents with early morning awakening and diminished libido.

There are a number of other features of pseudodementia that can be helpful in distinguishing it from dementia. Pseudodemented patients tend to answer, "I don't know" to many questions, tend to complain about their cognitive deficits and tend to have rather global impairment of memory, whereas demented patients tend to provide incorrect answers to many questions, tend to have greater impairment of short-term memory than long-term memory and tend to be less aware of their cognitive deficits than their pseudodemented counterparts (Wells, 1979). A therapeutic trial on an antidepressant may help to clinch the diagnosis of pseudodementia. Clearly, if the patient's cognitive problems completely resolve with treatment, the problem was almost certainly functional rather than organic. It is important to keep in mind, however, that demented patients can certainly suffer from depression and may sometimes exhibit some modest improvement in cognitive function with antidepressant treatment as well.

Delirium is probably the most important diagnosis for the psychiatric consultant to rule out when assessing a patient with impaired mental status. This is not always a simple task, but it is a crucial one, since many causes of delirium are reversible if treated and fatal if untreated.

The history can be invaluable in identifying a delirious patient. Delirium, unlike dementia, tends to have a rather abrupt onset, hours to days prior to the patient's initial presentation, while most patients with dementia have a history of symptoms dating back months to years, often with a history of insidious onset. In addition, a history of alcoholism should raise the psychiatrist's index of suspicion for delirium tremens, hepatic encephalopathy or Wernicke's encephalopathy. Likewise, a history of diabetes mellitus may suggest delirium secondary to hypoglycemia or diabetic ketoacidosis.

The mental status exam is also exceedingly important in identifying delirious patients. Delirious patients tend to have greater impairment of orientation and attention than of other cognitive functions. A fluctuating course is also characteristic of delirium, and although psychotic symptoms can certainly be seen in dementia, they are somewhat more common in delirium.

Finally, one should remember that delirium and dementia are not necessarily mutually exclusive. Indeed, demented patients appear to be somewhat more susceptible to delirium than the general population.

CORTICAL DEMENTIA AND SUBCORTICAL DEMENTIA

Many authors have divided dementing conditions into two camps. These two forms of dementia are considered to result from preferential neuronal loss in either cortical or subcortical areas. According to this schema, patients with subcortical dementia have preferential neuronal loss in such areas as the basal ganglia, brainstem, thalamus and subcortical white matter (Cummings and Benson, 1992; Huber, Shuttleworth, Paulson, et al, 1986), while patients with cortical dementia tend to have preferential neuronal loss in cortical areas. Some demented patients have a mixed picture with features of both cortical and subcortical dementia.

The clinical presentations of cortical and subcortical dementias can be contrasted on several levels. First, patients with cortical dementia tend to have more severe and more rapidly progressive dementia, and their memory deficits tend to result from difficulty learning new information, while patients with subcortical dementia tend to have less severely impaired cognitive function, and their memory deficits seem to be related to impaired retrieval of information (Cummings and Benson, 1992; Huber, Shuttleworth, Paulson, et al., 1986). In addition, patients with subcortical dementia tend not to exhibit such cortical findings as aphasia, agnosia and apraxia. Patients with subcortical dementia, on the other hand, tend to have dysarthric speech. From an affective standpoint, patients with subcortical dementia are more likely to appear depressed, manic, or apathetic than are patients with cortical dementia (Cummings and Benson, 1992). Finally, patients with subcortical dementia more typically suffer from movement disorders than do those with cortical dementia (Cadieux, 1989).

It should be emphasized, however, that the concepts of cortical dementia and subcortical dementia are rather controversial ones. For instance, some have questioned whether the "subcortical" dementia seen in Parkinson's disease is not simply due to the coincidental occurrence of Alzheimer's disease in patients with Parkinson's disease (Hakim and Mathieson, 1979). On the other hand, one might argue that patients with Alzheimer's disease, a well described cause of cortical dementia, have some features consistent with subcortical dementia, since these patients have degenerative changes in the nucleus basalis of Meynert, a subcortical structure, and can occasionally exhibit movement disorders (Cummings and Benson, 1984).

THE PSYCHIATRIC INTERVIEW

Despite the bewildering array of technologically sophisticated tests available to the consulting psychiatrist, the psychiatric interview remains the most useful tool in identifying the demented patient. No MRI, no CT scan, no battery of laboratory or neuropsychological tests can compare with the utility of a thorough clinical interview.

A careful history of present illness is essential. The clinician must remember that a history obtained solely from the patient is helpful but insufficient. Contacting a family member may provide valuable information regarding the severity and form of the patient's dementia. Such collateral information may not only help the clinician to identify the dementia syndrome, but also may point the clinician in the direction of a specific etiologic diagnosis.

Certain specific issues must be addressed in the history of present illness, such as the patient's social functioning, the patient's ability to perform activities of daily living, the presence or absence of incontinence, the presence or absence of behavioral dyscontrol, depression and psychosis, and the nature of the patient's supportive social network. The time course of the patient's symptoms can help to distinguish dementia from delirium and can also help to suggest the underlying cause of the patient's dementia. For example, patients with Alzheimer's disease tend to have a gradual, steady decline in their cognitive function, while those with multi-infarct dementia tend to have a more stepwise decline in function. The clinician may also find it useful to ask about other associated symptoms, such as problems with motor function.

Other aspects of the history may also provide helpful pieces to the diagnostic puzzle. Discussion of the patient's medications may provide the clinician with useful information, since many medications can cause cognitive impairment. Agents with anticholinergic potential are among the worst offenders in this regard, and it has been recently noted by Tune and associates (1992) that many commonly used medications which are not normally considered anticholinergic in fact do have anticholinergic potential. Family history is also very important since some dementing illnesses are familial.

The patient's past medical and psychiatric history are also essential pieces of information. Patients with histories of diabetes and hypertension, for example, are at increased risk of multi-infarct dementia. The patient's past psychiatric history may raise the clinician's index of suspicion for pseudodementia or may be particularly important if an elderly patient is experiencing psychotic symptoms, since functional psychotic disorders rarely have their initial presentation after age sixty-five (with psychotic depression being perhaps the major exception to this rule).

The mental status examination may be the most useful tool the psychiatric consultant has in the diagnostic process. Although a thorough history may be strongly suggestive of dementia, the psychiatric consultant must rely on objective findings to establish the diagnosis fairly unequivocally. What constitutes an adequate mental status examination is not as clear-cut as it may seem and may in fact vary from patient to patient. Patients with gross cognitive deficits may be easy to identify, while highly educated patients with subtle deficits may require a more thorough mental status assessment, such as that described in detail by Cummings and Benson (1992). In addition, a more thorough mental status examination may be necessary in order to identify a specific etiologic diagnosis. For the majority of patients, however, a more or less standard psychiatric mental status examination including the information shown in Table 2 should be adequate.

Table 2. The Mental Status Examination.

Appearance, Attitude and Behavior
Emotion (Mood and Affect)
Speech
Thought Process
Thought Content
Perception
Orientation
Attention
Memory (Short-term and Long-term)
Fund of Knowledge
Calculation
Language (Naming and Responses to Simple Commands)
Visuospatial Ability
Abstracting Ability
Judgement
Insight

Many clinicians find standardized dementia screening exams to be useful. One widely used screening exam is the Mini-Mental State Examination (Folstein, Folstein, McHugh, et al, 1975). This scale is reproduced in Table 3. Tombaugh and McIntyre (1992) recently reviewed the utility of the Mini-Mental State Examination. They recommended that three cut-off levels be employed to classify the severity of a patient's cognitive impairment (a score of twenty-four to thirty would indicate no cognitive impairment; a score of eighteen to twenty-three would indicate mild cognitive impairment, and a score of zero to seventeen would indicate severe cognitive impairment). They concluded that the Mini-Mental State Examination is useful as a brief screening test to assess cognitive impairment; however, they cautioned that the test should not be used to assess patients who are not fluent in English or who have less than an eighth grade education. They also pointed out that the diagnosis of dementia should not be based solely on the findings of the Mini-Mental State Examination.

Table 3. The "Mini-Mental State" Examination

Maximum Score	Score	
		ORIENTATION
5	( )	What is the (year)(season)(day)(month)?
5	( )	Where are we? (state)(country)(town)(hospital)(floor).
		REGISTRATION
3	( )	Name 3 objects: 1 second to say each. Then ask the patient all 3 after you have said them. Give 1 point for each correct answer. Then repeat them until he learns all 3. Count trials and record.
		ATTENTION AND CALCULATION
5	( )	Serial 7's. 1 point for each correct. Stop after 5 answers. Alternatively spell "world" backwards.
		RECALL
3	( )	Ask for the 3 objects repeated above. Give 1 point for each correct.

(Continued)

(Table 3. Continued)

LANGUAGE

9 ( ) Name a pencil, and watch (2 points).
Repeat the following "No ifs, ands or buts." (1 point)

Follow a 3-stage command: "Take a paper in your right hand, fold it in half, and put it on the floor" (3 points)

Read and obey the following:
CLOSE YOUR EYES (1 point)
Write a sentence (1 point)
Copy design (1 point)
Total score
(Assess level of consciousness along a continuum - alert/drowsy/stupor/coma)

INSTRUCTIONS FOR ADMINISTRATION OF MINI-MENTAL STATE EXAMINATION

ORIENTATION

(1) Ask for the date. Then ask specifically for parts omitted, e.g., "Can you also tell me what season it is?" One point for each correct.
(2) Ask in turn "Can you tell me the name of this hospital?" (town, country, etc.). One point for each correct.

REGISTRATION

Ask the patient if you may test his memory. Then say the names of 3 unrelated objects, clearly and slowly, about one second for each. After you have said all 3, ask him to repeat them. This first repetition determines his score (0-3) but keep saying them until he can repeat all 3, up to 6 trials. If he does not eventually learn all 3, recall cannot be meaningful tested.

ATTENTION AND CALCULATION

Ask the patient to begin with 100 and count backwards by 7. Stop after 5 subtractions (93, 86, 79, 72, 65). Score the total number of correct answers.
If the patient cannot or will not perform this task, ask him to spell the word "world" backwards. The score is the number of letters in correct order. E.g. dlrow=5, dlorw=3.

RECALL

Ask the patient if he can recall the 3 words you previously asked him to remember. Score 0-3.

LANGUAGE

Naming: Show the patient a wrist watch and ask him what it is. Repeat for pencil. Score 0-2.
Repetition: Ask the patient to repeat the sentence after you. Allow only one trial. Score 0 or 1.
3 - Stage command: Give the patient a piece of plain blank paper and repeat the command. Score 1 point for each part correctly executed.
Reading: On a blank piece of paper print the sentence "Close your eyes", in letters large enough for the patient to see clearly. Ask him to read it and do what it says. Score 1 point only if he actually closes his eyes.
Writing: Give the patient a blank piece of paper and ask him to write a sentence for you. Do not dictate a sentence, it is to be written spontaneously. It must contain a subject and verb and be sensible. Correct grammar and punctuation are not necessary.
Copying: On a clean piece of paper, draw intersecting pentagons, each side about 1 in., and ask him to copy it exactly as it is. All 10 angles must be present and 2 must intersect to score 1 point. Tremor and rotation are ignored.
Estimate the patient's level of sensorium along a continuum, from alert on the left to coma on the right.

From: Folstein MF, Folstein SE, McHugh PR: "Mini-mental state": a practical method for grading the cognitive state of patients for the clinician. Journal of Psychiatric Research 12: 189 - 198, 1975. Used with permission.

A number of other screening exams are in use as well. The Blessed Dementia Scale is one such test (Blessed, Tomlinson, Roth, 1968). This test has two components, one subjective and based on historical details, and one objective and based on the patient's performance on cognitive tasks. One standardized mental status examination widely used in the University of California, San Francisco system is the Neurobehavioral Cognitive Status Examination (Kiernan, Mueller, Langston, et al, 1987). This test involves a somewhat more extensive cognitive assessment than do the other screening tests discussed. For each cognitive function assessed, a screening question is presented to the patient initially. If the patient is unable to answer the screening question correctly, further questions are asked to assess the patient's deficits more thoroughly.

Although it is not a component of the psychiatric interview, a thorough physical examination is nonetheless a vital component of the diagnostic work-up of the demented patient. The neurologic examination is of particular importance, and may provide information helpful in making a specific etiologic diagnosis. The clinician is wise not to neglect the importance of the physical examination, and no discussion of this topic is complete without its mention.

To conclude our discussion of the clinical diagnosis of dementia, some mention of the role of neuropsychological testing is in order. Formal neuropsychological testing can be quite helpful in identifying marginally demented or pseudodemented patients. In addition, neuropsychological testing can sometimes shed light on a specific etiologic diagnosis. In many instances, however, it is not an essential component of the diagnostic work-up.

LABORATORY AND RADIOLOGIC ASSESSMENT OF THE DEMENTED PATIENT

Although laboratory and radiologic studies provide little information useful in identifying the dementia syndrome, they are an integral part of the diagnostic work-up of the demented patient and are particularly valuable in helping to identify specific etiologies of dementia. This is clearly more than a mere academic exercise, since some causes of dementia are treatable. It would be unforgivable, for example, to misdiagnose a patient with dementia secondary to hypothyroidism as having Alzheimer's disease.

The psychiatric consultant should consider certain laboratory tests as routine screening tests to be performed on virtually all patients found to be demented. These would include a complete blood chemistry and liver function panel, complete blood count, erythrocyte sedimentation rate, serologic testing for syphilis (preferably the MHA-TP test), thyroid function testing, Vitamin B12 and folate levels, and urinalysis. Other laboratory tests may prove valuable if there is some specific clinical indication for them. For example, it is not essential to perform a lumbar puncture on every demented patient, but if the patient has tested positive for syphilis, a lumbar puncture should be performed to rule out neurosyphilis. Likewise, routine HIV testing of all demented patients is probably overkill, but if a patients has a history of risk factors for HIV infection or clear evidence of compromised immune status, testing is clearly indicated.

Few consulting psychiatrists would fail to make use of radiologic imaging procedures if a patient is identified as being demented. Indeed, every newly identified demented patient should receive a CT Scan or MRI of the brain. The CT (computed tomography) scan is useful in making specific etiologic diagnoses, and more importantly, it can aid in identifying potentially treatable causes of dementia, such as tumors and normal pressure hydrocephalus. In general, patients should have a CT scan performed both with and without intravenous contrast dye. MRI (magnetic resonance imaging) is a brilliantly devised technique which does not utilize X-rays but, rather, relies upon the use of magnets and radiofrequency pulses to image tissue (Ramsey 1987). MRI has some advantages over CT scan; it gives a more accurate measurement of brain and CSF volume, gives somewhat better resolution of gray and white matter and seems more sensitive to structural changes due to ischemia (Steg, 1990).

It should be noted, however, that while these imaging procedures are generally extremely safe, they are not completely without risk. Patients undergoing CT scanning can suffer allergic reactions to the radiologic contrast dye or may suffer acute renal dysfunction from the nephrotoxic effects of the dye, particularly if there is a history of renal insufficiency. Patients should not be exposed to MRI if they have sizeable amounts of metal in their bodies (from a prior orthopedic procedure, for example). The magnet employed in MRI is extremely powerful and could conceivably injure the patient if the metal fragments were dislodged by the magnet.

Several other diagnostic tests are sometimes used in assessing demented patients. For example, some clinicians consider the electroencephalogram (EEG) to be an important component of the dementia work-up. Demented patients often exhibit mild diffuse slowing on EEG. Focal slowing on EEG may suggest stroke, brain abscess or tumor. (Steg, 1990)

Nuclear medicine studies have been used to assess demented patients, often in the context of research, but sometimes in the clinical setting as well. RISA (radioactive iodinated serum albumin) cisternography, for example, can be used in identifying normal pressure hydrocephalus. In this procedure, RISA is injected into the subarachnoid space, and the patient is serially scanned to assess CSF circulation and absorption. A characteristic dispersal pattern of the RISA is noted in patients with normal pressure hydrocephalus (Strub and Black, 1989).

PET (positron emission tomography) is a nuclear medicine imaging technique which is most commonly used to measure regional cerebral blood flow and regional cerebral metabolism. The technique generally involves the administration of a radionuclide labelled compound by either injection or inhalation. There are some practical problems with the use of PET in clinical practice. The cost is quite prohibitive, and an on-site cyclotron is required for the production of the radionuclide labelled compounds utilized. As such, PET is primarily a research tool at the present time.

SPECT (single photon emission computerized tomography) may prove to be of greater clinical value than PET. This technique is somewhat similar to PET in that it utilizes the administration of radionuclide labelled compounds in assessing cerebral blood flow. Unlike PET, however, it does not require the presence of an on-site cyclotron and is less expensive than PET. SPECT may be useful in distinguishing between multi-infarct dementia and Alzheimer's disease (Geaney and Abou-Saleh, 1990). In addition, other specific causes of dementia such as Pick's disease and Creutzfeldt-Jakob disease also seem to have distinctive patterns on SPECT. It also appears that SPECT may prove useful in identifying patients at risk for the future development of multi-infarct dementia (Devous, 1989).

ALZHEIMER'S DISEASE

Introductory Comments

Alzheimer's disease, a cortical dementia, is the most common cause of progressive dementia that the psychiatric consultant will encounter. It is disturbing to consider the prevalence of the disease. Approximately five percent of those older than sixty-five years old, and approximately twenty percent of those over eighty years old are affected. In addition, more than half of the nursing home patients in the United States suffer from Alzheimer's disease (Kaplan and Sadock, 1991).

Diagnosis

In the strictest sense, Alzheimer's disease can only be definitively diagnosed by brain biopsy or postmortem examination of the brain; however, a negative dementia work-up in an elderly patient with a history of gradually and steadily progressive cortical dementia is strongly suggestive of the diagnosis.

Clinical diagnostic criteria for the diagnosis of Alzheimer's disease have been established. DSM III-R provides criteria for the diagnostic category of Primary Degenerative Dementia of the Alzheimer Type; these criteria include the presence of dementia, insidious onset with a generally progressive deteriorating course, and exclusion of all other specific causes of dementia by history, physical examination and laboratory tests (American Psychiatric Association, 1987). Criteria for the clinical diagnosis of Alzheimer's disease have also been established by the National Institute of Neurological and Communicative Disorders and Stroke - Alzheimer's Disease and Related Disorders Association (NINCDS-ADRDA) Work Group. This joint effort resulted in diagnostic criteria which are considerably more extensive and detailed than those of DSM III-R (McKhann, Drachman, Folstein, et al, 1984). These criteria are shown in Table 4. Tierney and associates (1988) noted that the overall accuracy rate between the NINCDS-ADRDA criteria and neuropathologic classification was considerably higher than that noted in previous clinicopathologic studies, providing some validation of the quality of the Work Group criteria.

With respect to the diagnostic work-up, CT scan and MRI unfortunately have their greatest utility in ruling out other diagnoses, such as tumor or stroke. The presence of atrophy is not infrequently seen in elderly patients without dementia. In addition, the presence of high intensity signals in the white matter and periventricular regions on T_2-weighted MRI images is seen commonly in patients with Alzheimer's disease and in non-demented elderly patients (Harrell, 1991). On the other hand, SPECT may be more widely available to the clinician in the future and appears to be a rather sensitive and specific means of diagnosing Alzheimer's disease. In a recent review of the literature on the use of SPECT in evaluating demented patients, it was noted that SPECT can distinguish between Alzheimer's disease and multi-infarct dementia with eighty-two percent sensitivity and eighty-one percent specificity (Dewan and Gupta, 1992).

Clinical Features

The clinical course of Alzheimer's disease is usually relentlessly progressive. The disease typically has its onset after the age of fifty (and more characteristically after the age of sixty-five). Nonetheless, the disease can be seen occasionally in individuals younger

Table 4. Criteria for the Clinical Diagnosis of Alzheimer's Disease.

I. The criteria for the clinical diagnosis of PROBABLE Alzheimer's disease include:

dementia established by clinical examinations and documented by the Mini-Mental test, Blessed Dementia Scale, or some similar examination, and confirmed by neuropsychological tests;

deficits in two or more areas of cognition;

progressive worsening of memory and other cognitive functions;

no disturbance of consciousness;

onset between ages 40 and 90, most often after age 65; and

absence of systemic disorders or other brain diseases that in and of themselves could account for the progressive deficits in memory and cognition.

II. The diagnosis of PROBABLE Alzheimer's disease is supported by:

progressive deterioration of specific cognitive functions such as language (aphasia), motor skills (apraxia), and perception (agnosia);

impaired activities of daily living and altered patterns of behavior;

family history of similar disorders, particularly if confirmed neuropathologically; and

laboratory results of:

normal lumbar puncture as evaluated by standard techniques,

normal pattern or nonspecific changes in EEG, such as increased slow-wave activity, and

evidence of cerebral atrophy on CT with progression documented by serial observation.

III. Other clinical features consistent with the diagnosis of PROBABLE Alzheimer's disease, after exclusion of causes of dementia other Alzheimer's disease, include:

plateaus in the course of progression of the illness;

associated symptoms of depression, insomnia, incontinence, delusions, illusions, hallucination, catastrophic verbal, emotional, or physical outbursts, sexual disorders, and weight loss;

other neurologic abnormalities in some patients, especially with more advanced disease and including motor sign such as increased muscle tone, myoclonus, or gait disorder;

seizures in advanced disease; and

CT normal for age.

IV. Features that make the diagnosis of PROBABLE Alzheimer's disease uncertain or unlikely include:

sudden, apoplectic onset;

focal neurologic findings such as hemiparesis, sensory loss, visual field deficits, and incoordination early in the course of the illness; and

seizures or gait disturbances at the onset or very early in the course of the illness.

V. Clinical diagnosis of POSSIBLE Alzheimer's disease:

may be made on the basis of the dementia syndrome, in the absence of other neurologic, psychiatric, or systemic disorders sufficient to cause dementia, and in the presence of variations in the onset, in the presentation, or in the clinical course;

may be made in the presence of a second systemic or brain disorder sufficient to produce dementia, which is not considered to be the cause of the dementia; and

should be used in research studies when a single, gradually progressive severe cognitive deficit is identified in the absence of other identifiable cause.

VI. Criteria for diagnosis of DEFINITE Alzheimer's disease are:

the clinical criteria for probable Alzheimer's disease and histopathologic evidence obtained from a biopsy or autopsy.

VII. Classification of Alzheimer's disease for research purposes should specify features that may differentiate subtypes of the disorder. such as:

familial occurrence;

onset before age of 65;

presence of trisomy-21; and

coexistence of other relevant conditions such as Parkinson's disease.

Mckhann G, Drachman D, Folstein M, et al: Clinical diagnosis of Alzheimer's disease: report of the NINCDS-ADRDA work group under the auspices of Department of Health and Human Services task force on Alzheimer's disease. Neurology 34: 934 - 944, 1984. Used with permission.

than fifty as well. Life expectancy in Alzheimer's disease patients is quite variable, with some patients dying less than a year after diagnosis and some surviving up to twenty years (Cummings and Benson, 1992).

The clinical course of Alzheimer's disease may be divided into three phases, based on the clinical picture (Harrell, 1991). The *early phase* involves memory deficits (particularly short-term memory deficits), psychiatric symptoms and personality change, mild anomia and preservation of social skills. In this phase, the patient may continue to function fairly well and may live independently. Cognitive impairment may be so mild as to go un-noticed by the clinician if he or she neglects to assess mental status formally. The *middle phase* involves more profound cognitive impairment, as well as visuospatial disorientation, apraxia, agnosia, aphasia, problems with personal hygiene, agitation and psychosis. During this phase, the patient generally has easily recognized deficits. The patient may have long-term as well as short-term memory deficits and may begin to have difficulty recognizing friends and family. The *late phase* is characterized by mutism, profound dementia, and incontinence. The patient may eventually regress to a vegetative state and may lie in the fetal position on the bed. It is often during this phase that the patient meets death, usually resulting from the ravages of sepsis.

Psychiatric symptoms are common among Alzheimer's disease patients. The literature is somewhat unclear as to the prevalence of major depression in Alzheimer's disease; however, it is not felt to be particularly common (Cummings and Benson, 1992). The prevalence of psychotic symptoms is also somewhat unclear (Burns, 1992). Hallucinations have been noted in up to forty-nine percent of patients. Delusions are seen in anywhere from ten percent to seventy-three percent of patients (Birkett, 1972; Leuchter and Spar, 1985). Paranoid delusions are particularly common in patients with Alzheimer's disease and, unfortunately, are often quite problematic. From a somewhat psychodynamic standpoint, delusional thinking may be conceptualized as the patient's unconscious attempt to compensate for memory deficits and fill in information that he or she is unable to recall (Devanand, Sackeim, Mayeux, 1988). For example, if a patient cannot recall where she put her purse, she may accuse her son of stealing it. From a more neuropsychiatric standpoint, the delusions seen in Alzheimer's disease patients may result from temporal lobe and limbic system dysfunction (Burns, 1992).

Behavioral dyscontrol is a common problem for patients afflicted with Alzheimer's disease. Physical violence, wandering, and oppositional behavior are very distressing to the caregivers of such patients, perhaps more so than the cognitive deficits. Physical aggression is especially problematic. Indeed, it is often violent behavior that results in the placement of such patients into locked skilled nursing facilities.

A number of different clinical subtypes of Alzheimer's disease have been described. Some have divided Alzheimer's disease into two subtypes, based on whether the onset of the disease is senile (after age sixty-five) or pre-senile (before age sixty-five). Although patients with pre-senile onset have the same histopathological abnormalities as those with senile onset, there may be other differences between the two groups (Rossor, 1992). For example, Seltzer and Sherwin (1983) pointed out a greater prevalence of language deficits, an increased incidence of left handedness, and a shorter survival time in the pre-senile onset group.

There are a number of other systems that have been used to describe different clinical subtypes of dementia (Raskin, 1989; Ritchie and Touchon, 1992). Mayeux and associates (1985) described four subtypes; these included a subtype with extrapyramidal symptoms, severe intellectual decline and prominent psychotic symptoms, a subtype with myoclonus, severe intellectual decline, and frequent mutism, a subtype with minimal progression of symptoms over a four year period, and a subtype with gradual progression of cognitive impairment without other distinguishing features. Adams and Victor (1981) described five subtypes based on whether the patient presented with gait disturbance, amnesia, problems with spatial orientation, personality change with paranoia, or dysnomia.

Neuropathology and Pathophysiology of Alzheimer's Disease

The biology of Alzheimer's disease has been widely discussed in the literature. Indeed, our understanding of the disease has been enhanced considerably through the focused study of this topic.

The characteristic histopathologic changes seen in the brains of Alzheimer's disease patients include neurofibrillary tangles, senile (neuritic) plaques, and a general dropout of neurons and synapses. It should be noted, however, that neurofibrillary tangles and neuritic plaques can be seen in other conditions, as well as in non-demented elderly people (Cummings and Benson, 1992).

Neurofibrillary tangles are intraneuronal masses of aberrant filamentous proteins referred to as *paired helical filaments*. These paired helical filaments are comprised of the microtubule-associated protein *Tau* (Kowal and McKee, 1993). Certain areas of the brain seem to be particularly prone to the development of neurofibrillary tangles; these areas include portions of the hippocampal formation and parahippocampal gyrus, the amygdala, and certain hypothalamic and brainstem nuclei. Senile plaques are small, roughly spherical areas of neuronal degeneration which are seldom larger than two hundred microns in diameter. They are comprised of a cellular amyloid protein core surrounded by neuronal debris (Alafuzoff, 1992). Senile plaques are most highly concentrated in the temporal and parietal association areas (Arnold, Hyman, Flory, et al, 1991). Interestingly, the majority of studies indicate that the number of senile plaques does not correlate well with the severity of dementia, but the number of neurofibrillary tangles does correlate fairly well with the severity of dementia (the greater the number of neurofibrillary tangles, the more severe the dementia)(Kowall and Mckee, 1993).

In the past several years, there has been a veritable explosion of research examining the possible molecular mechanisms involved in the pathogenesis of Alzheimer's disease. It is felt that one very general mechanism involves disruption of the cytoskeleton (Lovestone and Anderton, 1992). It is felt that normal cytoskeletal structures within the neuron are eventually replaced by paired helical filaments, which ultimately accumulate and form neurofibrillary tangles (Perry, Kawai, Tabaton, et al, 1991). As mentioned, the major protein component of paired helical filaments is the microtubule associated protein *Tau* (Lovestone and Anderton, 1992). Under normal circumstances, *Tau* is felt to be instrumental in microtubule assembly (Goedert, Crowther, Garner, 1991); however, *Tau* protein found in paired helical filaments is not chemically identical to "normal" *Tau* and in fact appears to be a phosphorylated version of *Tau* (Lee, Balin, Otvos, et al, 1991). It may be that this phosphorylated version of *Tau* facilitates microtubule formation less effectively and instead results in paired helical filament formation (Lovestone and Anderton, 1992).

The role of amyloid beta protein (beta-amyloid) in the pathogenesis of Alzheimer's disease has also been the subject of considerable research. Senile plaques are partly comprised of extracellular deposits of amyloid beta protein, and amyloid beta protein is itself derived from the cleavage of a much larger protein, the beta-amyloid precursor protein (Hyman and Tanzi, 1992). The beta-amyloid precursor protein has a transmembranous segment, a segment which lies outside the neuron, and an intracellular segment. Amyloid beta protein is derived from part of the transmembranous segment as well as from part of the extracellular segment (Kang, Lemaire, Unterbech, et al, 1987). The precise role of amyloid in the pathogenesis of Alzheimer's disease is rather unclear, however. Murphy (1992) recently reviewed some of the suspected mechanisms, including direct neurotoxicity of amyloid beta protein and its potential role in acting as a facilitator of the neurotoxicity of amino acid neurotransmitters. It is far from certain, however, that amyloid beta protein has a specific causative role in the pathogenesis of Alzheimer's disease. In a recent discussion of the topic, for example, it was argued that amyloid beta protein may only play a role secondarily, as a protective reaction to neuronal injury by some other mechanism (Regland and Gottfries, 1992). It has also been suggested that beta-amyloid plays some role in the phosphorylation of the microtubule-associated protein *Tau*, although its precise role is, as yet, unclear.

Rather recently, it has been noted that apolipoprotein E (Apo E) may play some role in the pathogenesis of Alzheimer's disease. Travis (1993) has succinctly and eloquently summarized the recent research on Apo E. Apo E has been noted to bind tightly to amyloid beta protein, and in addition, it has been detected in the cerebral amyloid deposits and the neurofibrillary tangles found in the brains of Alzheimer's disease patients (Namba, Tomonaga, Kawasaki, et al, 1991). The precise role of Apo E, if any, is, as yet, unclear, but it is conceivable that it may somehow contribute to the deposition of amyloid beta protein (Travis, 1993).

The role of neurotransmitters, neuropeptides, and neuroendocrine influences is another richly researched topic in the pathogenesis of Alzheimer's disease. Perhaps the most important neurotransmitter system implicated in Alzheimer's disease is the cholinergic system. Early on, it was noted by Davies and Maloney (1976) that the brains of Alzheimer's disease patients had abnormally low levels of choline acetyltransferase. Subsequently, it was noted that by Whitehouse and associates that there was neuronal loss in the nucleus basalis of Meynert, which is felt to be a major cholinergic center in the brain and has extensive projections to the cerebral cortex. A central role of acetylcholine is by no means certain, however. Indeed, two recent reviews of the topic suggest that a cholinergic deficit may not be the primary neurotransmitter lesion in Alzheimer's disease (Fowler, O'Neill, Winblad, et al, 1992; Nordberg, 1992).

Other neurotransmitters have also been implicated in the pathogenesis of Alzheimer's disease. Vasopressin, for example, has been found in low concentrations in the hippocampus, nucleus accumbens and globus pallidus interna (Mazurek, Beal, Bird, et al, 1986). Since vasopressin may play a role in human memory function, these findings may well be relevant ones (Beckwith, Till, Scheider, 1984). Somatostatin deficits may also contribute to the disease process, as it has been noted that somatostatin levels in the parietal association cortex are much lower in Alzheimer's disease patients than in controls (Tamminga, Foster, Chase, 1985). In addition, there is evidence that somatostatin-containing neurons may be preferentially affected by neurofibrillary tangles (Roberts, Crow, Polak, 1985).

A number of biogenic amine neurotransmitter systems are also abnormal in patients with Alzheimer's disease. For example, neuronal loss has been noted in the locus ceruleus, a major adrenergic center (Tomlinson, Irving, Blessed, 1981). In addition, post-mortem studies of the brains of Alzheimer's disease patients have revealed low levels of dopamine, homovanillic acid, and norepinephrine (Adolfsson, Gottfries, Roos, et al, 1979).

A discussion of the pathogenesis of Alzheimer's disease would not be complete without at least some mention of the possible role of aluminum, and, indeed, there is at least some tenuous evidence to support this premise (Cummings and Benson, 1992). For instance, aluminum chloride has been noted to induce neurofibrillary tangle formation when injected into the brains of experimental animals (Wisniewski, Sturman, Shek, 1980). Trapp and associates (1978) noted that the brains of patients with Alzheimer's disease had higher levels of aluminum than those of controls. Other investigators, however, did not find a difference between Alzheimer's disease patients and controls (McDermott, Smith, Iqbal, et al, 1977). Candy and associates (1986) described the presence of aluminum in the core of neuritic plaques. A more recent study, however, indicated its absence (Landsberg, McDonald, Watt, 1992).

Brief mention of other theories of the pathogenesis of Alzheimer's disease should also be made at this point. It may be, for example, that some immunologic mechanism is at work in the development of the disease. A viral etiology has also been suggested (Cummings and Benson, 1992). Aberrant cellular regulation of potassium may also have some role in the pathogenesis of Alzheimer's disease, and it appears that findings in support of this theory may have paved the way to a future diagnostic skin test for Alzheimer's disease (Etcheberrigaray, Ito, Oka, et al, 1993).

The Role of Genetic Influences in Alzheimer's Disease

As with the explosion of research into the potential molecular mechanisms involved in Alzheimer's disease, genetics has similarly been a focus of much attention in recent years. Some of the studies done on this topic have focused more on cellular or molecular genetics, while others are more epidemiologic in nature.

Many astute observations have been made regarding the familial clustering of Alzheimer's disease. Early-onset familial Alzheimer's disease has been the focus of much of the research in this area. This disease is a relatively rare phenomenon, in which several members of a single family suffer from the disease and have onset of the disease prior to age sixty-five. In these families, approximately fifty percent of first degree relatives of the affected individual will develop the disease, suggesting an autosomal dominant mode of transmission. It certainly has been noted, however, that familial clustering may occur in the much more common late-onset form of Alzheimer's disease (Breitner, 1991). Indeed, there is some evidence suggesting an autosomal dominant mode of inheritance in such patients, but the pattern may be cloaked by the fact that many family members die before they are old enough to develop the disease (Mohs, Breitner, Silverman, et al, 1987).

Molecular genetics has provided some fascinating insights into the possible biological mechanisms involved in Alzheimer's disease. It has been noted, for example, that for at least some cases of early-onset familial Alzheimer's disease, the defective gene appears to be located on chromosome 21 (St. George-Hyslop, Tanzi, Polinsky, et al, 1987). This finding is particularly interesting since it is well known that patients with Down's syndrome, who have an extra copy of chromosome 21, frequently develop a clinical picture similar to Alzheimer's disease in the third to fourth decades of life (Franceschi, Comola, Piattoni, et al, 1990). In addition, the neuropathologic changes of Alzheimer's disease are also seen in such Down's syndrome patients (Burger and Vogel, 1973).

Some recent advances in the genetic understanding of Alzheimer's disease have involved the study of apolipoprotein E (Apo E). As it turns out, there are different isoforms of Apo E found in humans, and as such, there are different alleles of the Apo E gene corresponding to each of these isoforms (Travis, 1993). In a recent study, Saunders and associates (1993) noted that the allele for Apo E4 was much more common among patients with late-onset familial Alzheimer's disease or with sporadic cases of Alzheimer's disease (in which there is no family history) than among unaffected individuals. In another recent study involving individuals with a family history of Alzheimer's disease, it was noted that all individuals who had two copies of the allele for Apo E4 developed the disease by the age of eighty (Corder, Saunders, Strittmatter, et al, 1993).

NON-ALZHEIMER'S DEMENTIAS

Clearly there are myriad causes of dementia. The causes of dementia discussed in this chapter are certainly not the only ones in existence; however, they are among the most important ones for the psychiatric consultant to be familiar with. It should be noted that many of the disease processes discussed will not always present with dementia. Some will present in the form of delirium; others will present with psychiatric symptoms, and many will present with no significant cognitive or psychiatric sequelae at all, but with other manifestations.

Multi-Infarct Dementia

Multi-infarct dementia accounts for approximately fifteen percent of all cases of dementia in the elderly (Kaplan and Sadock, 1991). Patients with multi-infarct dementia, unlike those with Alzheimer's disease, tend to have a stepwise progression of cognitive impairment, presumably in synchrony with the occurrence of each newly sustained brain infarct. A number of criteria have been established to assist in the diagnosis of multi-infarct dementia. DSM III-R requires the presence of dementia, a stepwise course of deterioration with a patchy distribution of deficits early in the course, focal neurologic deficits, and tangible evidence of cerebrovascular disease (American Psychiatric Association, 1987). Hachinski and associates (1975) also have provided some widely utilized criteria for diagnosing multi-infarct dementia; these are summarized in Table 5. As indicated in the table, each criterion is assigned a numerical value, and a score of seven points or greater is indicative of a diagnosis of multi-infarct dementia.

Despite the usefulness of such criteria, however, the psychiatric consultant should keep in mind that distinguishing between multi-infarct dementia and Alzheimer's disease is not necessarily trivial. Indeed, both stroke and Alzheimer's disease occur rather frequently in the elderly population, and as such, they may both occur in the same patient by simple coincidence (Kase, 1986).

Multi-infarct dementia is actually only one of several forms of vascular dementia, although the two terms are often used as synonyms in the literature. In a review of the topic, Fourette and Boller (1991) broke down vascular dementia into several different subtypes, including multi-infarct dementia, lacunar dementia, Binswanger's subcortical encephalopathy, cerebral amyloid angiopathy, and single infarct dementia. A few of these subtypes should be further defined. Lacunar dementia involves the presence of lacunar infarctions, which are small, subcortical infarctions often visualized on CT as small lucencies. They are felt to result from the occlusion of small penetrating arteries, which in turn is felt to result from hypertensive cerebral vasculopathy (Gorelick and Mangone, 1991). Binswanger's subcortical encephalopathy (Binswanger's disease) involves dementia presumably stemming from periventricular white matter degeneration, sometimes referred to as *leukoariosis.* Binswanger's disease is also more commonly seen in hypertensive patients (Yao, Sadoshima, Ibayashi, et al, 1992).

Risk factors for vascular dementia, other than hypertension, include smoking and diabetes mellitus. In light of these risk factors, it has been strongly recommended that more research be done on the impact of controlling these variables on the course of multi-infarct dementia (Hachinski, 1992). Indeed, Meyer and associates (1986) noted that among hypertensive patients with multi-infarct dementia, control of systolic blood pressure to within 135 millimeters of mercury and 150 millimeters of mercury resulted in improved cognitive function in some patients. It was also noted, however, that if systolic blood pressure were lowered beyond this point, the clinical course of those patients tended to worsen.

Table 5. The Ischemic Score

Feature	Score
Abrupt onset	2
Stepwise deterioration	1
Fluctuating course	2
Nocturnal confusion	1
Relative preservation of personality	1
Depression	1
Somatic complaints	1
Emotional incontinence	1
History of hypertension	1
History of strokes	2
Evidence of associated atherosclerosis	1
Focal neurological symptoms	2
Focal neurological signs	2

From: Hachinski VC, Iliff LD, Zilhka E, et al: Cerebral blood flow in dementia. Archives of Neurology 32: 632 - 637, 1975. Used with permission.

Dementia and the Acquired Immunodeficiency Syndrome (AIDS)

The acquired immunodeficiency syndrome (AIDS) ia a devastating phenomenon involving a clinical picture of immune system dysfunction and other associated phenomena, including dementia. AIDS ultimately results from the ravages of the human immunodeficiency virus (HIV) on the patient's immune system. Risk factors for HIV infection are well known. Those individuals particularly at risk for infection with the virus include homosexual males and intravenous drug abusers. Heterosexual partners of infected individuals and frequent recipients of blood products (especially pooled blood products) are also at risk.

Because of the effect of HIV on the T-helper cells, patients are rendered vulnerable to a number of opportunistic infections, including oropharyngeal candidiasis, *Pneumocystis carinii* pneumonia, and toxoplasmosis. Patients are susceptible to central nervous system infection by opportunistic pathogens and are also susceptible to the development of a direct central nervous system infection by HIV itself. The AIDS dementia complex is a result of this direct CNS infection by HIV (Ho, Bredesen, Vinters, et al, 1989).

The AIDS dementia complex has fairly characteristic clinical features. It has the clinical picture of a subcortical dementia, and as such, cortical deficits, such as aphasia and apraxia, are relatively uncommon or appear late in the course of the AIDS dementia complex (Navia, Jordan, Price, 1986). Further, on neuropathologic examination of the brains of afflicted individuals, the structures most extensively involved tend to be subcortical ones (Cornford, Holden, Boyd, et al, 1992). The AIDS dementia complex tends to present late in the course of AIDS and is characterized by a number of features, including inattention, decreased concentration, forgetfulness, slowed movements, clumsiness, ataxia, apathy and personality change (Worley and Price, 1992). Late in the course of the AIDS dementia complex, patients may exhibit severe dementia, mutism and paraplegia.

While it is generally true that the AIDS dementia complex tends to occur after the onset of other signs and symptoms of AIDS, this is not universally true. In fact, the AIDS dementia complex can be the presenting feature of AIDS (Navia and Price, 1987). In addition, ten to twenty percent of apparently asymptomatic HIV-positive individuals appear to exhibit mild cognitive impairment on neuropsychological testing (Bornstein, Nasrallah, Para, et al, 1992).

On neuropathologic examination of the brains of such patients, the characteristic histopathological finding is the presence of focal grey and white matter microglial nodule inflammatory lesions associated with multinucleated giant cells (Cornford, Holden, Boyd, et al, 1992). It should be noted, however, that neuropathologic abnormalities are quite common among AIDS patients in general. Evidence of CNS opportunistic infections with cytomegalovirus, fungal and parasitic pathogens is common, as is the presence of CNS lymphomas (Ho, Bredesen, Vinters, et al, 1989). It should be kept in mind that such opportunistic infections or tumors can themselves result in cognitive impairment.

A number of laboratory findings have been noted in patients with HIV infection, aside from the positive ELISA test for HIV antibodies. Many neurologically normal HIV-positive individuals have abnormal CSF findings; more specifically, individuals with the AIDS dementia complex very often have an elevation of total protein and IgG. As such, although evaluation of the CSF cannot reliably diagnose the AIDS dementia complex, a lumbar puncture revealing completely normal CSF may help to rule out the diagnosis (McArthur, 1992).

Some clinicians have found CT and MRI to be somewhat useful in diagnosis of the AIDS dementia complex. CT scans often show evidence of cerebral atrophy and sometimes show decreased white matter density. Patients may have coincidental mass lesions, which may represent lymphomas or opportunistic pathogens. MRI is more sensitive than CT in detecting white matter degeneration in these patients (Ho, Bredesen, Vinters, et al, 1989).

Unfortunately, the prognosis of AIDS remains abysmal, with virtually all cases eventually ending in death. It has been noted, however, that azidothymidine (AZT) has been somewhat effective not only in prolonging survival in patients with AIDS, but also in the treatment of the AIDS dementia complex (McArthur, 1992). Indeed, there is some evidence of at least temporary improvement or stabilization of cognitive function with AZT therapy (Schmitt, Bigley, McKinnis et al, 1988). In addition, AIDS patients in general are at risk for affective disorders, anxiety disorders and psychosis, which may all respond to psychiatric intervention.

Parkinson's Disease

Parkinson's disease is an idiopathic neurologic disorder beginning in late adult life and afflicting approximately one in five hundred people (Kaplan and Sadock, 1991). The clinical picture of Parkinson's disease is one of a progressive worsening of a number of signs, including a resting "pill-rolling" tremor, shuffling gait, amd bradykinesia. Other clinical features include diminished blinking, masked facies, impaired postural reflexes, micrographia and hypophonia. Depression is also quite common, being seen in twenty-five percent of patients with the disease (Kaufman, 1990).

Dementia is also a common finding in Parkinson's disease patients. Biggins and associates (1992) recently reported that of eighty-seven patients with Parkinson's disease followed over a fifty-four month period, nineteen percent developed dementia. Nonetheless, reports of the frequency of dementia in Parkinson's disease vary widely, and it is felt that a large percentage of patients who do not meet criteria for dementia exhibit subtle evidence of cognitive impairment (Whitehouse, Friedland, Strauss, 1992).

The dementia seen in Parkinson's disease patients tends to be milder than that seen in Alzheimer's disease (Mayeux, Stern, Rosen, 1983). Clinical features of the dementia include memory impairment, poor wordlist generation, problem solving difficulties, impairment of visuospatial perception, slowed information processing, impaired set shifting and failure to initiate activities spontaneously (Cummings and Benson, 1992).

The dementia associated with Parkinson's Disease is generally considered to be of the subcortical variety. However, Mayeux and associates (1983) questioned that such a distinction should be made. In addition, others have suggested that the dementia seen in Parkinson's disease may be explained by the simultaneous occurrence of Alzheimer's disease (Hakim and Mathieson, 1979)). Others have pointed out that Parkinson's disease patients can exhibit apparent frontal lobe deficits on neuropsychological testing (Cools, Van Den Bercken, Horstink, et al, 1984).

There is a great deal known and a great deal unknown about the biology of Parkinson's disease. The nigrostriatal dopaminergic system seems to be the primary neurotransmitter system affected. Cell loss is noted in the substantia nigra, but other areas, including the locus ceruleus and the tenth cranial dorsal motor nuclei are also involved. Such areas contain Lewy bodies, which are seen as eosinophilic intracytoplasmic deposits upon histopathologic examination (Kaufman, 1990). As previously mentioned, some investigators have noted the characteristic histopathologic features of Alzheimer's disease in the brains of some demented patients with Parkinson's disease (Hakim and Mathieson, 1979). Cash and associates (1987) noted that demented Parkinson's disease patients had decreased locus ceruleus levels of norepinephrine, homovanillic acid, and 3-methoxy-4-hydroxyphenylethyleneglycol. More obvious neuropathologic changes seen in Parkinson's disease patients include cortical atrophy and depigmentation of the substantia nigra (Cummings and Benson, 1992). Indeed, shrinkage of the substantia nigra sometimes can be visualized on MRI (Duguid, De La Paz, Degroot, 1986).

The motor disturbances seen in Parkinson's disease can often respond dramatically to anticholinergic or dopaminergic agents, and, interestingly, cognitive impairment may also improve with treatment in some patients (Cummings and Benson, 1992).

Unfortunately, these improvements are not indefinitely sustained since the disease is a progressive one. The psychiatric consultant should also keep in mind that the use of anticholinergic agents and dopaminergic agents is, to some extent, a double-edged sword, since these agents can induce psychotic symptoms or worsen cognitive impairment in some patients.

Huntington's Disease

Huntington's disease is a devastating illness involving dementia, psychiatric symptoms and a movement disorder. The illness is hereditary, with an autosomal dominant inheritance pattern. As such, one of the most important pieces to the diagnostic puzzle is knowledge of a family history of the disease. The disease tends to have an insidious onset, with the age of onset usually ranging from thirty-five years old to forty-two years old; however, six percent of patients develop the disease before the age of twenty (LaCour, 1990). The prevalence of the disease appears to be approximately five to seven cases per one hundred thousand people, although estimates of this vary widely, and the disease can be much more common in specific isolated populations (Whitehouse, Friedland, Strauss, 1992; Folstein, 1989).

Folstein (1989) has eloquently described the movement disorder associated with Huntington's disease. The most characteristic feature is the presence of jerky involuntary movements affecting almost any part of the body; this phenomenon is referred to as *chorea*. Motor restlessness often precedes the onset of chorea; patients may often gesticulate frequently and have difficulty sitting still. Patients with the disease often exhibit dystonic posturing as well, and also have difficulty with fine motor coordination and gait. Dysarthria and dysphagia are also common findings.

Psychiatric symptoms are very commonly seen in Huntington's disease, and it is for this reason that the psychiatric consultant should be particularly aware of this disease. There is considerable controversy over the prevalence of psychiatric symptoms in Huntington's disease (Whitehouse, Friedland, Strauss, 1992). Suffice it to say, however, that psychosis and affective symptoms are both very common. In one retrospective study, depressive symptoms were noted in fifty-three percent of the patients studied, while psychotic symptoms were seen in thirty-four percent of patients (Pflanz, Besson, Ebmeier, et al, 1990). Hypomania and mania are also seen and, unfortunately, so is suicide (Folstein, 1989).

Dementia is, of course, an important feature of Huntington's disease. The dementia tends to be of the subcortical variety. As with Parkinson's disease, however, the subcortical nature of this dementia has also been questioned (Mayeux, Stern, Rosen, et al, 1983). In addition, evidence of apparent frontal lobe dysfunction has been noted in some patients with Huntington's disease (Cummings and Benson, 1992). Nonetheless, other studies do support the subcortical nature of the dementia seen in Huntington's disease (Huber, Shuttleworth, Paulson, et al, 1986). Cognitive deficits appear rather early in the course of the disease and progress with time. Memory deficits may be the most prominent neuropsychological feature of Huntington's disease, with greater impairment of retrieval of information than of recognition; concentration and visuospatial abilities are also impaired, while language is less affected (Whitehouse, Friedland, Strauss, 1992).

There is a great deal of literature on the biology of Huntington's disease. The major neurotransmitter system affected is that of gamma-aminobutyric acid (GABA), a major inhibitory neurotransmitter. Levels of GABA are diminished in the caudate, putamen, globus pallidus and substantia nigra (Quarrell, 1991). Neuropathologic changes seen in Huntington's disease include cortical atrophy, profound cell loss in the caudate nucleus, as well as atrophy of the putamen and globus pallidus (Cummings and Benson, 1992). The gene for the disease has been traced to the short arm of chromosome 4, and through the use of linkage analysis, it is now possible to identify afflicted individuals prior to the onset of symptoms (Harper, Morris, Tyler, 1991).

Unfortunately, Huntington's disease is a progressive and terminal condition. Nonetheless, palliative treatment is available. Neuroleptics are often used to treat the disabling involuntary movements these patients experience, and, of course, they are also helpful in alleviating psychotic symptoms (Folstein, 1989). The consulting psychiatrist plays a vital role in treating patients with psychosis or affective disorder. Indeed the role of the consulting psychiatrist should not be minimized, as cognitive function has been noted to improve significantly when patients receive treatment for their psychiatric symptoms (LaCour, 1990).

Pick's Disease

Pick's disease is a progressive dementing illness which, like Alzheimer's disease, typically produces a cortical dementia. The disease is much less common than Alzheimer's disease and typically has its onset during middle age.

The clinical features of Pick's disease tend to be somewhat different from those of Alzheimer's disease. For example, patients with Pick's disease tend to have relative preservation of memory, arithmetic and visuospatial skills, whereas language deficits are fairly pronounced (Cummings and Benson, 1992). In addition, patients with Pick's disease can sometimes exhibit features of the Kluver-Bucy syndrome, a behavioral syndrome involving hyperorality, emotional blunting, altered dietary habits, sensory agnosia, hypersexuality, and a tendency for patients to engage in tactile exploration of their surroundings (Cummings and Duchen, 1981).

Neuropathologic examination of the brains of these patients reveals atrophy of the frontal and anterior temporal lobes, with relative sparing of the parietal lobes (these changes can often be noted on CT or MRI) (Kaufman, 1990). Histopathologic examination reveals the presence of neuronal swellings and Pick bodies, which are argentophilic (silver staining) intracytoplasmic inclusions seen within the neuron. Perhaps more importantly, senile plaques and neurofibrillary tangles are not typically seen (Constantinidis, Richard, Tissot, 1974).

Alcohol Dementia

Alcohol abuse and dependence are quite common in our society, with a combined lifetime prevalence of eleven to sixteen percent in the United States (Larson, 1991). The medical sequelae of alcoholism are devastating and include liver disease, cardiomyopathy, hypertension, and peripheral neuropathy. Alcoholic patients are also at risk for seizures, subdural hematomas, delirium tremens and motor vehicle accidents.

Perhaps less well known is the tendency of alcoholics to become demented. As noted earlier in this chapter, alcohol dementia is different from Korsakoff's syndrome, which primarily involves memory deficits. The DSM III-R lists criteria for Dementia

Associated with Alcoholism, which include the presence of dementia which persists at least three weeks after the cessation of alcohol ingestion, and exclusion of all other causes of dementia by history, physical examination and laboratory tests (American Psychiatric Association, 1987).

Despite the prevalence of alcoholism in our society, there is a rather surprising lack of literature on the topic of alcohol dementia (by comparison with other causes of dementia). Several things can be said, however. In a review of the topic, Lishman reported that alcoholism accounts for seven to twenty-one percent of dementia cases (Lishman, 1981). Lishman also noted that many alcoholics exhibit dilated ventricles and sulcal widening on CT scan. In addition, Lishman pointed out that alcohol dementia may be underdiagnosed since many such patients have probably been misdiagnosed with Korsakoff's syndrome. On the other hand, it has been suggested that the CT scan findings just described may be secondary to fluid shifts related to alcoholism, rather than to actual neuronal loss. Indeed, these CT findings are not uncommonly reversed when the patient remains abstinent (Victor, Adams, Collins, 1989).

Many alcoholics exhibit deficits on neuropsychological testing. Tarter (1980), in a review of the topic, pointed out that these deficits may include impaired abstracting ability, impairment of spatial and perceptual skills, impaired performance on tasks of motor speed and dexterity, and impairment of memory. Some of these deficits have been noted to be more profound in patients with longer drinking histories. More importantly, it has also been noted that at least some of these deficits improve with sustained sobriety.

For the consulting psychiatrist, it is essential that the issue of alcohol abuse be addressed in such patients. Ideally, the patient should be referred to an inpatient chemical dependency treatment program once the patient's medical issues are adequately addressed. If the patient is being seen on an inpatient service, it is absolutely essential that the patient be placed on alcohol withdrawal precautions and provided with a PRN dose of a benzodiazepine to prevent withdrawal symptoms. It is also prudent to provide the patient with thiamine, folic acid, and a multivitamin. Thiamine is of particular importance since such patients are at risk for Wernicke's encephalopathy, and thiamine supplementation can help to prevent this devastating phenomenon.

Unfortunately, the demented patient may often have difficulty maintaining sobriety, since cognitive impairment often hinders the patient from adequately engaging in chemical dependency treatment. Family involvement can be very valuable in such situations; a supportive spouse, for example, can help the patient to remember to attend Alcoholics Anonymous meetings and can help to keep the patient away from alcohol.

Dementia Resulting from Traumatic Brain Injury

Head trauma is a relatively common phenomenon and is one of the most common causes of dementia in young and otherwise healthy people (Silver, Hales, Yudofsky, 1992). The facts speak for themselves. Seventy thousand to ninety thousand people each year sustain head injuries which result in chronic disabilities, and roughly twenty-five billion dollars per year are spent in the United States on the sequelae of traumatic brain injuries (Department of Health and Human Services, 1989).

When a patient sustains a head injury, the brain may be damaged by direct contusion at the point of impact, by a contrecoup mechanism on the side of the head opposite the point of impact, or by torsional forces while the head is recoiling from the impact. In addition, secondary damage can occur when there is hematoma formation, vasospasm or cerebral edema. In patients with severe head injuries, multifocal lesions are often seen, with evidence of contusion, intracranial hemorrhage and white matter degeneration (Strub and Black, 1988).

The cognitive sequelae of head injury may take many different forms. Aphasia occurs in up to thirty percent of patients who sustain serious head injuries, but many of these patients recover their language function with time. Other cognitive deficits include impairment of concentration, abstracting ability, calculation skills and memory (Silver, Hales, Yudofsky, 1992). Prediction tree techniques have been used to attempt to provide a prognosis for the recently injured patient. These analyses can be quite complex, with predictive accuracies as high as nearly eighty percent (Choi, Muizelaar, Barnes, 1991).

Psychiatric sequelae are not uncommon in patients with head injuries. Depression, mania, psychosis and personality change can all be seen. Many such patients exhibit personality changes consistent with frontal lobe damage; patients with orbitofrontal damage tend to exhibit impulsivity, disinhibition, hyperactivity and distractibility, while damage to the dorsolateral frontal area tends to induce apathy, passivity, emotional withdrawal and blunted affect (Silver, Hales, Yudofsky, 1992).

Normal Pressure Hydrocephalus

Normal pressure hydrocephalus is a well known cause of dementia. The classic clinical features of the syndrome are dementia, urinary incontinence, and gait disturbance. The phenomenon results from the impedance of CSF absorption through the arachnoid villi; this impaired absorption may result from meningitis, subarachnoid hemorrhage, or more commonly, from some unclear mechanism (Kaufman, 1990). There is considerable variation in the clinical features of the dementia caused by normal pressure hydrocephalus; however, it is sometimes classified as a subcortical dementia (Cummings and Benson, 1992).

Patients with normal pressure hydrocephalus are important to identify, since their dementia is at least potentially reversible. On CT scan, these patients are often noted to have enlargement of the ventricles out of proportion to the degree of cortical atrophy; however, CT (or MRI) is inadequate to make the diagnosis since this pattern is not always easily distinguished from that of simple cortical atrophy (Kaufman, 1990).

Although the CSF pressure is normal in these patients, it has been noted that these patients can show temporary improvement after lumbar puncture and removal of forty to fifty milliliters of CSF; indeed, it has been suggested that improvement after such a tap may help to predict which patients will respond favorably to a CSF shunting procedure, such as a ventriculoperitoneal shunt (Wikkelsø, Andersson, Blomstrand, 1982). As mentioned earlier in this chapter, RISA cisternography can be very helpful in the diagnosis of normal pressure hydrocephalus.

Patients with normal pressure hydrocephalus can respond favorably to surgical intervention. Meyer and associates (1985), for example, noted that the majority of patients in their study undergoing CSF shunting procedures exhibited improvement in cerebral blood flow, as well as improvement in gait, in activities of daily living and in cognitive function. Many of the patients regained their continence after such procedures as well.

Neurosyphilis

Infection of the central nervous system by *Treponema pallidum* has long been known to cause dementia. *Treponema pallidum* is a bacterial pathogen and can be transmitted by sexual contact, as well as by the transplacental route. Primary syphilis occurs two to three weeks after initial infection and is characterized by the presence of a genital lesion called a *chancre*. Secondary syphilis typically occurs four to ten weeks after the appearance of the chancre and is characterized by a diffuse rash. Tertiary syphilis occurs years after initial infection and can present with granuloma formation, cardiovascular symptoms, neurologic symptoms, psychiatric symptoms and dementia (Musher, 1992).

Dementia in tertiary syphilis can result from a number of different mechanisms but most commonly results from direct infection of the brain parenchyma by *Treponema pallidum*. This dementia tends to develop ten to twenty years after initial infection (but may occur much earlier in patients with HIV infection). Symptoms include memory impairment, impaired judgement and disorientation. A number of neurologic symptoms may also be present, including intention tremor, dysarthria, hyperreflexia, and Argyll-Robertson pupils (asymmetric, small pupils which do not react to light but do constrict with accommodation) (Coyle and Dattwyler, 1990). Psychiatric symptoms are well known and include mania, depression and psychosis (Kaplan, and Sadock, 1991).

It is essential that the psychiatric consultant be aware of neurosyphilis and its association with dementia, since neurosyphilis is a treatable condition. All patients with dementia should, of course, be tested for syphilis. The MHA-TP test is preferable to the RPR or VDRL, since the RPR and VDRL are often negative in patients with neurosyphilis (Hooshmand, Escobar, Kopf, 1972). If the patient has a positive MHA-TP test, a lumbar puncture must be done and the spinal fluid assessed for the presence of *Treponema pallidum* (Musher, 1992). An infectious disease specialist and a neurologist should be involved in the case if the question of neurosyphilis is entertained, and if it were decided that the patient should be treated for neurosyphilis, an aggressive antibiotic regimen would be necessary.

Hypothyroidism

Hypothyroidism can present with a number of signs, including brittle hair, dry skin, hoarseness and abnormal deep tendon reflexes with a delayed relaxation phase. The patient may complain of fatigue, constipation, weight gain, depressive symptoms, cognitive impairment or insensitivity to cool ambient temperatures. Additional clinical features may include hypertension, bradycardia, periorbital and peripheral edema and muscle cramps (Baker and McFarland, 1990).

Hypothyroidism is a well known cause of potentially reversible dementia. Unfortunately, it is also a rather uncommon cause of dementia, probably accounting for considerably less than two percent of all cases of dementia (Clarfield, 1988). The dementia seen in patients with hypothyroidism may involve deficits in abstraction, attention and recent memory (Whybrow, Prange, Treadway, 1969). Dementia may be seen in patients with only marginal cases of hypothyroidism involving only elevated levels of thyroid stimulating hormone (TSH) and no change in the level of free T4. (Haggerty, Evans, Prange, 1986). Psychiatric symptoms are commonly seen, particularly depressive symptoms and psychosis.

Assessment of thyroid function is a relatively simple matter, with measurement of TSH and free T4 being the only tests needed in the assessment of the demented patient. (In centers where the free T4 test in unavailable, a T4 level and T3 uptake will suffice). Treatment of hypothyroidism is relatively easily accomplished with administration of levothyroxine. Unfortunately, if the hypothyroidism is long-standing, the cognitive deficits seen may persist despite treatment (Whybrow, Prange, Treadway, 1969).

Additional Causes of Dementia

Vitamin deficiencies sometimes result in dementia. Most importantly, Vitamin B12 deficiency is not uncommon and is a potentially reversible cause of dementia. Vitamin B12 deficiency is readily treated with intramuscular supplementation.

Wilson's disease is an interesting hereditary disorder of copper metabolism and has an autosomal recessive pattern of inheritance. Patients with Wilson's disease may develop cirrhosis, dementia and psychiatric symptoms. Patients may exhibit an unusual movement disorder, with a so-called *wing beating* tremor. Patients also may have greenish deposits in the cornea termed *Kayser-Fleischer rings*. Most importantly, treatment with D-penicillamine can be quite effective in preventing progression of the disease. As such, early diagnosis is extremely important.

Creutzfeldt-Jakob disease is a devastating neurologic disorder caused by a proteinaceous infectious particle called a *prion*. This disease is often characterized by a rather rapidly progressive dementia typically associated with myoclonus. A number of cases of the disease are felt to have been iatrogenic, having resulted from the administration of infected cadaveric human growth hormone, corneal transplantation with infected corneal tissue, or the use of infected neurosurgical instruments (Webb, Leech, Brumback, 1990).

Perhaps one of the most important causes of dementia for the psychiatric consultant to keep in mind is medication-induced dementia. The classes of drugs most commonly implicated in causing cognitive dysfunction (particularly in the elderly) are benzodiazepines, tricyclic antidepressants, beta blockers, certain other antihypertensives, anticonvulsants and digitalis preparations (Lowenthal and Nadeau, 1991). It should be noted, however, that the cognitive changes resulting from medication side effects may often take the form of delirium rather than dementia.

PSYCHOSOCIAL ASPECTS OF TREATMENT

Much can be said about the plight of demented patients and their families. Demented patients are often difficult to live with. Not only are they frequently dependent on their family members for feeding, dressing and even toileting, but quite often, they are hostile and even violent. Indeed, it is often the family members who complain the most bitterly to the clinician, while the afflicted patients may seem largely unaware of their problems.

Practical Guidelines

A number of practical guidelines can be helpful in the treatment of the demented patient. These interventions can be of considerable benefit to the patient and the family, and although many may seem fairly trivial, they can have a considerable impact on the patient's ability to function.

Some interesting suggestions have been made regarding the living environment of the demented patient. Certain features of the environment may, for example, detract from the patient's attention span. Noise, crowding, glare and foul odors may all contribute to the patient's general level of confusion. The caregiver may find it helpful, therefore, to avoid exposing the patient to large family gatherings or crowded department stores (Hiatt, 1990).

Lighting and the strategic use of color may also be of considerable help to the patient. Adequate lighting can help to prevent nocturnal confusion ("sundowning"), and as such, the family or nursing staff may find it helpful to keep a light on in the patient's room at night. The use of color may be helpful to the patient in a number of ways. For example, giving a patient a blue shirt and trousers to put on may result in the patient mistaking the shirt for the trousers and vice-versa; however, giving the patient a white shirt and blue trousers may help the patient to distinguish between the two. If a patient has a problem with wandering out of the home, painting the exit doors the same color as the surrounding walls may prevent the patient from identifying the exits (Hiatt, 1990).

A number of other general recommendations can also be helpful. For example, a daily routine should be developed for the patient, to assist him or her with orientation to place, person, time and situation. On an inpatient service, it may be helpful to have the nursing staff orient the patient with each meal and to provide a clock and/or a calendar at the bedside. The patient should be encouraged to keep as active as possible with hobbies and other personal interests, and should be rewarded for positive behaviors, such as performance of activities of daily living (Hiatt, 1990).

Structured Interventions

The consulting psychiatrist may find various psychotherapeutic and psychoeducational approaches helpful in dealing with demented patients and their families. Behavioral approaches can be quite effective but, admittedly, are often difficult to implement. An example of such an approach might involve a system of rewarding patients with cigarettes or coffee when they perform positive behaviors (Gustafson, 1992).

Another technique, referred to as *reality orientation,* has also been utilized with at least some small benefits to patients. This approach involves small group meetings, in which the therapist not only orients the patients, but also discusses various topics, such as the weather and its relationship to the season; in this way, the therapist attempts to orient the patient in a more profound way than, for example, simply stating the date. The room in which the group meets is usually equipped with clocks, calendars and a blackboard (Powell-Proctor and Miller, 1982).

Another group therapy approach, termed *validation therapy,* has also been used. This approach operates under the assumption that the disorientation of the demented patient holds a somewhat symbolic meaning for the patient. As such, it is felt that focusing on the emotional content underlying the patient's disorientation may be helpful. For example, if a patient believes she is at home in her living room with her husband, rather than sitting in the group therapy room, the therapist might try to elicit her feelings about her husband. In actuality, validation therapy also serves a supportive function as well, and structured group activities, such as singing, are often incorporated into the therapy sessions (Bleathman and Morton, 1992).

In light of the tremendous amount of stress on the caregivers of demented patients, the psychiatric consultant should be mindful of their mental health needs as well. For most family members, referral to a support group is sufficient intervention, but for some, individual therapy or treatment with an antidepressant or anxiolytic may be necessary. Whatever the family's level of emotional distress, a clear line of communication between them and the psychiatrist (or primary care physician) is essential. The physician plays a key role as an educator and as a listener. Providing information about the patient's disease process and the treatments available can often be of considerable help to the distraught family member. Indeed, many family members have little knowledge of dementia and its manifestations, and they may feel bewildered and frightened by the patient's irrational behavior. With such individuals, it may be paradoxically reassuring for them to learn of a spouse's or parent's diagnosis.

Nursing Home Placement and Day Care

As an educator, the consulting psychiatrist should be aware of residential and day care options for the patient. Choosing a nursing home is clearly an individualized process. Indeed, some families may choose never to place a family member in a nursing home, while others will have a very low threshold for doing so.

Some general guidelines on finding a suitable nursing home may be much appreciated by the patient's family. A family visit to the facility should be arranged, and such issues as cleanliness, physical layout, quality of the meals and the attitudes of staff members should all be carefully scrutinized. The family members should be encouraged to discuss the selection process with members of their support group. Many of the support group members may themselves be quite knowledgeable about individual nursing homes and the selection process in general. It may be helpful for the psychiatrist to contact the social services department of a local hospital to obtain some names of reputable local facilities. Unfortunately, nursing home care is expensive, and a patient's assets may be rapidly depleted in the process of providing adequate care for the patient.

Adult day care may provide the patient's family with welcome relief from the burden of providing fulltime care for the patient. Such programs provide care for the patient for several hours a day, one to five days a week. The programs are rather variable with respect to their therapeutic orientations. Some are medically based, while others may be coordinated in conjunction with churches or other community organizations. Fees vary widely and may be prohibitive (Read, 1990).

Legal Issues

The consulting psychiatrist can often provide valuable information of a legal nature to the families of demented patients. At times, the demented patient may refuse essential medical treatment because of impaired judgement and insight. In such cases, the psychiatrist may be asked to render an opinion regarding the patient's competency to make medical decisions. Often, in such cases, a competency hearing must be arranged in order for a judge to declare the patient not to be competent to make such decisions.

In other instances, the psychiatrist may be consulted to assist in the protection of a demented patient's estate or to assist in the nursing home placement of an unwilling patient unable to function outside the setting of a nursing home. In such cases, the psychiatric consultant may be asked to initiate conservatorship proceedings. The details of these proceedings and the responsibilities of the conservator may vary somewhat from state to state. Suffice it to say, however, that the appointed conservator is usually given the authority to manage the patient's finances or to make medical decisions for the patient(or to do both) (Sandoe, 1988). As such, the patient's assets can be protected and adequate placement facilitated.

Some states mandate that newly diagnosed demented patients be reported to the local county health department. This is more than a meaningless bit of paperwork, since many demented patients continue to drive despite their physicians' warnings against this. The local health department should ensure that the Department of Motor Vehicles is notified of the patient's condition, so that the patient's license may be revoked. Lives may be saved by the clinician's compliance with such a mandate.

PHARMACOLOGIC INTERVENTIONS

Despite the efforts of a supportive family or a diligent nursing staff, many demented patients require some sort of psychopharmacologic treatment. A considerable number of demented patients are referred to the psychiatrist for pharmacologic management of behavior problems; however, depression is also quite common in some dementing disorders, and the potential benefits of antidepressant therapy should not be overlooked. A number of other drugs have been used, at least experimentally, to attempt to treat the cognitive impairment itself, rather than the behavioral manifestations assoicated with it.

Antidepressant Therapy

There is little magic in the application of antidepressant therapy to demented patients, but there *is* considerable controversy. For instance, some clinicians feel that tricyclic antidepressants (TCA's) are relatively contraindicated in elderly demented patients, particularly because of their tendency to worsen confusion; as such, it is felt by such clinicians that selective serotonin reuptake inhibitors (SSRI's), such as fluoxetine, are the first line drugs of choice in the demented. Other clinicians feel that the tricycic antidepressants are preferable to the SSRI's. Still others feel that trazodone is a reasonable first line antidepressant, particularly in agitated patients.

The psychiatric consultant should keep some general principles in mind when prescribing tricyclic antidepressants to demented patients. It is probably wise to avoid the tertiary amines, such as doxepin, imipramine and amitryptiline, because of their potential for causing confusion, sedation and orthostatic hypotension. These agents also tend to have greater cardiotoxicity as well; this is particularly problematic in the elderly demented population, since many of these patients have coexisting cardiac problems. In addition, orthostatic hypotension can be potentially deadly in elderly demented patients. For many such patients, an episode of orthostatic hypotension may result in the patient taking a fall. This fall may result in a hip fracture, which in turn may result in hospitalization, nosocomial infections and pulmonary emboli. When prescribing TCA's (and probably trazodone) for the elderly demented population, the psychiatric consultant should order an EKG prior to the initiation of the drug, to rule out the presence of conduction abnormalities or arrhythmias. As with most psychotropics, elderly demented patients should be started on lower dosages of TCA's, and dosage increases should be smaller and less frequent than those for younger patients.

The SSRI's are not without side effects, however, and should also be prescribed with care in the elderly demented population. The SSRI's can cause impaired hepatic metabolism of a number of commonly used medications, and as such, they can cause potentially toxic blood levels of these medications. In addition, in an elderly debilitated patient with compromised nutritional status, the nausea and anorexia sometimes induced by these agents may be problematic. The insomnia sometimes induced by these agents can potentially be problematic in patients who wander during the night.

Other agents are also available for the treatment of the depressed demented patient and also should be prescribed carefully in this population. Bupropion has virtually no anticholinergic or cardiotoxic effects; however, it can sometimes increase anxiety and impair sleep. More importantly, it has been noted to induce seizures in some patients, and because of this, it should not be prescribed in dosages exceeding 450 mg per day, and no single dose should exceed 150 mg. Indeed, it should probably be prescribed in much lower dosages in the elderly demented population, and it is best avoided entirely in patients with seizure disorders.

Trazodone is sometimes used in the treatment of depressed demented patients, especially if agitation and insomnia complicate the picture. Trazodone has little anticholinergic potential, but it can sometimes cause orthostatic hypotension and, on rare occasion, can be arrhythmogenic, particularly in patients with underlying cardiac disease. Trazodone should be prescribed with caution in males since it has been known (rarely) to induce priapism, sometimes resulting in impotence.

The monoamine oxidase inhibitors are occasionally used in the treatment of the depressed demented patient. Patients using these agents should follow a rather rigid diet in order to avoid tyramine-rich foods and must not use *any* medication without first consulting the psychiatrist. Tyramine-rich foods and many medications may precipitate hypertensive crises, which occasionally are fatal. Such a regimented lifestyle may be almost impossible to implement for many demented patients. One further problem with monoamine oxidase inhibitors is their potential for inducing orthostatic hypotension. As such, monoamine oxidase inhibitors are probably best avoided by most demented patients.

Pharmacologic Treatment of Cognitive Impairment

The development of agents to ameliorate the cognitive impairment of demented patients, especially those with Alzheimer's disease, has been an active area of research for several years. Admittedly, even the most optimistic studies are relative disappointing, and it is clear that this area of pharmacologic therapy is still in its infancy. Nonetheless, some interesting research findings have been made in recent years.

Many agents have been considered in treating demented patients. An ergoloid mesylate preparation (Hydergine [R]) has been among the most widely clinically used of these agents. Its efficacy has been questioned, however, and many consider it to be nothing more than a placebo. Nonetheless, there is considerable evidence in the literature that indicates a modest degree of efficacy, which may result from metabolic enhancement in the CNS (Hollister and Yesavage, 1984).

A number of other agents have also been considered. Vasopressin has been considered because of its apparent role in memory function, but appears to be of little value. Phosphatidylserine, which is felt to alter the functional state of the neuronal cell membrane, may be of some benefit. The so-called *nootropic* drug piracetam has long been considered in the treatment of dementia. The mechanism of action of piracetam and other nootropic agents is unclear, and it appears that they may not be particularly effective either (Gottfries, 1992).

Drugs which enhance cholinergic neurotransmission are among the most extensively studied in the pharmacologic treatment of cognitive dysfunction. Numerous studies have looked at such agents as choline, lecithin and physostigmine, with rather disappointing results overall. More recently, tetrahydroaminoacridine (tacrine) has been considered in the treatment of Alzheimer's disease, with somewhat more encouraging results (Volger, 1991).

A recent double-blind placebo-controlled study illustrates this point. In this study, an enrichment population design was used, in which patients who responded to tacrine in the initial phase of the study would be selected out for further study of their response to tacrine. Initially, it was noted that 215 of the original 632 patients in the study showed some response to tacrine. After this enrichment phase, it was noted that the patients who remained on tacrine did not show the same decline in cognitive function as those switched back to placebo (Davis, Thal, Gamzu, 1992).

Another recent study also suggests tacrine's efficacy and also illustrates some of its side effects. In this double-blind placebo-controlled parallel group study, 468 patients were given various dosages of tacrine, ranging from twenty mg per day to eighty mg per day, or were given placebo. Those patients taking eighty mg per day were noted to have a fifty-one percent response rate. Toxic effects were, however, fairly common in the patients taking tacrine. Alanine aminotransferase levels greater than three times normal were seen in twenty-five percent of patients, for example. In addition, other side effects included vomiting (eight percent), diarrhea (five percent), abdominal pain (four percent), dyspepsia (three percent), and rash (three percent). As such, the investigators suggested monitoring alanine aminotransferase levels weekly early in treatment, and at regular intervals thereafter. Fortunately, the hepatotoxicity seen was reversible with discontinuation of the drug (Farlow, Gracon, Hershey, 1992).

A few comments should be made concerning the mechanism of action of tacrine. As it turns out, its effect on the cholinergic system may actually be multifaceted in nature. It is not only a moderately long-acting cholinesterase inhibitor, but also may act as a partial agonist at muscarinic receptor sites, and may indirectly result in enhanced acetylcholine release into the synaptic cleft (Adem, 1992).

Finally, it should be noted that tacrine is almost certainly not a "wonder drug." Some clinicians question its future clinical value, and some studies do not support its efficacy (Volger, 1991). Nonetheless, the psychiatric consultant should be aware of tacrine, as psychiatrists may be called upon to prescribe it in the future. Indeed, it is one of the few agents that will be in future clinical use in the treatment of the cognitive impairment of Alzheimer's disease.

Treatment of the Agitated Demented Patient

Many different psychotropic drugs have been prescribed for the treatment of behaviorally disturbed demented patients. There has been considerable investigation into the use of these agents. The actual efficacy of many such drugs is not entirely clear; however, they can often be of considerable value and can sometimes keep a patient out of a nursing home or psychiatric unit. In addition, they can also help to prevent the use of prolonged physical restraint in the inpatient setting.

Antipsychotic agents are widely used for this purpose. Indeed, they are probably the first line agents of choice for most patients. They have a unique advantage over other agents in that they can treat not only agitation but also psychosis. A rather elegant meta-analytic review of the existing literature was provided by Schneider and associates (1990). This study revealed that neuroleptics are more effective than placebo but are nonetheless ineffective in a large percentage of patients. This study also indicated that no single neuroleptic had greater efficacy than any other.

Clinical wisdom, however, suggests that haloperidol may be the best choice for most patients, because of its side effect profile. Haloperidol has a relatively low potential for causing orthostatic hypotension, a relatively low anticholinergic effect and negligible cardiotoxicity. Unfortunately, however, it is one of the worst offenders with respect to extrapyramidal side effects. A reasonable starting dose for the elderly demented patient is 0.5mg BID, with gradual titration upwards as needed for control of symptoms. The dose necessary for control of behavior varies considerably from patient to patient. Some elderly patients respond to very low doses, while young patients may require fifteen mg per day or more. In elderly patients, it is best to avoid a daily dose greater than approximately seven to eight mg.

Carbamazepine is another agent used in the treatment of agitated patients. Carbamazepine, an anticonvulsant, has an advantage over neuroleptics in that it does not cause extrapyramidal symptoms; it can, however, cause sedation, ataxia, hepatotoxicity, and in rare instances, agranulocytosis or aplastic anemia. For this reason, a baseline CBC and liver function tests should be performed on all patients starting on carbamazepine and should be repeated at regular intervals following its initiation. The starting dose of carbamazepine may vary with the patient's age; elderly patients should probably be started on fifty to one hundred mg BID, while younger patients may be started on 200mg BID. Blood levels should be followed closely, with the target range being approximately eight to twelve micrograms per milliliter.

Propranolol, a nonselective beta blocker, is another fairly popular agent. Indeed, some proponents feel that it is highly effective but also point out that it often takes up to four to six weeks to have its full effect (Yudofsky, Silver, Hales, 1990). Yudofsky and associates recommend rather high doses, with a target range of two hundred to eight hundred mg per day, in divided doses. Side effects noted include hypotension, confusion, depression, bradycardia and impotence. Patients should ideally have a screening EKG, and patients with a history of COPD, asthma, insulin-dependent diabetes mellitus, hyperthyroidism, congestive heart failure or peripheral vascular disease should not receive propranolol. The clinician should keep in mind also that propranolol can increase the plasma levels of neuroleptics and anticonvulsants.

Trazodone also appears to be somewhat effective in the treatment of the agitated demented patient. Trazodone can be started at a dose of fifty mg per day in elderly patients and fifty mg BID in younger demented patients, with a target dose of two hundred to four hundred mg per day (Salzman, 1987). Trazodone generally has a fairly mild side effect profile, with gastrointestinal upset and sedation being the most common side effects. Nonetheless, orthostatic hypotension is not uncommon, and arrhythmias can also be seen, as can priapism.

Buspirone, a non-benzodiazepine anxiolytic, is becoming increasingly popular in the treatment of agitated demented patients. Its primary advantage over the other agents discussed is its relatively benign side effect profile. It also often exhibits a four to six week latency of onset of its therapeutic effect (Yudofsky, Silver, Hales, 1990). In elderly patients, it should be initiated at a dosage of five mg BID or TID, with an ultimate target dosage of approximately thirty mg per day, although some patients may require up to sixty mg per day. The side effects of buspirone include dizziness, nausea, headaches and paradoxical anxiety.

A host of other drugs have been used in the treatment of agitated demented patients. These include valproic acid, fluoxetine, L-deprenyl, lithium and various benzodiazepines. An extensive discussion of these agents and their efficacies is beyond the scope of this chapter.

CONCLUSION

Precious few demented patients can be cured of their dementing conditions, and many patients have a relentlessly progressive course. It is quite appropriate for the psychiatric consultant to feel frustrated when working with such patients. It is not appropriate, however, for the psychiatrist to feel helpless. Indeed, the psychiatric consultant, being both an empathic listener and a medical scientist, is uniquely suited to dealing with these patients and their families. The psychiatrist can make helpful interventions as as educator, as a therapist and as a clinical pharmacologist. In addition, it is clear that the biological understanding of the dementing disorders is constantly expanding. New diagnostic procedures are certainly on the horizon, and it is not inconceivable that highly effective treatments for many dementing disorders will someday be available.

REFERENCES

Adams RA and Victor M: Principles of Neurology. McGraw - Hill, New York, 1991

Adem A: Putative mechanisms of action of tacrine in Alzheimer's disease. Acta Neurologica Scandinavica 139 (Suppl.): 69 - 74, 1992

Adolfsson R, Gottfries CG, Roos BE, et al: Changes in the brain catecholamines in patients with dementia of the Alzheimer Type. British Journal of Psychiatry 135: 216 - 223, 1979

Alafuzoff I: The pathology of dementias: an overview. Acta Neurologica Scandinavica Suppl. 139: 8 - 15, 1992

American Psychiatric Association: Diagnostic and Statistical Manual of Mental Disorders, Third Edition, Revised. American Psychiatric Association, Washington, D.C., 1987

Arnold SE, Hyman BT, Flory J, et al: The topographical and neuroanatomical distribution of neurofibrillary tangles and neuritic plaques in the cerebral cortex of Alzheimer's disease. Cerebral Cortex 1: 103 - 116, 1991

Bachman DL, Wolf PA, Linn RT, et al: Incidence of dementia and probable Alzheimer's disease in a general population: the Framingham study. Neurology 43: 515 - 519, 1993

Baker C, McFarland KF: Endocrinology in Rakel RE (ed.): Textbook of Family Practice, 4th Ed. WB Saunders Company, Philadelphia, 1990, 1149 - 1202

Bannister R: Brain and Bannister's Clinical Neurology, 7th Ed. Oxford Medical Publications, New York, 1992

Beckwith BE, Till RE, Scheider W: Vasopressin analogue (DDAVP) improves memory in human males. Peptides 5: 819 - 822, 1984

Biggins CA, Boyd JL, Harrop FM, et al: A controlled longitudinal study of dementia in Parkinson's disease. Journal of Neurology, Neurosurgery, and Psychiatry 55: 566 -571, 1992

Birkett D: The psychiatric differentiation of senility and arteriosclerosis. British Journal of Psychiatry 120: 321 - 325, 1972

Bleathman C and Morton I: Validation therapy: extracts from 20 groups with dementia sufferers. Journal of Advanced Nursing 17: 658 - 666, 1992

Blessed G, Tomlinson BE, Roth M: The association between quantitative measures of dementia and of senile change in the cerebral grey matter of elderly subjects. British Journal of Psychiatry 114: 797 -811, 1968

Bornstein RA, Nasrallah HA, Para MF, et al: Neuropsychological performance in asymptomatic HIV infection. The Journal of Neuropsychiatry and Clinical Neurosciences 4: 386 - 394, 1992

Breitner JC: Clinical genetics and genetic counseling in Alzheimer disease. Annals of Internal Medicine 115: 601 - 606, 1991

Burger PC, Vogel FS: The development of the pathologic changes of Alzheimer's disease and senile dementia in patients with Down's syndrome. American Journal of Pathology 73: 457 - 476, 1973

Burns A: Psychiatric phenomena in dementia of the Alzheimer's type. International Psychogeriatrics 4 (Suppl. 1): 43 - 54, 1992

Cadieux RJ: Early differentiation of senile dementias. Hospital Practice 24: 77 - 94, 1989

Candy JM, Klinowski, Perry RH: Aluminosilicates and senile plaque formation in Alzheimer's disease. The Lancet 1: 354 - 357, 1986

Cash R, Dennis R, L'Heureux R, et al: Parkinson's disease and dementia: norepinephrine and dopamine in locus ceruleus.
Neurology 37: 42 - 46, 1987

Choi SC, Muizelaar JP, Barnes TY, et al: Prediction tree for severely head-injured patients. Journal of Neurosurgery 75: 251 - 255, 1991

Clarfield AM: The reversible dementias: do they reverse?
Annals of Internal Medicine 109: 476 - 486, 1988

Constantinidis J, Richard J, Tissot R: Pick's disease: histological and clinical correlations.
European Neurology 11: 208 - 217, 1974

Corder EH, Saunders AM, Strittmatter WJ, et al: Gene dose of apolipoprotein E type 4 allele and the risk of Alzheimer's disease in late onset families.
Science 261: 921 - 923, 1993

Cools AR, Van Den Bercken JH, Horstink MW, et al: Cognitive and motor shifting aptitude disorder in Parkinson's disease.
Journal of Neurology, Neurosurgery, and Psychiatry 47: 443 - 453, 1984

Cornford ME, Holden JK, Boyd MC, et al: Neuropathology of the acquired immune deficiency syndrome (AIDS): report of 39 autopsies from Vancouver, British Columbia.

The Canadian Journal of Neurological Sciences 19: 442 - 452, 1992

Coyle PK and Dattwyler R : Spirochetal infection of the central nervous system. Infectious Disease Clinics of North America 4: 731 - 746, 1990

Cummings JL, Benson DF: Subcortical dementia: review of an emerging concept. Archives of Neurology 41: 874 - 879, 1984

Cummings JL and Benson DF: Dementia: A Clinical Approach, 2nd Ed.
Butterworth - Heinemann, Boston, 1992

Cummings JL and Duchen LW: Kluver-Bucy syndrome in Pick disease: clinical and pathologic correlations.
Neurology 31: 1415 - 1422, 1981

Davis KL, Thal LJ, Gamzu ER, et al: A double-blind, placebo-controlled multicenter study of tacrine for Alzheimer's disease.
The New England Journal of Medicine 327: 1253 - 1259, 1992

Davies P and Maloney AJ: Selective loss of central cholinergic neurons in Alzheimer's disease.
The Lancet 2: 1403, 1976

Department of Health and Human Services: Interagency head injury task force report.
U.S. Government Printing Office, Washington, D.C., 1989

Devanand DP, Sackeim HA, Mayeux R: Psychosis, behavioral disturbance, and the use of neuroleptics in dementia.
Comprehensive Psychiatry 29: 387 - 401, 1988

Devous MD: Imaging brain function by single-photon emission computer tomography in Andreasen NC (ed.): Brain Imaging: Applications in Psychiatry. American Psychiatric Press, Inc., Washington, D.C., 1989, 147 - 234

Dewan MJ and Gupta S: Toward a definitive diagnosis of Alzheimer's disease. Comprehensive Psychiatry 33: 282 - 290, 1992

Duguid JR, De La Paz R, DeGroot J: Magnetic resonance imaging of the midbrain in Parkinson's disease.
Annals of Neurology 20: 744 - 747, 1986

Etcheberrigaray R, Ito E, Oka K, et al: Potassium channel dysfunction in fibroblasts identifies patients with Alzheimer's disease.
Proceedings of the National Academy of Sciences 90: 8209 - 8213, 1993

Farlow M, Gracon SI, Hershey LA, et al: A controlled trial of tacrine in Alzheimer's disease.
JAMA 268: 2523 - 2529, 1992

Folstein SE: Huntington's Disease: A Disorder of Families.
The Johns Hopkins University Press, Baltimore, 1989

Folstein MF, Folstein SE, McHugh PR: "Mini-mental state": a practical method for grading the cognitive state of patients for the clinician.
Journal of Psychiatric Research 12: 189 - 198, 1975

Forette F and Boller F: Hypertension and the risk of dementia in the elderly.
The American Journal of Medicine 90 (Suppl. 3A): 3A-14S - 3A-19S, 1991

Fowler CJ, O'Neill C, Winblad B, et al: Neurotransmitter, receptor and signal transduction disturbances in Alzheimer's disease.
Acta Neurologica Scandinavica Suppl. 139: 59 - 62, 1992

Franceschi M, Comola M, Piattoni, et al: Prevalence of dementia in adult patients with trisomy 21.
American Journal of Medical Genetics 7: 306 -308, 1990

Geaney DP and Abou-Saleh MT: The use and applications of single-photon emission computerised tomography in dementia.
British Journal of Psychiatry 157 (Suppl. 9): 66 - 75, 1990

Goedert M, Crowther RA, Garner CC: Molecular characteristics of microtubule-associated proteins Tau and MAP2.
Trends in Neuroscience 14: 193 -199, 1991

Gorelick PB and Mangone CA: Vascular dementias in the elderly.
Clinics in Geratric Medicine 7: 599 - 614, 1991

Gottfries CG: Review of treatment strategies.
Acta Neurologica Scandinavica Suppl. 139: 63 - 68, 1992

Gustafson R: Operant conditioning of activities of daily living on a psychogeritric ward: a simple method.
Psychological Reports 70: 603 - 607, 1992

Hachinski VC, Iliff LD, Zilhka E, et al: Cerebral blood flow in dementia.
Archives of Neurology 32: 632 - 637, 1975

Hachinski VC: Preventable senility: a call for action against the vascular dementias.
The Lancet 340: 645 - 648, 1992

Haggerty JJ, Evans DL, Prange AJ: Organic brain syndrome associated with marginal hypothyroidism.
American Journal of Psychiatry 143: 785 -786, 1986

Hakim AM and Mathieson G: Dementia in Parkinson disease: a neuropathologic study.
Neurology 29: 1209 - 1214, 1979

Harper PS, Morris M, Tyler A: Predictive tests in Huntington's disease in Harper PS (ed.): Huntington's Disease. WB Saunders Company, Philadelphia, 1991, 373 - 413

Harrell LE: Alzheimer's disease.
Southern Medical Journal 84 (Suppl. 1): 1S-32 - 1S-40, 19

Hiatt LG: Design of the home environment for the cognitively impaired person in Mace NL (ed.): Dementia Care - Patient, Family and Community.
The Johns Hopkins University Press, Baltimore, 1990, 231 - 242

Ho DD (moderator), Bredesen DE, Vinters HV, Daar ES (discussants): The acquired immunodeficiency syndrome (AIDS) dementia complex (UCLA Conference).
Annals of Internal Medicine 11: 400 - 410, 1989

Hollister LE and Yesavage J: Ergoloid mesylates for senile dementia: unanswered questions.
Annals of Internal Medicine 100: 894 - 898, 1984

Hooshmand H, Escobar MR, Kopf SW: Neurosyphilis: a study of 241 patients.
JAMA 219: 726 - 729, 1972

Huber SJ, Shuttleworth EC, Paulson GW, et al: cortical vs. subcortical dementia - neuropsychological differences.
Archives of Neurology 43: 392 - 394, 1986

Hyman BT and Tanzi RE: Amyloid, dementia and Alzheimer's disease.
Current Opinion in Neurology and Neurosurgery 5: 88 - 93, 1992

Ineichen B. Measuring the rising tide. How many dementia cases will there be by 2001?
British Journal of Psychiatry 150: 193 - 200, 1987

Kang J, Lemaire HG, Unterbeck A, et al: The precursor of Alzheimer's disease amyloid A4 resembles a cell surface receptor.
Nature 325: 733-736, 1987

Kaplan HI, Sadock BJ: Synopsis of Psychiatry: Behavioral Sciences, Clinical Psychiatry, 6th Ed. Williams and Wilkins, New York, 1991

Kase CS: "Multi-infarct" dementia - a real entity?. Journal of The American Geriatrics Society 34: 482 - 484, 1986

Kaufman DM: Clinical Neurology for Psychiatrists, 3rd Ed. W.B. Saunders Company, Philadelphia, 1990

Kowall NW and McKee AC: The histopathology of neuronal degeneration and plasticity in Alzheimer disease in Seil FJ (ed.): Advances in Neurology, Vol. 59. Raven Press Limited, New York, 1993, 5 - 33

Kiernan RJ, Mueller J, Langston JW, et al: The Neurobehavioral cognitive status examination: a brief but differentiated approach to cognitive assessment. Annals of Internal Medicine 107: 481 - 485, 1987

LaCour FA: Huntington's disease. Alabama Medicine, The Journal of MASA 16: 20 - 25, 1992

Landsberg JP, McDonald B, Watt F: Absence of aluminum in neuritic plaque cores in Alzheimer's disease (letter). Nature 360: 65 - 68, 1992

Larson EW: Alcoholism: the disease and the diagnosis. The American Journal of Medicine 91: 107 - 109, 1991

Leibovici A, Tariot PN: Agitation associated with dementia: A systematic approach to treatment. Psychopharmacology Bulletin 24: 49 - 53, 1988

Lee VM, Balin BJ, Otvos L, et al: A68: A major subunit of paired helical filaments and derivatized forms of normal Tau. Science 251: 675 - 678, 1991

Leuchter A and Spar J: The late onset psychoses: Clinical and diagnostic features. Journal of nervous and mental disease 173: 488 - 499, 1985

Lishman WA: Cerebral disorder in alcoholism. Brain 104: 1 - 20 , 1981

Lovestone S and Anderton B: Cytoskeletal abnormalities in Alzheimer's disease. Current Opinion in Neurology and Neurosurgery 5: 883 - 888, 1992

Lowenthal DT and Nadeau SE: Drug-induced dementia. Southern Medical Journal 84 (Suppl. 1): 1S-24 - 1S-31, 1991

Mazurek MF, Beal MF, Bird ED, et al: Vasopressin in Alzheimer's disease: a study of postmortem brain concentrations. Annals of Neurology 20: 665 - 670, 1986

McArthur JC: Neurologic complications of human immunodeficiency virus infection in Gorbach SL, Bartlett JG, Blacklow NR (eds.): Infectious Diseases. WB Saunders Company, Philadelphia, 1992, 956 - 971

Meyer JS, Kitagawa Y, Tanahashi N, et al: Evaluation of treatment of normal-pressure hydrocephalus.
Journal of Neurosurgery 62: 513 - 521, 1985

Mayeux R, Stern Y, Spanton S: Heterogeneity in dementia of the Alzheimer type: evidence of subgroups.
Neurology 35: 453 - 461, 1985

McDermott JR, Smith AI, Iqbal K, et al: Aluminum and Alzheimer's disease.
The Lancet 2: 710 - 711, 1977

Mayeux R, Stern Y, Rosen J, et al: Is "subcortical dementia" a recognizable clinical entity?.
Annals of Neurology 14: 278 - 283, 1983

Mckhann G, Drachman D, Folstein M, et al: Clinical diagnosis of Alzheimer's disease: Report of the NINCDS-ADRDA work group under the auspices of Department of Health and Human Services task force on Alzheimer's disease.
Neurology 34: 934 - 944, 1984

Meyer JS, Judd BW, Tawaklna T, et al: Improved cognition after control of risk factors for multi-infarct dementia.
JAMA 256: 2203 -2209, 1986

Mohs RC, Breitner JC, Silverman JM, et al: Alzheimer's disease - morbid risk among first-degree relatives approximates 50% by 90 years of age.
Archives of General Psychiatry 44: 405 - 408, 1987

Murphy M: The molecular pathogenesis of Alzheimer's disease: Clinical prospects.
The Lancet 340: 1512 - 1515, 1992

Musher DM: Syphilis in Gorbach SL, Bartlett JG, Blacklow NR (eds.): Infectious Diseases. WB Saunders Company, Philadelphia, 1992, 822 - 827

Namba Y, Tomonaga M, Kawasaki H, et al: Apolipoprotein E immunoreactivity in cerebral amyloid deposits and neurofibrillary tangles in Alzheimer's disease and kuru plaque amyloid in Creutzfeldt-Jakob disease.
Brain Research 541: 163 - 166, 1991

Navia BA, Jordan BD, Price RW: The AIDS dementia complex: I. clinical features. Annals of Neurology 19: 517 - 524, 1986

Navia BA and Price RW: The acquired immunodeficiency syndrome dementia complex as the presenting or sole manifestation of human immunodefiency virus infection. Archives of Neurology 44: 65 - 69, 1987

Nordberg A: Biological markers and the cholinergic hypothesis in Alzheimer's disease. Acta Neurologica Scandinavica Suppl. 139: 54 - 58, 1992

Perry G, Kawai M, Tabaton M, et al: Neuropil threads of Alzheimer's disease show a marked alternation of the normal cytoskeleton.
Journal of Neuroscience 11: 1748 - 1755, 1991

Pflanz S, Besson JA, Ebmeier FP: The clinical manifestation of mental disorder in Huntington's disease: a retrospective case record study of disease progression.
Acta Psychiatrica Scandinavica 83: 53 - 60, 1990

Powell-Proctor L and Miller E: Reality orientation: a critical appraisal.
British Journal of Psychiatry 140: 457 - 463, 1982

Quarrell O: The neurobiology of Huntington's disease in Harper PS (ed.): Huntington's Disease. WB Saunders Company, Philadelphia, 1991, 141-178

Ramsey RG: Neuroradiology, 2nd Ed. W.B. Saunders Company, Philadelphia, 1987

Raskin MA: Organic mental disorders in Busse EW and Blazer DG (eds.): Geriatric Psychiatry. American Psychiatric Press, Inc., Washington, D.C., 1989, 313 - 368

Read S: Community resources in Cummings JL and Miller B (eds.): Alzheimer's Disease - Treatment and Long-term Management. Marcel Dekker, Inc., New York, 1990, 235 - 244

Rossor M: Alzheimer's disease. Postgraduate Medical Journal 68: 528 - 532, 1992
Rheaume YL, Lasch KE (eds.): Clinical Management of Alzheimer's Disease. Aspen Publishers, Inc., Rockville, 1988, 53 - 73

Regland B and Gottfries C: The role of amyloid beta-protein in Alzheimer's disease. The Lancet 340: 467 - 469, 1992

Reifler BV: Arguments for abandoning the term pseudodementia.
Journal of the American Geriatrics Society 30: 665 -668, 1982

Reynolds CF, Hoch CC, Kupfer DJ, et al: Bedside differentiation of depressive pseudodementia from dementia.
American Journal of Psychiatry 145: 1099 - 1103, 1988

Ritchie K and Touchon J: Heterogeneity in senile dementia of the Alzheimer type: individual differences, progressive deterioration or clinical sub-types.
Journal of Clinical Epidemiology 45: 1391 - 1398, 1992

Roberts GW, Crow TJ, Polak JM: Location of neuronal tangles in somatostatin neurones in Alzheimer's disease (letter).
Nature 314: 92 -94, 1985

Salzman C: Treatment of the elderly agitated patient. Journal of Clinical Psychiatry 48 (5, Suppl.): 19 - 22, 1987

Sandoe A: Legal considerations in Alzheimer's disease in Volicer L, Fabiszewski KJ,

Saunders AM, Strittmatter WJ, Schmechel MD, et al: Association of apolipoprotein E allele $\epsilon 4$ with late - onset familial and sporadic Alzheimer's disese.
Neurology 43: 1467 - 1472, 1993

Schmitt FA, Bigley JW, McKinnis R, et al: Neuropsychological outcome of zidovudine (AZT) treatment of patients with AIDS and AIDS-related complex.
New England Journal of Medicine 319: 1573, 1988

Schneider LS, Pollock VE, Lyness SA: A metaanalysis of controlled trials of neuroleptic treatment in dementia.
Journal of the American Geriatrics Society 38: 553 - 563, 1990

Seltzer B and Sherwin I: A comparison of clinical features in early and late-onset primary degenerative dementia - one entity or two?
Archives of Neurology 40: 143 - 146, 1983

Silver JM, Hales RE, Yudofsky SC: Neuropsychiatric aspects of traumatic brain injury in Yudofsky SC and Hales RE (eds.): Textbook of Neuropsychiatry. American Psychiatric Press, Washington, D.C., 1992, 363 - 396

Steg RE: Determining the cause of dementia.
Nebraska Medical Journal 75: 59 - 63, 1990

St. George-Hyslop PH, Tanzi RE, Polinsky RJ, et al: The genetic defect causing familial Alzheimer's disease maps on chromosome 21.
Science 235: 885 - 889, 1987

Strub RL and Black FW: Neurobehavioral Disorders: A Clinical Approach. F.A. Davis Company, Philadelphia, 1989

Tamminga CA, Foster NL, Chase TN: Reduced brain somatostatin levels in Alzheimer's disease (letter).
The New England Journal of Medicine 313: 1294 - 1295, 1985

Tarter RE: Brain damage in chronic alcoholics: a review of the psychological evidence in Richter D (ed): Addiction and Brain Damage. University Park Press, Baltimore, 1980, 267 - 296

Tierney MC, Fisher RH, Lewis AJ, et al: The NINCDS-ADRDA criteria for the clinical diagnosis of probable Alzheimer's disease: a clinicopathologic study of 57 cases.
Neurology 38: 359 - 364, 1988

Tombaugh TN, McIntyre NJ: The Mini-mental state examination: a comprehensive review.
Journal of the American Geriatrrics Society 40: 922-935, 1992

Tomlinson BE, Irving D, Blessed G: Cell loss in the locus ceruleus in senile dementia of the Alzheimer type.
Journal of The Neurological Sciences 40: 419 - 428, 1981

Trapp GA, Miner GD, Zimmerman RL, et al: Aluminum levels in brain in Alzheimer's disease.
Biological Psychiatry 13: 709 - 718, 1978

Travis J: New pieces in the Alzheimer's disease puzzle.
Science 261: 828 - 829, 1993

Tune L, Carr S, Hoag E, et al: Anticholinergic effects of drugs commonly prescribed for the elderly: potential means for assessing risk of delirium.
American Journal of Psychiatry 149: 1393 - 1394, 1992

Victor M, Adams RD, Collins GH: The Wernicke-Korsakoff Syndrome and Related Neurologic Disorders Due to Alcoholism and Malnutrition, 2nd Ed. F.A. Davis Company, Philadelphia, 1989

Volger BW: Alternatives in the treatment of memory loss in patients with Alzheimer's disease.
Clinical Pharmacy 10: 447 - 456, 1991

Wells CE: Pseudodementia.
American Journal of Psychiatry 136: 895 - 900, 1979

Whitehouse PJ, Friedland RP, Strauss ME: Neuropsychiatric aspects of degenerative dementias associated with motor dysfunction in Yudofsky SC and Hales RE (eds.): Textbook of Neuropsychiatry. American Psychiatric Press, Washington, D.C., 1992, 585 - 604

Whitehouse PJ, Price DL, Struble RG, et al: Alzheimer's disease and senile dementia: loss of neurons in the basal forebrain.
Science 215: 1237 -1239, 1982

Webb RM, Leech RW, Brumback RA: Spongiform encephalopathies: the physician's responsiblity.
Southern Medical Journal 83: 141 - 145, 1990

Whybrow PC, Prange AJ, Treadway CR: Mental changes accompanying thyroid gland dysfunction: a reappraisal using objective psychological measurement.
Archives of General Psychiatry 20: 48 - 63, 1969

Wikkelsø C, Andersson H, Blomstrand C, et al: The clinical effect of lumbar puncture in normal pressure hydrocephalus.
Journal of Neurology, Neurosurgery, and Psychiatry 45: 64 - 69, 1982

Wisniewski HM, Sturman JA, Shek JW. Aluminum choride induced neurofibrillary changes in the developing rabbit: a chronic animal model.
Annals of Neurology 8: 479 - 490, 1980

Worley JM and Price RW: Management of neurologic complications of HIV-1 infection and AIDS in Sande MA and Volberding PA (eds.): The Medical Management of AIDS, 3rd Ed. WB Saunders Company, Philadelphia, 1992, 193 - 217

Wragg RE, Jeste DV: Neuroleptics and alternative treatments - management of behavioral symptoms and psychosis in Alzheimer's disease and related conditions.
Psychiatric Clinics of North America 11: 195 - 213, 1988

Yao H, Sadoshima S, Ibayashi S, et al.: Leukoaraiosis and dementia in hypertensive patients.
Stroke 23: 1673 - 1677, 1992

Yudofsky SC, Silver JM, Hales RE: Pharmacologic management of aggression in the elderly.
Journal of Clinical Psychiatry 51 (10, Suppl.): 22 - 28, 1990

PSYCHOTHERAPY SOLUTIONS IN THE MEDICAL SETTING

Stuart J. Eisendrath, M.D.

Associate Professor of Clinical Psychiatry
Director, Psychiatric Consultation-Liaison Program
University of California, San Francisco
Langley Porter Psychiatric Institute
401 Parnassus Avenue, Box F-0984
San Francisco, CA 94143-0984

ABSTRACT

Consultation-Liaison psychiatrists are often faced with helping their patients cope with difficult medical problems. Solution-oriented psychotherapeutic techniques provide brief interventions that consulting psychiatrists can effectively employ. These solutions provide "skeleton keys" that can be used in a broad patient population. These solutions include reframing, projection of the problem, role reversal, clarifying the meaning of the medical illness, and face-saving techniques. This paper examines these interventions and gives case examples of each.

INTRODUCTION

Consultation-Liaison (C-L) psychiatrists are often faced with helping their patients cope with difficult medical problems. In many instances the consultant is in an excellent position to provide psychotherapeutic interventions. Recent advances in understanding psychotherapeutic techniques offer C-L psychiatrists enhanced ways of helping their patients deal with their patients' psychological problems with brief and effective techniques. These techniques are based upon solution-oriented theories. These techniques provide solutions to problems patients frequently encounter in coping with their medical illness.

The basic concept of solution-oriented psychotherapy is that there are certain interventions that are like "skeleton keys" that work with a wide variety of patients (1). These solutions do not require an in-depth psychiatric assessment of the individual patient's psychological development. They do require a positive relationship between patient and consultant and the physician's empathic awareness of the patient's current view of his or her situation. Solution-oriented approaches differ from psychoanalytically-derived

Consultation-Liaison Psychiatry: 1990 and Beyond
Edited by H. Leigh, Plenum Press, New York, 1994

techniques which require the consultant to have an awareness of the patient's psychological development--in other words, a sense of where the patient has been (2)(3)(4). Solution-oriented approaches require a knowledge of where the patient is and where he or she wishes to go. In a literal geographic example, if an individual was currently located in Los Angeles and wished to go to San Francisco, the solution-oriented technique would only require that the consultant attempting to aid the individual know the way to San Francisco and not where the patient had been before arriving in Los Angeles. Psychoanalytically-derived approaches might depend on understanding how the patient had come to arrive in Los Angeles.

This latter approach is often time consuming and many junior psychiatric residents performing C-L rotations, have not been trained in psychoanalytically-derived approaches. Solution-oriented approaches can be learned and applied quite readily and is ideal in the training setting. It can provide therapeutic tools for even the beginning consultant who wishes to provide emotional support for his/her patients. Several of these techniques will now be examined in detail.

Reframing

Many clinicians are already familiar with some aspects of reframing (5). For example, a consultant who explains that a noncompliant patient is suffering from an organic brain syndrome rather than a personality disorder, may help reframe the patient in the nursing staff's view. The staff may then feel less angry and better able to cope with the patient. Although diagnostic reframing can be extremely useful, this paper will be discussing reframing in the therapeutic sense. Watzlawick (6) had described therapeutic reframing as a "means to change the conceptual and/or emotional setting or viewpoint in relation to which a situation is experienced and to place it in another frame which fits the facts of the same concrete situation equally well or even better, and thereby change its entire meaning". Reframing techniques allows an individual to look at their situation from a previously unconsidered viewpoint. It is designed to alter the opinion a person has about a situation. As such it is particularly useful with a medical condition that is unlikely to be altered immediately. When the consultant utilizes reframing with the medically ill patient, he may first clarify how a patient sees his situation. The consultant may then utilize elements of suggestion and persuasion to present the patient with a different viewpoint of his situation.

Case Example. A fifty-one year old black male carpentry foreman was admitted to the Coronary Care Unit (CCU) for classical symptoms of a myocardial infarction. His clinical picture, electrocardiogram, and laboratory findings suggested a massive infarction. When this information was conveyed to him, he became less compliant with his medical care. In fact, he got out of his hospital bed and demonstrated that he could do just as many pushups as he could before entering the hospital. He even raised the idea of signing out of the hospital against medical advice. His attending physician requested a psychiatric consultation and the consultant spoke with the patient and his family. The consultant learned that the man took tremendous pride in his physical strength and was an amateur weightlifter. The consultant interpreted that the patient perceived the myocardial infarction and the necessary stay in the CCU as a threatened loss of his manhood. The consultant then reframed the situation for the patient by saying: "It takes a strong man to put up with what the cardiologists are asking of you." Coping with the passivity of bedrest were pictured as requiring a great deal of manhood. The patient accepted this view of his situation and complied with the remainder of treatment in the CCU.

Case Example. A thirty-two year old male with ulcerative colitis underwent a colectomy after ten years of medical treatment. Postoperatively the patient became depressed about having a permanent disfiguring ileostomy that had been required due to the extent of his disease. His surgeon requested a psychiatric consultation. In reviewing the patient's history with him, the psychiatrist noted that the patient had suffered fatigue, frequent hospitalizations, and the need to plan his day around the location of bathrooms. The psychiatrist suggested that the patient might see his situation as not just a loss of his bodily integrity, but rather as an improvement. His preoperative symptoms were all expected to resolve and he no longer had a significant risk of cancer. The alternative view of the ileostomy as an enhancement to the patient's health, rather than a major loss, helped the patient resolve his depression.

Because reframing may involve an element of persuasion, it can be considered a form of manipulation. Although manipulation has been considered pejoratively as a psychotherapeutic technique by some, this view is short-sighted (7). Manipulation, in the sense it is utilized for reframing, implies a goal of achieving what is in the patient's best interest. For example, reframing a frightening medical situation or procedure so that a patient can tolerate it more easily is clearly in the patient's best interest.

Projection of the Problem/Role Reversal

Many patients have difficulty viewing their situation with objectivity or as much compassion as they might allow others. Projection of the problem allows the individual to view their problem differently by encouraging them to project their problem onto someone else, either a friend or stranger; this often allows them to gain a more reasonable perspective. For some patients, asking them to project their situation onto a spouse, in essence imagining a role reversal, can be especially useful in clarifying their views. Viewing their problem in someone else may allow patients to see their situation more adaptively than they previously had.

Case Example. A sixty year old accountant had angina and underwent a coronary artery bypass graft. His cardiologist noted depression and requested a psychiatric consultation. The consultant found that the depression was primarily related to the fact that the patient believed he was "weak" in feeling fearful about his medical condition and surgery. He felt he should have been able to handle his distress in a more manly fashion. The consultant asked how the patient would feel about a friend of his expressing the level of distress that the patient had exhibited; in particular, the consultant asked whether the friend would have seemed less manly for having done so. The patient replied that he would have seen his friend's response as reasonable and perhaps even a sign of strength in being able to express his feelings so openly. The consultation concluded with the patient feeling more permissive towards his own feelings about his frightening medical experience.

Case Example. A forty-one year old woman was undergoing a bone marrow transplant for leukemia. During her chemotherapy she began to voice a desire to terminate her treatment. Her oncologist found that she was quite depressed and requested psychiatric consultation. The consultant learned that her depression was focused on her sense that she was a burden to her husband and children, despite the potential cure she might expect after her bone marrow transplant. The consultant asked her how she would feel about the situation if her husband was the one with leukemia--would she want him to undergo the treatment or would she feel it to be too much of a burden. She immediately replied that she would want him to undergo the treatment and she could see that he felt the same way about her. Her depression and desire to terminate her treatment resolved after this discussion.

Case Example. A thirty-five year old woman underwent a mastectomy for breast cancer. After her surgery she described feeling depressed to her surgeon who then obtained a psychiatric consultation. Upon exploration the consultant learned that the woman was concerned about how her husband would accept her physical condition. The consultant asked her how she would feel if her husband had an amputation of a limb. She replied that she would still love him. The consultant suggested that the husband might have a similar response to her surgery. The patient felt reassured but somewhat uncertain still about the husband's response. The consultant suggested that she ask her husband about his feelings. She did so. The husband told her that he considered her to be more than a breast and that he was happy to have her be alive. Her depression resolved.

Clarifying the Meaning of Illness

Clarifying the unique meaning to an individual of their disease often leads to decreased distress . Learning who else the patient knows who had the disease, where in the life trajectory the illness is affecting the person, or what fears the patient has about the illness are crucial to understanding the meaning (8). Knowing the meaning an illness has for an individual may allow the consultant to intervene directly. In some instances clarifying the patient's view allows the consultant to reframe the situation as described above. In other circumstances, clarifying the meaning allows the patient to feel they are genuinely understood by their consultant. In some instances clarifying the meaning allows the consultant to resolve the situation.

Case Example. An eighty year old male was admitted to the vascular surgery service for peripheral vascular disease leading to a below-the-knee amputation. Despite an excellent physical recovery postoperatively the patient appeared severely depressed and psychiatric consultation was obtained. In discussing the reason for the patient's mood, the consultant focused on the assumed concerns the patient had about his mobility with the amputation and the change in his body image. These discussions did not produce any lessening of the patient's depressive symptoms. Finally, the consultant asked the patient what was he most worried about in terms of dealing with the amputation. The patient replied that he was most concerned whether he would be able to fulfill his "conjugal duties". Once this issued was clarified, a conjoint meeting was held with the patient and his wife to openly discuss his concerns with the consultant. This meeting discussed the likelihood that the patient should continue to be able to fulfill his duties, particularly after the wife offered to try various sexual positions should the need arise. The patient responded to the meeting by becoming less depressed and more hopeful about his future.

Face-Saving Techniques

Individuals who have developed some forms of abnormal illness behavior--conversion reactions and factitious disorders--often become trapped in their symptoms (9). They have no way to relinquish their symptom without demonstrating that their symptom was psychogenic, and thereby proving detractors correct. Many of these patients have considerable trouble in viewing their problem from a psychological perspective and are averse to psychiatric treatment. Techniques that offer the patient a face-saving way to relinquish their symptom may be extremely useful especially after a confrontation for a conversion or factitious disorder has already proven ineffective or humiliating for a patient.

When these techniques are used in the context of maintaining a somatic approach to treatment, they allow patients to progress in a manner they are comfortable with. Face-saving approaches include modalities such as biofeedback, relaxation training, or self hypnosis. Some patients may protest that these techniques only work with patients with psychological problems. Patients need to be educated that these interventions can work with a variety of conditions, even those that are seemingly purely organic in origin such as hypnosis for cancer pain.

In order for these techniques to work, the consultant must feel comfortable in avoiding a confrontation with the patient. Some caregivers feel a sense of obligation to inform the patient that their problems are purely psychological in origin. This approach often accomplishes little except angering the patient and typically result in the patient searching for a new caregiver. A face-saving approach involves informing the patient that there is no major or irreversible illness, but the consultant nevertheless believes the suffering is quite real. The consultant can then suggest various techniques to help the patient gain control of their symptoms.

Case Example. A thirty year-old male was evaluated at an epilepsy center with simultaneous electroencephalogram telemetry/video observation for his four year history of medically refractory seizures. Some previous physicians had accused him of pseudoepileptic seizures since there were several psychological factors, as well as his atypical seizure symptoms, suggestive of this possibility and he had responded so poorly to conventional treatments. At times he had been offered psychiatric treatment, but had vehemently refused. His evaluation at the center confirmed the diagnosis of pseudoepileptic seizures. In view of his past resistance to psychiatric intervention, he was offered a face- saving way to control his symptom. He was told that there although there were no definite electrical abnormalities associated with his seizures, he could learn a technique that would help him gain control of his brain wave patterns. He was referred for EEG biofeedback so that he could learn to control and prevent his seizures. Over the course of a ten-week program, his seizure frequency was reduced from three per week to zero. Over this interval he spontaneously began to describe an association between psychological stressors and his seizures.

DISCUSSION

The solution-oriented approaches can work with a broad variety of patients. They require little background in depth psychology such as psychoanalytic concepts and thus are easily learned by beginning psychiatric residents. They can be applied quite readily with some practice. The techniques don't always work, however. For example, a Sikh Indian underwent an emergency colectomy and had an ileostomy. When depressed postoperatively, he clarified that he believed he would no longer be acceptable to his wife who was in Europe at the time. When asked if he would reject his wife if she had undergone similar surgery, he definitively stated he would reject her because of his religious beliefs related to handling of human waste. The patient's cultural context prevented the role reversal from being effective. Similarly, reframing doesn't always work and we cannot expect it to; for example, many losses must be grieved rather than reframed.

Nonetheless for many patients, these solution-oriented techniques can be extremely useful and applied quite readily. The consultant who masters these techniques will be in a better position to help patients cope with their medical problems. Indeed, in some instances, these techniques may help conserve resources, such as by shortening hospital stays or decreasing frequency of office visits (10)(11)(12).

All of the previously described techniques involve certain common elements. These techniques are built upon the consultant developing an empathic awareness of the patient's current situation. They do not require an extensive knowledge of the patient's prior psychological development. These techniques help patients to feel more in control at times when their disease may be making them feel helpless (13). The techniques work best when they are used in conjunction with other interventions that physicians commonly employ such as reassurance and clear communication with their patients. The techniques can convey a strong sense of support to the patient. They help provide the patient with a tool to use in their coping with their medical problem. They also provide a sense of hope and collaboration with their consultant in coping with their illness.

REFERENCES

1. De Shazer S: Keys to Solution in Brief Therapy. New York. W.W. Norton 1985.

2. O'Hanlon WH, Weiner-Davis M: In Search of Solutions: A New Direction in Psychotherapy.
New York. W.W. Norton, 1988.

3. Wahl CW: The Technique of Brief Psychotherapy with Hospitalized Psychosomatic Patients.
International Journal of Psychoanalytic Psychotherapy 1:69-82, 1972.

4. Blacher, RS: The Briefest Encounter: Psychotherapy for Medical and Surgical Patients. General Hospital Psychiatry: 6:226-232,1984.

5. Eisendrath SJ: Reframing Techniques in the General Hospital.
Family Systems Medicine. 4:91-95, 1986.

6. Watzlawick P: The Gentle Art of Reframing.
In P. Watzlawick, J. Weakland, and R. Fisch (Eds.) Change-Principles of Problem Formation and Problem Resolution. New York: Norton, 1974.

7. Briggins C, Zinberg N: Manipulation and Its Clinical Application.
American Journal of Psychotherapy. 23:198-206, 1969.

8. Viederman M, Perry S: Use of a Psychodynamic Life Narrative in the Treatment of Depression in the Physically Ill. General Hospital Psychiatry. 3:177-185, 1980.

9. Eisendrath SJ: Factitious Physical Disorder: Treatment without confrontation.
Psychosomatics 30:383-87, 1989.

10. Viney LL, Clarke AM, Bunn TA, Benjamin YN: The Effect of a Hospital-Based Counseling Service on the Physical Recovery of Surgical and Medical Patients.
General Hospital Psychiatry 7:294-301, 1985.

11. Fulop G, Strain JJ, Vita J, et al: Impact of Psychiatric Comorbidity on Length of Hospital Stay for Medical/Surgical Patients: A Preliminary Report. American Journal of Psychiatry. 144:878-882, 1987.

12. Levitan SJ, Kornfeld DS: Clinical and Cost Benefits of Liaison Psychiatry. American Journal of Psychiatry. 138:790-795, 1981.

13. Eisendrath SJ: Issues of Control in the General Hospital Surgical Setting. International Journal of Psychosomatics. 34:3-5, 1987.

PHYSICAL FACTORS AFFECTING PSYCHIATRIC CONDITION: A PROPOSAL FOR A FUTURE DSM

Hoyle Leigh, MD

Professor and Vice Chairman
Department of Psychiatry
University of California, San Francisco
Director, Fresno Division and Chief of Psychiatry
Fresno VA Medical Center

INTRODUCTION

The advent of DSM III and DSM III-R has improved psychiatric nomenclature considerably in terms of precision and clarity (1-2). The multiaxial system has been very useful in educating nonpsychaitrists that psychiatric conditions often co-exist with medical conditions, or are secondary to them as in organic mental disorders. Consultation-liaison psychiatrists often encounter situations, however, for which there is no appropriate diagnostic entity in DSM III-R. While the diagnosis of Adjustment Disorder might be appropriate for some of these conditions, DSM III-R specifically excludes from the adjustment disorder any condition that has a duration of more than six months. Furthermore, DSM III-R excludes from adjustment disorders syndromes that meet the diagnostic criteria of other major psychiatric disorders such as mood disorders and anxiety disorders.

I therefore propose that a new diagnostic entity be included in the DSM IV called "Physical Factors Affecting Psychiatric Condition", and, further, that the adjustment disorders include a new subcategory called "Chronic Adjustment Disorder". I propose that following the diagnosis of "Physical factors affecting psychiatric condition:" (fictious DSM IV code 999.xx:, the last digits could specify chronicity and degree of contribution). This diagnosis would end with a colon, after which the Axis I or II diagnosis is specified, and the physical condition should be specified following a hyphen (e.g. for moderate major depression precipitated and maintained by lung cancer would be: 999.23: 296.22-lung ca). For "Chronic adjustment disorder" (fictitious DSM IV code 888), I propose that the DSM III-R convention of specifying the type as an extension of the code, which is followed by a hyphen and the physical illness (e.g. chronic adjustment disorder with anxious mood precipitated and maintained by lung cancer would be: 999.21: 888.24-lung ca.) ICD 10 diagnostic code might be used following the hyphen in lieu of spelling out the physical illness as necessary.

Consultation-Liaison Psychiatry: 1990 and Beyond
Edited by H. Leigh, Plenum Press, New York, 1994

CASE EXAMPLES

Case I. A 46 year old married man with a nine year history of multiple sclerosis was referred to the psychiatrist for suspected depression. The patient became progressively depressed since losing his job three years ago because of increasing disability, which resulted in his being wheel-chair bound. Currently, the patient feels hopeless, worried, has low self-esteem, but has no neurovegetative symptoms of depression. The patient has become irritable of late, with angry outbursts from time to time. Since the loss of his job, he has been mostly staying at home, resulting in marital discord with his wife who also stays at home. He is not currently receiving any medications.

Discussion: In this case, the patient clearly shows some elements of depression without fulfilling the criteria for major depression. The presence of a psychosocial stressor (diagnosis of multiple sclerosis, physical disability) might argue for an adjustment disorder, but DSM III-R specifically excludes this diagnosis if the reaction has persisted for longer than six months. One might stretch the point a bit and argue that as the stressor (multiple sclerosis) is continuing, the patient might still be adjusting, but DSM III-R indicates that even when stressors are continuing, a new level of adjustment is expected within 6 months. While organic affective syndrome might be considered, the patient's symptoms are more likely a reaction to the consequences of the physical illness (disability, inability to work, etc.) rather than a direct effect of multiple sclerosis on the brain. Proposed diagnosis: Physical Factors Affecting Psychiatric Condition: Chronic Adjustment Disorder with depressive features- Multiple Sclerosis (999.23: 888.00-Multiple Sclerosis).

Case 2. A 35 year old single employed woman with ulcerative colitis of many years' duration was referred to the psychiatrist for suicidal ideation. The patient showed depressed mood, hopelessness, helplessness, low self-esteem, psychomotor retardation, anhedonia, sleep disturbance, and weight loss (which might have been related to ulcerative colitis as well). She felt despondent about her poorly controlled medical condition. She refused to undergo total colectomy. On careful questioning, it was established that she had developed symptoms of depression each time there was an exacerbation of her colitis. There was no family history of mood disorders.

Discussion: Her current symptomatology met all the diagnostic criteria for major depression. Of course, it could be argued that the depressive episode was initiated by the exacerbation of her ulcerative colitis, but, again, the depression was a psychological reaction to it rather than a direct effect of ulcerative colitis on the brain (although ensuing fatigue, electrolyte imbalance, etc., may have secondarily contributed to the depressive syndrome). While adjustment disorder may again be considered, DSM III-R clearly excludes from adjustment disorder syndromes that meet the diagnostic criteria for mood disorder. Thus, the precise diagnosis for this syndrome would be Depressive Episode that is an emotional reaction to an exacerbation of a physical condition (ulcerative colitis). A better diagnosis would be : Physical Factors Affecting Psychiatric Condition: Depressive Syndrome- Ulcerative Colitis (999.23: 296.33-Ulcerative Colitis). In using the term, "Depressive Syndrome", I am adopting the notion of a psychiatric syndrome as a final common pathway (3).

Case 3. A 57 year old married man was referred to the psychiatrist for suspected depression. The patient had suffered a myocardial infarction three years ago. Although he recovered from the MI, he continued to have rather severe angina pectoris, inadequately controlled by medications. Shortly after the MI, he sold his prosperous business, became a "hermit", spending most of his days watching videotapes. For three years, he related very little with his family and friends. On psychiatric examination, the patient was discouraged about his continuing angina that he felt would eventually kill him. Of note is that his father also had angina, and died at the age of 59 of an MI.

Discussion: While there were clearly depressive features, the patient's symptomatology did not meet the criteria for major depression. He was worried and generally upset, but the anxiety features did not warrant the diagnosis of a specific anxiety disorder. More striking was his personality change --- from an active, outgoing one to a recluse. I believe this is an example of "Physical Factors Affecting Psychiatric Condition: Chronic Adjustment Disorder with personality change and depressive symptoms- angina pectoris (999.23: 888.40-Angina Pectoris)".

Case 4. A 68 year old woman was referred to a psychiatrist for general anxiety and "panic attacks" following a fainting episode some eight months ago. The patient developed increasingly frequent syncopal episodes, which contributed to her fears of dropping dead, with increasing frequency of the panic episodes, resulting in her being confined at home with fear of being outside alone. The panic attacks occurred at least two or three times a week now, and included the associated symptoms of sweating, shortness of breath, numbness, fear of dying, trembling and shaking, and some dizziness. The panic attacks were not usually associated with the syncopal episodes. A careful medical workup revealed Stokes Adams syndrome.

Discussion: The patient's symptomatology met all the diagnostic criteria of panic disorder with agoraphobia. Nevertheless, the age of onset and the course of the anxiety disorder clearly indicate that the symptoms of Stokes Adams syndrome were instrumental in the patient's psychiatric symptomatology while the atrioventricular node dysfunction by itself was not the physiologic cause of the psychiatric symptoms. Adjustment disorder would not be an appropriate diagnosis as the criteria for another axis I diagnosis (Panic Disorder with Agoraphobia). Proposed diagnosis: Physical Factors Affecting Psychiatric Condition: Panic Disorder with agoraphobia - Stokes Adams syndrome (999.23: 300.21-Stokes Adams Syndrome).

Case 5. A 70 year old man on the surgical unit was referred to the psychiatrist for suspected depression. The patient was admitted to the hospital about two months ago with a hip fracture and underwent hip replacement surgery. His postoperative course was complicated with fever, anorexia, weight loss, and dysphagia. He had lost approximately thirty pounds during the hospitalization. The consultation was precipitated by the patient's refusal to swallow food. He was now afebrile and there was no apparent cause for the severe anorexia. The only way the patient was sustained at this point was by tube-feeding. On psychiatric examination, the patient stated that he had choked several times in the previous weeks as he attempted to swallow food. Part of the problem, as it turned out, was that his dentures no longer fit because of his weight loss, which made it painful for him to chew adequately. As he attempted to swallow the inadequately chewed food, he choked. After several attempts of this kind, the patient woke up several times at night in terror as he felt himself choking on his saliva. He had, in fact, developed a phobia of swallowing, including liquids and water. There was no evidence of depression.

Discussion: The patient fulfilled all the diagnostic criteria for a simple phobia, including intense anxiety when asked to swallow, avoidance of any situations requiring swallowing, necessitating tube-feeding and continuing to be hospitalized, and he recognized that his fear was excessive and unreasonable. In this case, the patient's phobia was directly related to his expriences of choking, that were, in turn, caused by weight loss that caused his dentures not to fit properly. Desensitization treatment and new dentures were curative of the patient's phobia in several months. The appropriate diagnosis for this patient would be: Physical Factors Affecting Psychiatric Condition: Simple Phobia of Swallowing-Mascatory difficulty due to ill fitting dentures (999.14: 300.29-Masticatory difficulty due to ill-fitting dentures)

DISCUSSION AND CONCLUSION

DSM III-R has a very useful diagnostic category --- Psychological Factors Affecting Physical Condition. DSM III-R is deficient in that it does not have a comparable nomenclature for physical factors affecting mental condition. I believe that the addition of the category "Physical Factors Affecting Psychiatric Condition" will not only provide a nice symmetry, but also emphasize the fact that physical conditions often affect the mental and emotional states of patients in ways different from Organic Mental Disorders, and in the full spectrum of psychiatric symptomatology from minor adjustment disorders to specific major psychiatric syndromes on Axis I or II.

Similarly, the category of adjustment disorders should be broadened to include chronic adjustment to chronic or recurring stressors. The category of adjustment disorder in DSM III-R is a time-limited and a subthreshold disorder. I believe that there is clearly a subset of adjustment disorders that are not time-limited. On the other hand, I believe that the subthreshold nature of adjustment disorders should be preserved in DSM IV, i.e., adjustment disorder should not be diagnosed if the disturbance meets the diagnostic criteria for a specific mental disorder such as anxiety or mood disorder. Once a disorder meets the diagnostic criteria for a specific syndrome, there is usually an autonomous course that must be treated with specific treatments, no matter what may contribute to the etiology. Thus, a depressive syndrome (major depression) is a final common pathway entity that call for careful evaluation and usually psychopharmacologic treatment, whether it is caused by an environmental stresssor such as bereavement, adjustment to recurrent physical illness, or severe genetic loading.

My proposal is conceptually similar to Fogel's (4) to indicate the psychiatric syndrome in Axis I, and to indicate the specific contributing physical condition in Axis III, but goes further by creating a separate category in Axis I, "Physical Factors Affecting Psychiatric Condition", and by indicating both the physical factors and the psychiatric conditions in axis I.

The utility of giving the dual diagnoses of "Physical Factors Contributing to Psychiatric Condition" and the Axis I or II diagnosis, and specifying the association between the psychiatric syndrome and the physical illness by a hyphen will facilitate research, especially in consultation-liaison settings. The research questions would include: what physical illness contributes to which Axis I and II conditions, and to what degree? What are the best pharmacologic, psychologic, and environmental treatment modalities for these specific conditions? In what way is chronic adjustment disorder to one physical illness different from another? etc.

For those psychiatric symptoms and conditions that do not meet the criteria for specific mental disorder, the diagnosis of Adjustment Disorder would be appropriate. However, adjustment to physical disease/disability, which is often chronic or episodic, deserves separate consideration from adjustment to an external psychosocial stressor. In fact, some such adjustment reactions to physical conditions may be unavoidable, and even adaptive, unlike in adjustment disorders to external stressors. Making the diagnosis of "Physical Factors Affecting Psychiatric Condition", and specifying the condition to be Chronic Adjustment Disorder, and further specifying the physical illness as a part of the diagnosis will enhance the objectives of the DSM IV approach of precision, in chronicity, severity, and the relationship between the psychiatric and physical illnesses.

Should Axis III include the physical illness specified in Axis I? I believe the answer is yes. Axis III should include all medical illness, whether it contributes to the Axis I psychiatric diagnosis or not. Axis III simply provides information concerning the biological/medical dimension of the patient, which serves as a consideration in managing the patient. The physical illness specified after a hyphen in Axis I, however, should be integrated in the treatment plan of the psychiatric disorder.

What about a patient who has both a major psychiatric disorder and adjustment problems to a physical illness? If a major psychiatric disorder develops within a specified period of the onset of a chronic physical illness, the index of suspicion for "Physical Factors Affecting Psychiatric Condition" should be raised. Since my proposal lists both diagnoses, the presence of the major psychiatric syndrome will be apparent even if there may be some disagreement among clinicians concerning just how much contribution the physical factors make to the major psychiatric syndrome.

What about patients who have pre-existing major psychiatric disorder such as bipolar major depression, who develops a physical illness that, in turn, contributes to the psychiatric symptomatology which may or may not be identical to the pre-existing ones (e.g. severe anxiety and change in behavior in addition to depression)? My proposal will clearly indicate this relationship by first listing the pre-existing psychiatric diagnosis, followed by the "Physical factors..." diagnosis, e.g., Bipolar disorder, depressed, Physical Factors Affecting Psychiatric Condition: Chronic Adjustment Disorder with Mixed Disturbance of Emotions and Conduct- Multiple Sclerosis (296.52, 999.23: 888.40-Multiple Sclerosis). In this case, this patient would have both a specific psychiatric disorder and an adjustment disorder diagnoses, which are clearly justified because of the specific nature of the patient's present conditions.

What about patients with chronic neurological disease (e.g. Parkinson's disease), in which the distinction between organic mood disorder and mood disorder due to adjustment difficulty may be difficult or impossible to make? My proposal would call for making both diagnoses. Recognition of the potential etiologic role of the neurologic condition would lead to vigorous treatment of the underlying condition, while recognizing the adjustment difficulties to the chronic condition would lead to mobilization of supportive resources and rehabilitation efforts.

The multiaxial approach of DSM III helped clinicians veer away from an either-or approach, and encouraged physicians to understand that psychiatric conditions often co-exist with physical illness. In DSM IV, I believe we should advance one more step by specifying the relationship between a psychiatric syndrome and a physical illness when such a relationship exists. The recognition that adjustment disorders can be chronic, and the creation of a new category, "Physical Factors Affecting Psychiatric Condition" would be one such step.

Note: This chapter is a slightly modified version of a paper, entitled, "Physical factors affecting psychiatric condition: A proposal for DSM-IV," which appeared in General Hospital Psychiatry, volume 15, pages 155-159, 1993. Reprinted with permission.

REFERENCES

1. American Psychiatric Association: Diagnostic and Statistical Manual of Mental Disorders (Third Edition-Revised), American Psychiatric Association, Washington, DC, 1987

2. Leigh H, Price L, Ciarcia J, Mirassou MM: DSM III and Consultation-Liaison Psychiatry: Toward a Comprehensive Medical Model of the Patient. General Hospital Psychiatry. 4:283-289, 1982

3. Leigh H, Reiser, MF: *The Patient, Biological, Psychological, and Social Dimensions of Medical Practice, 2nd Ed,* Plenum Press, New York, 1985

4. Fogel BS: Major depression versus organic mood disorder: A questionable distinction J Clin Psychiatry 51:53-56, 1990

TRAINING IN MEDICAL PSYCHIATRY

Scott Ahles, M.D.

Associate Clinical Professor of Psychiatry
University of California, San Francisco
Chief of Psychiatry, Valley Medical Center
445 South Cedar Ave
Fresno, CA 93703

I. INTRODUCTION

The "re-medicalization of psychiatry" is a phrase which has been heard frequently in recent years. In using this phrase, psychiatrists are usually referring to the advances in psychopharmacology over the last couple of decades which have led to new medical treatments for many psychiatric disorders. Not all changes in psychiatry however, are consistent with the concept of the re-medicalization of psychiatry. Witness for example, the expansion of free-standing psychiatric hospitals which have taken psychiatrists away from a close association with the rest of their medical colleagues. Re-medicalization of psychiatry should refer to more than just treating psychiatric patients with medication; it should include the ability of a psychiatrist to work in a general medical hospital relating to non-psychiatric physicians and treating patients with combined medical and psychiatric problems. The goal of this paper is to describe a program of training in medical psychiatry which has been developed in the Psychiatry Residency Training Program at the University of California, San Francisco-Fresno Division.

II. OVERVIEW

The psychiatry residency training program at UCSF, Fresno consists of five modules of training which occur over a four year program. The first module during the first six months of training in the PGY-I year consists of the internship experience. The PGY-I residents rotate through four months of internal medicine and two months of neurology.

Table 1. Clinical and Didactic Curriculum.

	Internship PG Ia	Inpatient Year PG Ib, IIa	General Hospital Psychiatry Year PG IIb, IIIa	Outpatient Year PG IIIb, IVa	Elective PG IVb
Clinical Rotations					
	Medicine Neurology	2 Inpatient settings Substance abuse	Consultation-Liaison Emergency Psychiatry Psychiatry Consultation Clinic	Adult Outpatient Child Outpatient Community Psychiatry	Chief Resident Research Other Elective
Didactic Curriculum					
Psycho-Pharmacology and Biological Psychiatry	Neurobiology Internal Medicine Series	Psychopathology Psychopharmacology Neuropsychiatric Aspects of AIDS	Biopsychiatry Biopsychosocial Rounds	Behavioral Neurology Psychiatric Therapeutics	Specific Seminars
Psycho-therapy and Psycho-dynamics		Psychiatric Interviewing Introduction to Psychotherapy Basic Psychological Theory Short-term Psychotherapy Learning theory and Behavioral Therapy	Advanced Psychodynamics Psychodynamic Case Conference	Psychodynamic Reading Seminar Psychotherapeutic Techniques Cognitive/Behavioral Therapyt Videotape Seminar Observational Seminar Psychoanalytic Therapy Group Therapy Family/Marital Therapy Interpersonal Therapy Social Skills Training	
Subspecialty and Special Topics		Psychodiagnostics Introduction to Psychiatric Consultation Chemical Dependency Community Orientation Computers in Practice and Research Ethics History of Psychiatry Forensic Psychiatry	Consultation-Liaison Emergency Psychiatry Transcultural Psychiatry Community Rounds Geriatric Psychiatry	Child Development/ Psychopathology Child Psychotherapy & Psychopharmacology Community Psychiatry Forensic Psychiatry	Private Practice Seminar Admin Psych Seminar

Longitudinal Experiences

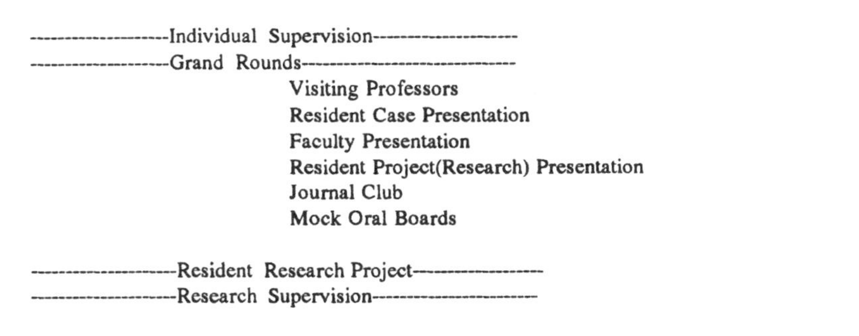
--------------------Individual Supervision--------------------
--------------------Grand Rounds--------------------
Visiting Professors
Resident Case Presentation
Faculty Presentation
Resident Project(Research) Presentation
Journal Club
Mock Oral Boards

--------------------Resident Research Project--------------------
--------------------Research Supervision--------------------

The next year of training during the second half of the PGY-I year and first half of the PGY-II year is the inpatient module. The residents gain experience in inpatient psychiatry rotating at a community hospital inpatient service, a VA Hospital inpatient service and an inpatient substance abuse and dual diagnosis program.

The third module of training occurs during the second half of the PGY-II year and the first half of the PGY-III year and is an experience in medical psychiatry or general hospital psychiatry. The rotations during this year include a rotation on the Consultation-Liaison Psychiatry Service, on an Emergency Psychiatry Service and in a Psychiatry Consultation Clinic. The program of this year of training is described in more detail below.

Across all years of the program there exists a comprehensive didactic curriculum. The didactic curriculum consists of courses which are arranged into three separate tracts as outlined in Table 1. The first tract contains seminars in biopsychiatry and psychopharmacology. The second tract includes seminars in psychodynamics and psychotherapy. The third tract contains seminars in various subspecialty areas.

The fourth module of the residency training program is the outpatient year which occurs during the latter half of the PGY-III year and the first half of the PGY-IV year. Residents have in fact, begun to treat outpatients on a longitudinal basis in the early years of the program. During this year however, they receive concentrated experience in treating outpatients of a multitude of diagnoses and using a variety of treatment techniques.

The last module of the program is the elective experience which occurs during the last six months of the program. Residents may choose between a chief residency experience in which they work with junior residents and faculty, a concentrated forensic experience at a state forensic hospital, or advanced training in child and adolescent psychiatry.

III. THE MEDICAL PSYCHIATRY YEAR

Training in the medical psychiatry year in the UCSF-Fresno Psychiatry Residency Training Program occurs at Valley Medical Center in Fresno. Valley Medical Center is a large county hospital which provides care for an indigent population in the Central Valley of California. The Department of Psychiatry at Valley Medical Center is administratively separate, interestingly, from Fresno County's Mental Health Department which provides community health services for Fresno county residents. The goal of the Department of

Psychiatry at Valley Medical Center is to provide psychiatric services for the patients of the general medical hospital population. This administrative separation has allowed the VMC Department of Psychiatry to focus on this task.

The two major goals of the Departemnt are clinical care and education. With respect to clinical care, a wide variety of patients are seen on our services. Many of them would be much less frequently seen on standard psychiatric inpatient units and in mental health clinics. The first group would include patients who have a primary psychiatric disorder who present in the medical setting. Examples of this might include patients with depressive disorders or adjustment disorders who present with suicide attempts; patients with anxiety disorders who present with symptoms that mimic medical illnesses such as panic attacks mimicking myocardial infarctions; and patients with disorders such as schizophrenia who happen to get admitted with an unrelated medical problem but who need treatment for their psychiatric disorder while their medical problems are being evaluated and treated.

The second group would be patients who manifest psychological reactions to their medical illness. This would include patients with severe medical problems whose lives have been significantly disrupted by their illness and who are having a hard time adjusting and reconstructing their lives. This would include patients with spinal cord injuries and amputations; patients with chronic renal failure who are on dialysis; cancer patients; patients with severe cardiopulmonary disease and so on.

The third group would be patients with psychosomatic disorders or what in DSM-III is classified under the category "Psychological Factors Affecting Physical Illness". Besides the classical psychosomatic illnesses, this would include any patients in whom psychological factors or social factors are interferring with their medical treatment. For example, we frequently see diabetic patients whose diabetes is difficult to control either because of their denial of their illness or because of their complex social situation.

The fourth group of patients would include patients with somatoform disorders such as conversion disorders, Briquet's Syndrome or hypochondriasis. These patients typically present with medical complaints for which no underlying organic pathology can be discovered. It is frequently much easier to treat these patients if the psychiatric services are available in the general medical hospital rather than in a situation where the patient has to be shunted off to some separate mental health facility.

The final group of patients are patients with neuropsychiatric disorders. These are disorders in which some organic disturbance has led to psychiatric symptoms. For example, because our hospital is a regional trauma center, we see significant numbers of patients who have organic, affective, personality or psychotic disorders as a result of their head injury. Other categories would include patients with endocrionopathies which affect their CNS function, patients with CNS tumors or patients with CNS infections. This latter category is becomming increasingly common as the incidence of AIDS escalates. Another group of patients in this category would be patients with various forms of dementias with whom we would deal with various issues of diagnosis, treatment, and behavioral management as well as legal issues such as consent and conservatorship.

The educational program for the residents is set up such that the residents spend six months rotating on the Psychiatry Consultation-Liaison Service, three months on the Emergency Psychiatry Service and three months in the Psychiatry Consultation Clinic. Much emphasis is placed on education and the residents receive close supervision of all their clinical work. Significant effort is put into helping the residents shore up their identity not only as a psychiatrist but also as a medical physician and finally as a specialist who has something unique to offer in the medical setting. Throughout our services we stress the interaction between the psychiatric residents and the residents of all the other departments. In their interactions with the medical housestaff, the psychiatry residents are encouraged to not just make recommendations about the treatment of patients that are seen, but also to actively participate in that treatment and to provide education to the housestaff on the psychiatric symptomology that is being manifest by the patient who is being seen.

At the beginning of the medical psychiatry residency year the residents are provided with an orientation manual which describes all of the services as well as the policies of the department. Part of the manual includes a section on goals and objectives. Specific goals and objectives are outlined for each of the three services -- consultation-liaison, emergency psychiatry and psychiatry consultation clinic.

A computerized log system has been developed so that data from each patient that a resident sees is entered into the computer and logs are printed out. This allows us to review the caseloads of the residents to assure adequate depth and breadth.

Besides the supervision that the residents receive from core faculty at Valley Medical Center, they also meet weekly with psychotherapy supervisors because they will, during this year, continue to follow outpatients on a longitudinal basis.

Residents may participate in medical student education. We've developed a core third year medical student rotation on the Consultation-Liaison Service, which is at times subscribed to by students from UC, San Francisco. From time to time we also have fourth year students from a variety of medical schools rotating on our services and in those situations, the residents act as primary teachers for the students.

The residents all participate in our monthly quality assurance meeting. They are also given four exams throughout the year. Two of these are written exams which test comprehension of material from the various didactic seminars. The other two are oral exams which are of the ABPN Board Exam format. Finally we have developed a library in the department. The library contains numerous books and journals in the field of psychiatry with particular emphasis on topics related to medical psychiatry.

IV. THE CONSULTATION-LIAISON ROTATION

This is a six month rotation in which residents gain experience in both consultation and liaison psychiatry. Residents consult on patients throughout all of the general medical and surgical wards of the hospital. For the most part patients are seen on the day that the consultation is requested. Each resident also has specific liaison assignments.

The typical day would begin with liaison rounds in which the psychiatry resident would talk to the admitting team from the night before to ascertain whether there were any patients admitted who might require our interventions. The next part of liaison rounds would include the resident going to their assigned liaison units. Rather than spending large amounts of time rounding with the teams in the units, the residents instead make contact with the unit teams to either discuss patients we have already seen in those units or to gather information on new patients whom we have been requested to see. Next, the resident would proceed to follow-up rounds in which they would go see the patients on whom they have already done consults. Follow-up rounds include not only interacting with the patients but interacting with the physicians and nursing staff and often social work staff who are involved in the care of that patient. Once follow-ups have been seen, the residents would proceed to the evaluation of new consultations. At 11:30 each morning the residents from the Consultation Service as well as Emergency Psychiatry and Psychiatry Consultation Clinic all meet for the daily seminar. Following the seminar and following lunch, the residents on the Consultation Service meet with the attending for Consultation-Liaison teaching rounds. During the rounds, follow-up of patients active on the service would be discussed and new patients would be presented. Following the presentations the attending and the group of consultation-liaison residents go to see,interview and discuss the new patients that were seen that day, as well as any follow-up patients who need to be seen. After the consultation-liaison teaching rounds the residents have time to write their notes as well as to complete any interactions with patients, patient's families, treating physicians and/or nursing staff.

Once a consultation request is received, the resident contacts the requesting physician to discuss the case and clarify the consultation question. Next the resident gathers history from the patient's chart, nurses, family, any available mental health records and any other pertinent collateral historians. Following a discussion of the case during the consultation-liaison teaching rounds the resident provides feedback concerning diagnosis, assessment and treatment to the treating team including physician staff and nursing staff. A consultation note is placed in the chart and then the resident provides regular follow-up for the patient and documentation of the follow-up throughout the duration of the patient's hospital stay. Finally, the resident makes a psychiatric disposition if needed at the time of discharge.

We have developed a Consultation-Liaison form for documentation of our consultations. This is a three page form which includes a page for history, a page for the mental status exam and a page for diagnosis/assessment and recommendations. The recommendations section is divided into biological, psychological and social interventions. Biological recommendations might include suggestions for psychotropic medications or further medical diagnostic work-up. Psychological recommendations might include recommendations for psychotherapy, for more extensive mental status evaluation/psychological testing or recommendations for specific ways which the treating team might better interact with the patient. Social recommendations might include suggestions for specific social service interventions, family interventions or recommendations concerning issues of conservatorship and consent. The final part of the consultation-liaison form provides a space for a reference article which we frequently provide along with a copy of the consultation. We maintain a file of frequently used articles to hand out to the treating team for their further education.

The specific units on which we have liaisons include the Medical Intensive Care Unit, Coronary Care Unit, Surgical Intensive Care Unit, Burn Unit, Dialysis Unit, as well as the Diabetes Service and the AIDS team. Residents on the Consultation-Liaison Service will be assigned to various of these units.

Components of the liaison experience include the liaison rounds in the mornings which were described above, as well as the provision of consultations on patients in these various units along with the associated follow-up. With each of the liaisons there is a multi-disciplinary team meeting which includes the medical treating team, nursing staff, psychiatry, social work and dietary. We have been available and have frequently participated in group meetings with the medical and nursing staff. These frequently have been organized around a discussion of the difficult patient but at times have been organized around interactional problems among the staff themselves. We also have frequently been involved in meetings with the family particularly in situations where interaction with the family is of significant importance for the treatment of the patient. Finally, we have always been available to our liaison units and consulting teams to provide educational seminars on psychiatric topics which they request.

V. EMERGENCY PSYCHIATRY SERVICE

The Emergency Psychiatry Service (EPS) has been established in the emergency room of Valley Medical Center and in close cooperation with the Emergency Medicine Department. Residents assigned to the Emergency Psychiatry Service are supervised by a full-time psychiatrist assigned to the emergency room. The residents also work in conjunction with the emergency medicine staff and housestaff. We have striven over the years to develop a close collaborative working relationship between psychiatry and emergency medicine. The psychiatry residents and psychiatry attending will usually start the day at 7:30 A.M., meeting with the emergency medicine team for their morning report. At this time the emergency medicine team briefly runs through all the patients who are currently in the emergency room. This morning report provides an opportunity for psychiatry to get feedback on patients who we have already seen and to receive information on patients we are being requested to see.

Following the morning report, the residents will meet with the psychiatry attending to discuss and interview patients. The psychiatry attending is available to the emergency room psychiatry resident throughout the day and is frequently present in the emergency room for further consultation and interactions with patients.

The patients seen by the Emergency Psychiatry Service may be patients who are in the emergency room at large or patients who have been admitted to an area in the emergency department called the Behavioral Care Unit (BCU), which is an area designated for patients who are on psychiatric holds.

There are several types of patients who are seen by the emergency psychiatry service. One type may be these patients who are brought in on legal holds for evaluation for admission to our acute psychiatry unit. These patients will be evaluated by the psychiatry resident for admission and either admission will be arranged or some other appropriate disposition will be arranged. Other common problems seen by the Emergency Psychiatry Serivce are patients who come in either with suicidal ideation or with a suicide attempt; patients with the various manifestations of alcohol and drug abuse problems; and patients with the various manifestations of dementia. We may also consult on patients who come in with medical symptoms but whom the treating emergency medicine physician feels have an underlying psychiatric disorder such as conversion or one of the other somatoform disorders. A very common type of patient seen by the emergency psychiatry service is the patient who presents with altered mental status of undetermined etiology. In these cases, the Emergency Psychiatry Service works together very closely with the Emergency Medicine Service to conjointly work up the patients and try to determine the etiology of the patient's altered mental status and then plan appropriate treatment.

An Emergency Psychiatry Service form has been developed for recording historical information, mental status exam, diagnosis and treatment recommendations. This form also contains a section for orders for patients who are admitted to the BCU. These might include vital sign orders, level of observation orders and restraint orders which would be carried out and documented by the BCU nurse in conjunction with security if necessary.

The residents generally work two days per week on the Emergency Psychiatry Service and participate in this service in conjunction with their participation in the Psychiatry Consultation Clinic other days of the week over a six month period.

VI. PSYCHIATRY CONSULTATION CLINIC

The Psychiatry Consultation Clinic has been organized within the administrative structure of the medical and surgical clinics of the general medical hospital and is separate from other mental health clinics within the county system. Most of the referrals to the clinic come from the various medical and surgical clinics at Valley Medical Center. Some of the referrals come from our inpatient Psychiatry Consultation Service or from the Emergency Psychiatry Service. The clinic is staffed by a half-time psychiatrist, a clerk and psychiatry residents who rotate through the clinic on a part-time basis for a period of six months, while they are also rotating on the Emergency Psychiatry Service part-time.

The patient population varies significantly from a typical mental health population. For example we have very few patients with schizophrenia and bipolar disorders. We have on the other hand, patients with physical illnesses who are experiencing grief, depression or anxiety in reaction to their physical illness; we see patients with somatoform disorders and psychosomatic disorders as well as various forms of organic mental syndromes. Increasingly we are seeing a geriatric population and hope to eventually develop some liaisons with the nursing homes that many of these patients reside in. We also see patients with chronic pain problems and work closely with physicians in the medicine clinic who are conjointly seeing these patients.

We have begun to work on liaisons with other clinics within the hospital clinic structure. At the present time, the faculty psychiatrist and the residents meet on a regular basis with the faculty and residents of the Family Practice Clinic and of the Internal Medicine Clinic to discuss psychiatric issues as well as patients who are followed conjointly.

The goals of the clinic are to offer clinical services to patients as well as to provide training for residents. At times the clinic functions on a strictly consultation model in which a patient is referred by a physician who wants information on how he should treat his patient. Commonly, this might be a request from a pysician with a patient with depression who he would like to treat. In that case we would make recommendations and refer the patient back to the treating physician. In a majority of the cases, however, the patients are referred for consultation and follow-up. Treatment modalities would include pharmacology, relaxation therapy, hypnosis and psychodynamic psychotherapy. Many of the residents who pick up patients for psychotherapy during their clinic rotation will continue to follow them beyond the time that they leave the clinic. Another service of the clinic is referral. We provide referral for patients who need services that we can't provide such as substance abuse rehabilitation or day treatment services.

Group therapy is another modality which we have utilized in the clinic. We currently have two ongoing groups which are each co-led by a faculty member and a resident. One group is for patients with physical illnesses who are having difficulty coping with the disability imposed by their physical illnesses. The other group is for patients who have somatoform disorders. This is a difficult group of patients to treat and we've been surprised that many of these patients seem to do better in the group format as opposed to the individual format.

VII. DIDACTICS

While the residents rotate through the medical psychiatry year, they receive a comprehensive didactic series which is geared toward expanding their knowledge in various areas of medical psychiatry as well as furthering their development as psychiatrists in general. There are five seminar series, one of which meets each day from 11:30 to 12:30, Monday through Friday. The first is the Consultation-Liaison Seminar Series. The schedule for the seminar series is attached (Appendix 1). As can be seen from the schedule, the series is broken down into six parts. Part One is on Assessment and Treatment. It includes topics such as consultation-liaison process, consultation write-up, biopsychosocial apporach, neuropsychiatric mental status exam, as well as topics on the diagnosis and treatment of some of the basic problems that come up on the consultation-liaison service. Part Two of the Consultation-Liaison Seminar Series is entitled "Psychiatric Disorders in the Medical Setting". This section discusses the diagnosis and treatment of various psychiatric disorders which patients may have in conjunction with the medical disorder that leads to their admission. Topics include anxiety disorders, personality disorders, schizophrenia and eating disorders. Part Three of the series is entitled "Psychological Reactions to Physical Illness". This series of lectures deals with how patients cope with physical illness and includes topics such as illness process, grief, adjustment and depression, death and dying, as well as topics germain to specific setting such as the intensive care unit, burn unit and dialysis unit and specific diseases such as cancer, spinal cord injuries and AIDS. Part Four of the C-L series includes a discussion of the Somatoform Disorders such as somatozation disorder, conversion, hypochondriasis, body dysmorphic disorder and psychogenic pain. Also included in this section are discussions of factitious disorder, Munchausen syndrome and malingering. Part Five of the C-L series is the section on Psychosomatic Disorders and includes an historical review of psychosomatic medicine as well as discussions on current aspects of psychosomatic medicine such as stress and psychoendoimmunology. Specific organ systems are discussed including the cardiovascular system, pulmonary system, gastrointestinal system and male and female reproductive systems. Also further discussed are the problems of acute and chronic pain. Part Six, the final section of the C-L series, is the section on Neuropsychiatry. This includes discussions of neuromedical disorders which may cause psychiatric symptoms. Included in this section are the topics of delirium and dementia as well as the psychiatric sequelae of such things as seizure disorder, head trauma, stroke, metaboic disorders, vitamin deficiency states, movement disorders, inflammatory and infectious disorders of the CNS, endocrine disorders and brain tumors.

Each resident receives a syllabus of readings that are indexed to the lectures in the C-L seminar series. The bibliography of the syllabus is attached (Appendix 2). The next seminar series is entitled "Emergency Psychiatry Seminar" series. This is a series which is split between didactic presentations and case discussions.

The didactic topics include decision making in emergency psychiatry, assessing suicidality, organic vs functional, dealing with violent patients in the emergency room, substance abuse syndromes, the evaluation of the child in the emergency room, forensic aspects of emergency psychiatry, geriatric patients in the emergency room, crisis intervention, mental retardation and amytal interviews (Appendix 3). Alternating with the didactic topics are case discussions. These include two types of case discussions. One is the Biopsychosocial Rounds which is a case discussion of the patient seen in the emergency room which is geared toward clarifying diagnosis and discussing treatment from a biopsychosocial aspect. Another part of this series is the Psychodynamics Case Conference which is interspersed throughout this series during the year. This is an in-depth discussion of a patient that one of the residents is following in psychotherapy and includes a discussion of the psychodynamics of the case as well as the psychotherapy technique most appropriate for that patient.

The next seminar series is the one that includes the Transcultural Seminar and the Geriatric Seminar. In Fresno we see patients from diverse ethnic backgrounds including patients from Mexico and other Central American countries, as well as an increasing population from several of the Southeast Asian countries, particularly Hmongs.

A Transcultural Seminar has been developed which presents many of the transcultural issues and helps residents to deal with the many unique clinical problems that come up in these diverse populations. Following the Transcultural Seminar in this series is the Geriatric Seminar. Since we have a fairly large elderly population, this seminar is designed to help residents treat this group of patients. Topics include things such as the psychiatric interview in geriatric patients, laboratory evaluation of dementia, differential diagnosis and classification of dementia, use of psychotropic medications in the elderly, psychotherapy in the elderly as well as issues such as community care, diet and nutrition and exercise.

Interspersed among the transcultural and geriatric lectures are a Journal Club which meets approximately once a month as well as a visiting professor small group discussions. The visiting professor small group discussions are luncheon meetings in which the residents will meet with a visiting professor who is in town for grand rounds and discuss a case. The Journal Club is designed to help residents learn how to critically read research articles. We have developed a form, which is filled out in preparation for discussion of an article.

The next series consists of two seminars, the Biopsychiatry Seminar and the Behavioral Neurology Seminar. The Biopsychiatry Seminar has lectures under various topics including lectures on neurotransmitters and receptors; endocrine aspects of psychiatric disorders; brain imaging in psychiatry; chronobiology; genetic studies in psychiatric disorders and the biopsychiatry of various disorders including panic disorders, obsessive-compulsive disorder, schizophrenia and so on. The Behavioral Neurology Seminar is a seminar which is designed to look at the brain and try to understand how the brain processes information and how malfunctioning of the brain leads to various forms of pathology. Topics include neuroanatomy, attention, neglect, the limbic system, memory and learning, aphasia and alexia, disorders of auditory visual and somatosensory processing, kindling, frontal and temporal lobe syndromes and cerebral lateralization.

The final seminar series is the Advanced Psychodynamics Seminar series. This is a series which dovetails with some of the psychodynamic and psychotherapy courses earlier in the residency program. The psychodynamics series is important as residents do continue to follow patients long term longitudinally throughout their third year of training.

VIII. OTHER POTENTIAL EDUCATIONAL EXPERIENCES

There are other clinical services that might be developed that could serve as significant additional educational experiences for training in medical psychiatry. Several hospitals have opened medical-psychiatry wards which serve diverse groups of patients. There has been increasing interest in and awareness of patients who present with psychiatric symptomatology related to brain disease. Many of these wards treat these types of patients whom are becoming increasingly common with the escalating numbers of patients with dementia. This type of ward could serve as a setting for an excellent educational experience in the diagnosis and management of complex medical-psychiatric cases.

Other educational experiences that might be developed to promote training in medical psychiatry would be various fellowships. Consideration can certainly be given to fellowships in Consultation-Liaison Psychiatry, Emergency Psychiatry and Geriatric Psychiatry. Several centers have already developed these training experiences.

IX. SUMMARY/CONCLUSIONS

Described above is a training program in medical psychiatry. There are certainly many different ways that residents could receive training in medical psychiatry. The important point is that residents do receive training that helps them shore up an identity not only as a psychiatrist, but also as a physician; and as a physician, one who has something special and unique to contribute to the care of patients in a medical setting.

APPENDIX 1

UCSF-FRESNO
Psychiatry Residency Training Program
Third-Year Curriculum

CONSULTATION-LIAISON
SEMINAR SERIES SCHEDULE
ACADEMIC YEAR 1992-1993

PART I: ASSESSMENT AND TREATMENT

WEEK 1	Overview of Consultation/Liaison Psychiatry, the Consultation Process, the Consultation Writeup
WEEK 2	The Biopsychosocial Approach
WEEK 3	The Neuropsychiatric Mental Status Exam
WEEK 4	Differential Diagnosis of Neuropsychiatric Disorders
WEEK 5	Evaluation of Alcoholism in the Medical Setting
WEEK 6	Psychiatric Symptoms Secondary to Medical Drugs/Drug Interactions
WEEK 7	Differential Diagnosis of the Acutely Psychotic Patient in the Medical Setting
WEEK 8	Medico-Legal Evaluation -- Consent, 5150, Conservatorship
WEEK 9	EEG and CAT in the Differential Diagnosis of Neuropsychiatric Disorders
WEEK 10	Psychopharmacology in the Medically Ill
WEEK 11	Cardiovascular Effects of Tricyclic Antidepressants
WEEK 12	Psychotherapy in the Medically Ill
WEEK 13	Hypnosis/Relaxation

PART II: PSYCHIATRIC DISORDERS IN THE MEDICAL SETTING

WEEK 14	Anxiety Disorders in the Medical Setting
WEEK 15	Personality Disorders in the Medical Setting
WEEK 16	Problem Patients
WEEK 17	The Schizophrenic Patient on the Hospital Ward

WEEK 18 Eating Disorders

PART III: PSYCHOLOGICAL REACTIONS TO PHYSICAL ILLNESS

WEEK 19 The Illness Process

WEEK 20 Coping With Illness

WEEK 21 Grief, Adjustment Reaction, Depression

WEEK 22 Death and Dying

WEEK 23 The Setting of Intensive Care

WEEK 24 Life Prolonging Procedures--Dialysis/Transplant

WEEK 25 Cancer

WEEK 26 Spinal Cord Injury

WEEK 27 Burn Injury

WEEK 28 AIDS

PART IV: THE SOMATOFORM DISORDERS

WEEK 29 Somatization as a Way of Life/Conversion Disorders

WEEK 30 Briquet's Syndrome/Hypochondriasis

WEEK 31 Factitious Disorder (Munchausen's Syndrome)/Malingeering

WEEK 32 Other Somatoform Disorders

PART V: PSYCHOSOMATIC DISORDERS

WEEK 33 History of Psychosomatic Medicine

WEEK 34 Stress/Psychoendoimmunology

WEEK 35 Psychosomatic Aspects of Cardiovascular Disease

WEEK 36 Psychosomatic Aspects of Pulmonary Disease

WEEK 37 Psychosomatic Aspects of Gastrointestinal Disease

WEEK 38 Psychosomatic Aspects of OB/Gyn and Urology

WEEK 39 Chronic Pain

WEEK 40 Acute Pain

PART VI: SOMATOPSYCHIC DISORDERS/NEUROPSYCHIATRY

WEEK 41 Delirium

WEEK 42 Dementia

WEEK 43 Psychiatric Aspects of Seizure Disorders

WEEK 44 Head Trauma and Stroke: Psychiatric Sequelae

WEEK 45 Neuropsychiatric Sequelae of Metabolic Disorders and Vitamin Deficiency States

WEEK 46 Neurobehavioral Aspects of Movement Disorder

WEEK 47 Neuropsychiatric Aspects of Inflamatory and Infectious Disease

WEEK 48 Neuropsychiatric Aspects of Endocrine Disease

WEEK 49 Neuropsychiatric Aspects of Brain Tumors

APPENDIX 2

UCSF-Fresno
Psychiatry Residency Training Program
Third-Year Curriculum

CONSULTATION-LIAISON
SEMINAR SERIES BIBLIOGRAPHY
ACADEMIC YEAR 1992-1993

PART I: ASSESSMENT AND TREATMENT

WEEK 1 Overview of Consultation/Liaison Psychiatry; the Consultation Process; the Consultation Write-up

1. Lipowski, Z. J. and Lipsitt, D. R.,**"Consultation-Liaison Psychiatry: An Overview,"** Psychosomatic Medicine - Current Trends and Clinical Applications. New York:Oxford University Press, 1977.(Chapter 21, pp. 373-385).

2. **"Consultation Process,"** An outline.

3. Strain, J. and Grossman, S., **"Psychiatric Assessment in the Medical Setting,"** Psychological Care of the Medically Ill. NewYork: Appleton-Century-Crofts, 1974. (Chapter 2, pp. 11-22).

4. Garrick, T.R., M.D. and Stotland, N.L., M.D., **"How to Write a Psychiatric Consultation,"** The American Journal of Psychiatry, 139:7, July 1982, pp. 849-855.

5. **"The Basic Mental Status Examination,"** Handout.

WEEK 2 The Biopsychosocial Approach

6. Green, S. A., **"Biopsychosocial Medicine,"** Mind and Body: The Psychology of Physical Illness. Washington DC: American Psychiatric Press, Inc., 1985. (Chapter 1, pp. 3-7).

7. Reiser, D. E. and Rosen, D.H., **"Clinical Application of the Biopsychosocial Model,"** Medicine as a Human Experience Baltimore: University Park Press, 1984. (Chapter 2,pp.43-60).

* References without numbers are in the MGH Handbook of General Hospital Psychiatry (3rd edition), and not in this syllabus.

8. Reiser, D. E. and Rosen, D. H., **"Care of the Patient: Art or Science?,"** Medicine as a Human Experience Baltimore: University Park Press, 1984. (Chapter 3, pp. 61-72).

WEEK 3 The Neuropsychiatric Mental Status Exam

9. Cummings, J. L., **"The Neuropsychiatric Interview and Mental Status Examination,"** Clinical Neuropsychiatry. Orlando: Grune & Stratton, Inc., 1985. (Chapter 2, pp. 5-16).

10. Gross, D.A., M.D., **"The Bedside Neuropsychological Examination,"**Psychiatry Letter, Vol. III, Issue 11, November, 1985, pp. 61-66.

11. Handout: **VMC Neuropsychiatric MSE Checklist**

WEEK 4 Differential Diagnosis of Neuropsychiatric Disorders

12. Cummings, J. L., **"Disorders of Verbal Output: Mutism, Aphasia, and Psychotic Speech,"** Clinical Neuropsychiatry. Orlando: Grune & Stratton, Inc., 1985. (Chapter 3, pp. 17-35).

13. Cummings, J. L., **"Amnesia, Paramnesia and Confabulation,"** Clinical Neuropsychiatry. Orlando: Grune & Stratton, Inc., 1985. (Chapter 4, pp. 36-47).

14. Cummings, J. L.,**"Visuospatial and Visual Perceptual Disturbances,** Clinical Neuropsychiatry. Orlando: Grune & Stratton, Inc., 1985. (Chapter5,pp.48-56).

15. Cummings, J. L.,**"Dissociative States, Depersonalization, Multiple Personality, and Episodic Memory Lapses,"** Clinical Neuropsychiatry.Orlando: Grune & Stratton, Inc., 1985. (Chapter 10, pp. 117-126).

16. Cummings, J. L.,**"Hallucinations,"** Clinical Neuropsychiatry. Orlando: Grune & Stratton, Inc., 1985. (Chapter 16, pp. 221-233).

WEEK 5 Evaluation of Alcoholism in the Medical Setting

* Cassem, N. H., **"Alcoholism: Acute and Chronic States,"** Massachusetts General Hospital: Handbook of General Hospital Psychiatry (Third Edition). Saint Louis: The C.V.Mosby Co., 1991. (Chp. 2, pp 9-22).

17. Gill, D.J., M.D.,**"Alcoholism and the Consultation Liaison Psychiatrist,"** Psychiatric Clinics of North America, Vol. 10, No. 1, March, 1987, pp. 129-139.

WEEK 6 Psychiatric Symptoms Secondary to Medical Drugs/Drug Interactions

18. Extein, I. and Gold, M. S.,**"Medication-Induced and Toxin-Induced Psychiatric Disorders,"** Medical Mimics of Psychiatric Disorders. Washington: American Psychiatric Press, Inc., 1986. (Chapter 7, pp. 165-198).

19. **"Drugs That Cause Psychiatric Symptoms,"** The Medical Letter, Vol. 31, Issue 808, December 29, 1989, pp. 113-118.

20. Rizack, M. and Hillman, C, **"Psychotropic vs. Other Medicine Interactions,"** The Medical Letter Handbook of Adverse Drug Interactions. New York: The Medical Letter, 1987. (Segments from).

WEEK 7 Differential Diagnosis of the Acutely Psychotic Patient in the Medical Setting

* Cassem, N. H.,**"Psychotic Patients,"** Massachusetts General Hospital: Handbook of General Hospital Psychiatry (Third Edition). Saint Louis: C. V. Mosby Co., 1991. (Chapter 11, pp.217-236).

WEEK 8 Medico-Legal Evaluation/Consent, 5150, Conservatorship

* Cassem, N. H.,**"Legal Aspects of Consultation,"** Massachusetts General Hospital: and book of General Hospital Psychiatry (Third Edition). Saint Louis: C. V. Mosby Co., 1991. (Chapter 29, pp. 619-638).

21. **"Conservatorship Procedure,"** Handout

22. **"Consent to Treatment and 72-Hour Holds,"** Handout

23. Consent to Medical Treatment, Letter From County Counsel to Judge Keyes.

24. Dependent Adult and Elder Abuse/Child Abuse Reporting Laws.

25. Durable Power of Attorney

26. Probate Conservatorship

WEEK 9 EEG and CAT in the Differential Diagnosis of Neuropsychiatric Disorders

27. Hughes, J. R. and Wilson, W. P., **"EEG in Organic Brain Syndrome,"** EEG and Evoked Potentials in Psychiatry and Behavioral Neurology. Boston: Butterworths, 1983. (Chapter 1, pp. 1-24).

28. Ramsey, R.G.,**"Introduction and Normal Anatomy,"** Computed Tomography of the Brain Advanced Exercises in Diagnostic Radiology-9. Philadelphia: W.B. Saunders Co., 1977. (Chapter 1, pp. 1-23).

WEEK 10 Psychopharmacology in the Medically Ill

* Cassem, N. H.,**"Psychotropic Drug Prescribing,"** Massachusetts General Hospital: Handbook of General Hospital Psychiatry (Third Edition). Saint Louis: C.V. Mosby Co., 1991. (Chapter 26, pp. 527-570).

WEEK 11 Cardiovascular Effects Of Tricyclic Antidepressants

29. Jefferson, James W., M.D., **"Cardiovascular Effects and Toxicity of Anxiolytics and Antidepressants,"** Journal of Clinical Psychiatry, 50:10, October 1989, pp. 368-378.

WEEK 12 Psychotherapy in the Medically Ill

30. Stein, E. H. et al, **"Brief Psychotherapy of Psychiatric Reactions to Physical Illness,"** American Journal of Psychiatry, 125:8, February 1969, pp. 1040-1047.

* Cassem, N.H.,**"Brief Psychotherapy,"** Massachusetts General Hospital: Handbook of General Hospital Psychiatry (Third Edition). Saint Louis: C. V. Mosby Co., 1991. (Chapter 16,pp.321-342).

31. Van Dyke, C. et al,**"Psychotherapeutic Approaches to Physically Ill Patients,"** Emotions in Health and Illness-Applications to Clinical Practice. Florida: Grune & Stratton, Inc., 1983. (Chapter 12, Pp. 187-197).

32. Green, S.A.,**"Treating Mind and Body,"** Mind & Body: The Psychology of Physical Illness. Washington DC: American Psychiatric Press, Inc., 1985. (Chapter 9, pp.157-198).

WEEK 13 Hypnosis/Relaxation

33. Guggenheim, F. G. and Weiner, M.F.,**"Hypnosis on the Medical Wards,"** Manual of Psychiatric Consultation and Emergency Care. NewYork: Jason Aronson, Inc., 1984. (Chapter 35, pp. 353-361).

34. Ferguson, J. M. et al, **"A Script for Deep Muscle Relaxation,"** Disease of the Nervous System, Vol. 38, No. 9, September 1977, pp. 703-708.

35. **"Hypnotic Suggestions,"** Handout.

PART II: PSYCHIATRIC DISORDERS IN THE MEDICAL SETTING

WEEK 14 Anxiety Disorders in the Medical Setting

* Cassem, N. H., **"Anxiety,"** Massachusetts General Hospital: Handbook of General Hospital Psychiatry (Third Edition). Saint Louis: C. V. Mosby Co., 1991. (Chapter 9, pp. 159-190.

WEEK 15 Personality Disorders in the Medical Setting

* Cassem, N. H., **"Patients with Borderline Personality Disorders,"** Massachusetts General Hospital: Handbook of General Hospital Psychiatry (Third Edition). Saint Louis: C. V. Mosby Co., 1991. (Chapter 10, pp. 191-216).

36. Kahana, R. J. and Bibring, G. L., **"Personality Types in the Medical Management,"** pp. 109-123.

WEEK 16 Problem Patients

37. Hackett, T. P. and Cassem, N. H., **"Disruptive States,"** Massachusetts General Hospital: Handbook of General Hospital Psychiatry (Second Edition). Saint Louis: C.V. Mosby Co., 1987. (Chapter 12, pp.231-249).

38. Groves, J. E., **"Taking Care of the Hateful Patient,"** New England Journal of Medicine, 298: 883-887, 1978.

WEEK 17 The Schizophrenic Patient on the Hospital Ward

39. Gelenberg, A. J., **"The Catatonic Syndrome,"** The Lancet, June 19, 1976, pp. 1339-1340.

40. Manschreck, A. J. and Petri, M., **"The Paranoid Syndrome,"** The Lancet, July 29, 1978, pp. 251-253.

41. Krauthammer, O., M.D., and Klerman, G. L., M.D., **"Secondary Mania,"** Archives of General Psychiatry, Vol. 35, November 1978, pp. 1333-1339.

WEEK 18 Eating Disorders

42. Herzog, D. B., **"Focus on Eating Disorders."**

PART III: PSYCHOLOGICAL REACTIONS TO PHYSICAL ILLNESS

WEEK 19 The Illness Process

43. Strain, J. and Grossman, S., **"Psychological Reactions to Medical Illness and Hospitalization,"** Psychological Care of the Medically Ill. New York :Appleton Century Crofts, 1975. (Chapter 3,pp.23-36).

44. Moos, R. H., **"The Crisis of Physical Illness: An Overview and Conceptual Approach,"** Coping with Physical Illness 2: New Perspectives. New York: Plenum Medical Book Co., 1984. (Chapter 1, pp. 3-25).

WEEK 20 Coping with Illness

45. Lipowski, Z.J. et al, **"Physical Illness, The Individual and the Coping Processes,"** Psychiatry in Medicine, Vol. 1, April 1970, pp. 91-102.

* Cassem, N.H., **"Coping with Illness,"** Massachusetts General Hospital: Handbook of General Hospital Psychiatry (Third Edition). Saint Louis: C. V. Mosby Co., 1991. (Chapter 15, pp. 309-320).

WEEK 21 Grief, Adjustment Reaction, Depression

* Cassem, N. H., **"Depression,"** Massachusetts General Hospital: Handbook of General Hospital Psychiatry (Third Edition). Saint Louis: C. V. Mosby Co., 1991. (Chapter 12, pp. 237-268).

46. Strain, J.J. and Grossman, S., **"Evaluating Depression in the Medical Patient,"** Psychological Care of the Medically Ill. New York: Appleton Century Crofts, 1975. (Chapter 6, pp.64-75.)

WEEK 22 Death and Dying

* Cassem, N.H., **"The Dying Patient,"** Massachusetts General Hospital: Handbook of General Hospital Psychiatry (Third Edition). Saint Louis: C.0 V. Mosby Co., 1991. (Chapter 17, pp. 343-372).

WEEK 23 The Setting of Intensive Care

* Cassem, N. H., **"The Setting of Intensive Care,"** Massachusetts General Hospital: Handbook of General Hospital Psychiatry (Third Edition). Saint Louis: C. V. Mosby Co., 1991. (Chapter 18, pp. 373-400).

* Cassem, N. H., **"The Surgical Patient,"** Massachusetts General Hospital: Handbook of General Hospital Psychiatry (Third Edition). Saint Louis: C. V. Mosby Co., 1991. (Chapter 5, pp. 69-88).

WEEK 24 Life Prolonging Procedures -- Dialysis/Transplant

* Cassem, N. H., **"Hemodialysis and Renal Transplantation,"** Massachusetts General Hospital: Handbook of General Hospital Psychiatry (Third Edition). Saint Louis: C. V. Mosby Co., 1991. (Chapter 19, pp. 401-430).

47. Calland, C. H., M.D., **"Iatrogenic Problems in End-Stage Renal Failure,"** New England Journal of Medicine, Vol. 287, No. 7, August 17, 1982, pp. 334-336.

WEEK 25 Cancer

48. Fawzy, I. F. et al, **"Psychosocial Management of Cancer,"** Psychiatric Medicine, Vol. 1, No. 2, 1983, pp. 165-179.

49. Moos, R. H., **"Bearing Cancer,"** Coping with Physical Illness 2: New Perspectives. New York: Plenum Medical Book Co., 1984. (Chapter 5, pp. 59-72).

WEEK 26 Spinal Cord Injury

50. Judd, Fiona K. and Burrows, G. D., **"Liaison Psychiatry in a Spinal Injuries Unit,"** 1986 International Medical Society of Paraplegia, pp. 6-19.

WEEK 27 Burn Injury

* Cassem, N.H., **"Psychiatric Care of the Burn Victim,"** Massachusetts General Hospital: Handbook of General Hospital Psychiatry (Third Edition) Saint Louis: C. V. Mosby Co., 1991. (Chapter 22, pp. 465-476).

WEEK 28 AIDS

51. Faulstich, M.E., Ph.D. **"Psychiatric Aspects of AIDS,"** American Journal of Psychiatry, 144:5, May 1987, pp. 551-556.

52. Kelly, K., M.D., **"AIDS and Ethics: An Overview,"** General Hospital Psychiatry, 9:331-340, 1987.

PART IV: THE SOMATOFORM DISORDERS

WEEK 29 Somatization as a Way of Life/Conversion Disorders

53. Ford, C. V., **"Disease, Illness, and Health,"** The Somatizing Disorders-Illness as a Way of Life. New York: Elsevier Biomedical, 1983. (Chapter 2, pp. 7-23).

54. Ford, C. V., **"The Sick Role,"** The Somatizing Disorders - Illness as a Way of Life. New York: Elsevier Biomedical, 1983. (Chapter 3, pp. 24-35).

WEEK 30 Briquet's Syndrome/Hypochondriasis

55. Ford, C. V., **"Hysteria,"** The Somatizing Disorders Illness as a Way of Life. New York: Elsevier Biomedical, 1983. (Chapter 5, pp. 49-75).

56. Ford, C. V., **"Hypochondriasis,"** The Somatizing Disorders - Illness as a Way of Life. New York: Elsevier Biomedical, 1983. (Chapter 6, pp. 76-97).

WEEK 31 Factitious Disorder (Munchausen's Syndrome) - Malingering

57. Ford, C. V., M.D. **"Factitious Illness,"** The Somatizing Disorders - Illness as a Way of Life. New York: Elsevier Biomedical, 1983. (Chapter 9, pp. 135-154).

58. Ford, C. V., **"The Munchausen Syndrome,"** The Somatizing Disorders - Illness as a Way of Life. NewYork: Elsevier Biomedical, 1983. (Chapter 10, pp. 155-175).

59. Ford, C. V., **"Malingering,"** The Somatizing Disorders- Illness as a Way of Life. New York: Elsevier Biomedical, 1983. (Chapter 8, pp. 127-134).

WEEK 32 Other Somatoform Disorders

60. Ford, C. V., **"Disability Syndromes,"** The Somatizing Disorders - Illness as a Way of Life. NewYork: Elsevier Biomedical, 1983. (Chapter 11, pp. 176-202).

PART V: PSYCHOSOMATIC DISORDERS

WEEK 33 History of Psychosomatic Medicine

61. Sheehan, D. V. and Hackett, T. P., **"Psychosomatic Disorders,"** The Harvard Guide to Modern Psychiatry Cambridge's the Belknap Press, 1978. (Chp 16,pp. 319-353).

62. Stoudemire, Alan M.D. and Hales, Robert E. M.D. **Psychological and Behavioral Factors Affecting Medical Conditions and DSM - IV: An Overview** Psychosomatics - Volume 32, Number 1, Winter 1991 Pages 5 - 13

WEEK 34 Stress/Psychoendoimmunology

63. Calabrese, J.R. et al, **"Alterations in Immunocompetence During Stress, Bereavement, and Depression: Focus on Neuroendocrine Regulation,"** The American Journal Of Psychiatry, 144:9, September 1987, pp. 1123-1134.

64. Dorian, B. and Garfinkel, P. E., **"Stress, Immunity and Illness -A Review,"** Psychological Medicine 17, 1987, pp. 393-407.

WEEK 35 Psychosomatic Aspects of Cardiovascular Disease

65. Young, L. D., M. D., **Psychiatric Syndromes and Psychological Symptoms Associated with Organic Heart Disease,"** Psychiatric Medicine, Vol. 1, No. 2, 1983, pp. 181-204.

66. Swift, R. M., Ph.D. and Black, H. R., M.D., **"Essential Hypertension: Psychiatric Aspects and Use of Psychotropics,"** No.1 in a series, Vol.25, No. 10, October 1984, pp. 737-745.

WEEK 36 Psychosomatic Aspects of Pulmonary Disease

67. Fann, W.E. et al, **"Pulmonary Disorders and Psychosocial Stress,"** Phenomenology and Treatment of Psychophysiological Disorders. England: MTP Press Limited, 1982. (Chapter 2, pp. 15-33).

WEEK 37 Psychosomatic Aspects of Gastrointestinal Disease

68. Fann, W.E. et al, **"Psychological Elements of Gastrointestinal Disorders,"** Phenomenology and Treatment of Psychophysiological Disorders. England: MTP Press Limited, 1982. (Chapter 1, pp. 1-13).

WEEK 38 Psychosomatic Aspects of OB/Gyn and Urology

69. Nadelson, C.C. et al, **"Psychosomatic Aspects of Obstetrics and Gynecology,"** Psychosomatics, Vol 24,No.10, October 1983, pp. 871-884.

WEEK 39 Chronic Pain

70. Melzack, R., Ph.D. and Taenzer, P., B. Sc.,**"Concepts of Pain Perception and Therapy,"** Geriatrics, November 1977, pp. 44-48.

* Cassem, N. H., **"The Pain Patient: Evaluation and Treatment,"** Massachusetts General Hospital: Handbook of General Hospital Psychiatry (Third Edition). Saint Louis: C. V. Mosby Co., 1991. (Chapter 4, pp. 39-68).

WEEK 40 Acute Pain

71. Perlman, S. L., M.D., **"Modern Techniques of Pain Management,"** The Western Journal of Medicine, Vol. 148, No. 1, January 1988, pp. 54-61.

PART VI: SOMATOPSYCHIC DISORDERS/NEUROPSYCHIATRY

WEEK 41 Delirium

72. Lipowski, S. J., **"Delirium Updated,"** Comprehensive Psychiatry, Vol. 21, No. 3, May/June 1980, pp. 190-196.

WEEK 42 Dementia

73. Cummings, J. L., **"Dementia,"** Clinical Neuropsychiatry. Orlando: Grune & Stratton, Inc., 1985. (Chapter 8, pp. 75-94).

WEEK 43 Psychiatric Aspects of Seizure Disorders

74. Strub, R. L. and Black, F. W.,**"Epilepsy,"** Organic Brain Syndromes: An Introduction to Neurobehavioral Disorders. Philadelphia: F. A. Davis Co., 1982. (Chapter 11, pp. 335-368).

WEEK 44 Head Trauma and Stroke: Psychiatric Sequelae

75. Strub, R. L. and Black, F.W., **"Closed Head Trauma,"** Organic Brain Syndromes: An Introduction to Neurobehavioral Disorders. Philadelphia: F. A. Davis Co., 1982. (Chapter 8, pp. 269-297).

76. Hales, R.E. & Yudofsky, S.C. (eds.) **"Neuropsychiatric Aspects of Cerebrovascular Disease,** Textbook of Neuropsychiatry. Washington DC: American Psychiatric Press, Inc., 1987. (Chapter 11, pp. 191-208).

WEEK 45 Neuropsychiatric Sequelae of Metabolic Disorders and Vitamin Deficiency States

77. Hales, R.E. & Yudofsky, S.C. (eds.) **"Neuropsychiatric Aspects of Metabolic Disease,** Textbook of Neuropsychiatry. Washington DC: American Psychiatric Press, Inc., 1987. (Chapter 16, pp. 287-306).

78. Hales, R.E. & Yudofsky, S.C. (eds.) **"Neuropsychiatric Aspects of Vitamin Deficiency States,** Textbook of Neuropsychiatry. Washington DC: American Psychiatric Press, Inc., 1987. (Chapter 18, pp.327-338).

WEEK 46 Neurobehavioral Aspects of Movement Disorder

79. Cummings, J.L., **"Neuropsychiatric Aspects of Movement Disorders,"** Clinical Neuropsychiatry. Orlando: Grune & Stratton, Inc., 1985. (Chapter 12, pp. 140-162).

WEEK 47 Neuropsychiatric Aspects of Inflamatory and Infectious Disease

80. Hall, R. C.W. and Stickney, S. K., **"Medical And Psychiatric Features of Systemic Lupus Erythematosus"**, Psychiatric Medicine, Vol. 1, No. 3, 1984, pp. 287-301.

81. Ling, M.H.M. et al, **"Side Effects of Corticosteroid Therapy,"** Archives of General Psychiatry, Vol. 38, April 1981, pp. 471-477.

82. Hales, R.E. & Yudofsky, S.C. (eds.) **"Neuropsychiatric Aspects of Infectious and Inflammatory Diseases of the Central Nervous System"**, Textbook of Neuropsychiatry. Washington DC: American Psychiatric Press, Inc., 1987. (Chapter 19, pp. 339-350).

WEEK 48 Neuropsychiatric Aspects of Endocrine Disease

83. Leigh, H.,M.D. and Kramer, S.I., **"The Psychiatric Manifestations of Endocrine Disease,"** Year Book Medical Publishers, Inc., 1984, pp. 413-u445.

WEEK 49 Neuropsychiatric Aspects of Brain Tumors

84. Hales, R.E. & Yudofsky, S.C. (eds.)**"Neuropsychiatric Aspects of Brain Tumors,** Textbook of Neuropsychiatry. Washington DC: American Psychiatric Press, Inc., 1987. (Chapter 20, pp. 351-364).

APPENDIX 3

UCSF-FRESNO

Psychiatry Residency Training Program
Third-Year Curriculum

EMERGENCY PSYCHIATRY
SEMINAR SCHEDULE
ACADEMIC YEAR 1992-1993

WEEK 1	Introduction to Emergency Psychiatry
WEEK 2	BIOPSYCHOSOCIAL ROUNDS
WEEK 3	Decision Making in Emergency Psychiatry
WEEK 4	BIOPSYCHOSOCIAL ROUNDS
WEEK 5	Assessing Suicidality
WEEK 6	BIOPSYCHOSOCIAL ROUNDS
WEEK 7	What is Organic vs Functional
WEEK 8	BIOPSYCHOSOCIAL ROUNDS
WEEK 9	Violent Patients
WEEK 10	BIOPSYCHOSOCIAL ROUNDS
WEEK 11	Psychodynamics Case Conference
WEEK 12	Psychodynamics Case Conference
WEEK 13	Substance Abuse
WEEK 14	BIOPSYCHOSOCIAL ROUNDS
WEEK 15	Psychodynamics Case Conference
WEEK 16	Psychodynamics Case Conference
WEEK 17	Children
WEEK 18	BIOPSYCHOSOCIAL ROUNDS
WEEK 19	Psychodynamics Case Conference

WEEK 20	Psychodynamics Case Conference
WEEK 21	Forensics in the E.R.
WEEK 22	Psychodynamics Case Conference
WEEK 23	Psychodynamics Case Conference
WEEK 24	BIOPSYCHOSOCIAL ROUNDS
WEEK 25	Geriatrics in the E.R.
WEEK 26	BIOPSYCHOSOCIAL ROUNDS
WEEK 27	Psychodynamics Case Conference
WEEK 28	Psychodynamics Case Conference
WEEK 29	Crisis Intervention
WEEK 30	BIOPSYCHOSOCIAL ROUNDS
WEEK 31	Psychodynamics Case Conference
WEEK 32	Psychodynamics Case Conference
WEEK 33	Mental Retardation
WEEK 34	BIOPSYCHOSOCIAL ROUNDS
WEEK 35	Psychodynamics Case Conference
WEEK 36	Psychodynamics Case Conference
WEEK 37	Amytal Interview
WEEK 38	BIOPSYCHOSOCIAL ROUNDS
WEEK 39	Psychodynamics Case Conference
WEEK 40	Psychodynamics Case Conference
WEEK 41	BIOPSYCHOSOCIAL ROUNDS
WEEK 42	Psychodynamics Case Conference
WEEK 43	Psychodynamics Case Conference
WEEK 44	E.R. Research
WEEK 45	BIOPSYCHOSOCIAL ROUNDS

WEEK 46 Psychodynamics Case Conference

WEEK 47 Psychodynamics Case Conference

CONSULTATION-LIAISON IN CHILD PSYCHIATRY: CONTINUITY AND CHANGE IN THE PAST DECADE

David A. Fox, M.D.

Department of Developmental and Behavioral Pediatrics
Valley Children's Hospital
Fresno, CA 93703

INTRODUCTION

An analytical study of developments in child psychiatric consultation in the 1980s must take into account changes in the knowledge base of child psychiatry, including psychopathology and expectable development in infants, children, and adolescents, and the changing social, economic, political, and professional contexts in which consultation takes place. Because consultation-liaison work is often at the furthest reach of applications of new research, changes in practice often occur slowly. Conversely, interdisciplinary interaction and cross-fertilization between child psychiatry and pediatrics is a stimulus for change and often provides new models for assessment and treatment. Since child psychiatrists are rarely the sole providers of professional care for a child and family, all types of clinical practice are, in effect, consultative, in nature. The explicitness and design of the consultative relationship, whether planful or unwitting, will be examined in relation to changes on both sides of the professional interchange.

Very few of the changes to be described are well documented; much of the supporting data is anecdotal; and many of the links between sources of change in the environment of consultation practice and actual shifts in practice are inferential. Nevertheless, in this review I will attempt to provide a model of systematic changes and some predictions for the next decade.

SOURCES OF CHANGE IN PEDIATRIC CONSULTATION-LIAISON PRACTICE

The practice of child consultation-liaison psychiatry depends on the application *of* data on diagnostic and interventive strategies *across* a diverse set of pathological circumstances *within* a largely externally determined system of care *by* professionals *with* defined roles and self-definitions. Changes in each of these parameters over the past decade will be explored.

Consultation-Liaison Psychiatry: 1990 and Beyond
Edited by H. Leigh, Plenum Press, New York, 1994

Influential New Research Findings

The impact of a decade of research on mother-infant interaction and heightened awareness of the sensitivity of infants to the affective state of their primary caretaker (Tronick,1983; Greenspan, 1981) has influenced the human environment of Neonatal Intensive Care units and to a lesser extent care in hospital nursery units. Efforts to identify and intervene with severely impaired parents of newborns are frequently built into the program design of such units. Similarly, understanding of the development of attachment behaviors (Ainsworth et al, 1978; Bowlby, J.,1969) has lead to earlier efforts to promote parental care of compromised infants. The demonstration of infant sensory and autoregulatory characteristics to their parents has proven a powerful tool in facilitating early interaction (Brazelton,1973).

Research on individual differences in temperament (Thomas et al, 1963; Carey, 1970) and coping styles (Murphy and Moriarty, 1976; Murphy, 1981) have taken much longer to be integrated into consultation-liaison practice. New understandings of cognitive and language development (Yates, 1991; Baker and Cantwell, 1991) have more frequently been translated into clinical practice by pediatric psychologists and behavioral pediatricians than by child psychiatrists.

Changes in the social environment and new understandings of traumatizing situations have played a major role in shaping the in-patient and out-patient consultative situations during the 1980s. The pioneering studies of Terr (1979, 1981, 1983) and Pynoos (Pynoos and Eth, 1986; Pynoos et al, 1987) have quickly been translated into assessment and interventive efforts in multiple types of acute and chronic trauma. Awareness of the frequency of physical and sexual abuse of children and adolescents has altered the approach of teachers, pediatricians and their child psychiatrist consultants to a wide variety of symptom presentations (Browne and Finklehor, 1986; Green, 1978c; Brant and Tisza, 1977; Yates, 1982; McLeer et al, 1988).

The comprehensive exploration of children's reaction to parental separation and divorce by Wallerstein and her colleagues (Wallerstein and Corbin, 1991) has provided a framework for examining the complex interactions between parental and child stress, applicable to family disruption, chronic illness, and developmental disorders. The exposition of findings of these studies in non-professional literature and electronic media has changed the consultative interaction in many instances. Families and consultants are more likely to begin their interaction with a shared and more sophisticated frame of reference about family dynamics than in the past.

Research findings in childhood psychopharmacology have played a significantly lesser role in consultative practice than have comparable findings in adults. Because of stringent restrictions on research with children and the greater difficulty of carrying out psychopharmacological research in children, studies are more likely to be open clinical trials with small numbers of children. As a result the development of clinical consensus regarding drug treatment is slow. With a few exceptions, clinical research with children has been an extension of adult studies. The prime exception to this trend is the series of studies on the effects of clonidine on Giles de la Tourette syndrome and hyperactivity (Hunt et al, 1985; Cohen et al, 1980), the use of naltrexone in autistic children (Campbell et al, 1989), and the application of tricyclic antidepressants to attentional disorders (Garfinkle et al, 1983).

Several other developments in pediatric psychopharmacology have begun to have an effect on consultative practice. The clarification of bipolar illness in childhood and use of lithium and carbamazine (Meltzer,1987; Green,1991) has allowed many severely ill children to remain in community settings. The rapid introduction of clomipramine has testified to its dramatic clinical effectiveness in obsessive compulsive disorders in childhood (Flament et al,1985).

Research in psychotherapy has played a relatively minor role in influencing new directions of child and adolescent psychiatric consultation. Recent reviews of individual psycho-therapy and play therapy with children (Lewis, 1991; Coppolillo, 1991) indicate that the pace of research in these areas is disappointingly slow. Of studies reviewed by Lewis only 23 of 68 were published in the previous decade. In Coppolillo's review only 3 of 22 studies cited were published in the 1980s. While the pace of development in cognitive and behavior therapy has been greater, much of the expertise in these areas has been developed by child psychologists and behavioral pediatricians rather than child psychiatrists.

Developments in family and group therapy have played a significantly larger role in both in-patient and out-patient settings, especially in relation to chronic illness, psychosomatic disorders, post-traumatic syndromes, and substance abuse. New models of treatment have been defined, techniques clarified, and the range of application extended (Reiss, 1981; Minuchin and Fishman, 1981; Wallerstein and Kelly, 1980; Stanton et al, 1982; Green, 1978c; Cramer-Azima, 1991).

Effects Of Changing Psychopathology

Many of the changes in consultative practice in children and adolescents have been the result of significant shifts in individual, family, and social pathology. The increasing incidence of some types of traumatizing events has lead to clearer syndrome definition and recognition, and has been a spur to the development of new strategies of intervention. Many of these changes are substantially interconnected, often in complex relationships, and the symptomatic presentation of children and adolescents as well as family resources for treatment are multiply affected. Among these changes in family and social systems, which includes increases in poverty in families with young children, physical and sexual abuse, family dissolution, exposure to family violence, exposure to community violence, children being reared by someone other than their parents, pre-natal risks and low birth weight, and AIDS, the far-reaching impact of substance abuse casts a long shadow.

In inner city populations of children and adolescents it has become increasingly rare in the past decade for substance abuse not to be incurred as a primary or secondary consideration in psychiatric consultations. The effects of prenatal drug exposure on prematurity, low birth-weight, pre-natal addiction, cognitive impairment, hyperactivity, and behavioral pathologies have become dramatically prominent. Throughout their development these children are more likely to be seen for consultation within the health care, educational, foster care, and judicial systems (Zagar et al,1989).

Low birth-weight infants with prolonged NICU stays or AIDS have added risks of parental abandonment before release from the hospital, and much higher risk of subsequent abandonment to either extended family or the social service system. Perinatal risks are also increased by the decreased frequency of prenatal care by substance abusing mothers. While community educational efforts have had an impact on reducing substance abuse during pregnancy, relapse of drug abuse occurs post-natally, increasing the risk of parental abuse and abandonment. Infants who are temperamentally difficult (irritable, irregular in biological rhythms, negative in interpersonal interactions, highly intense, or under-responsive) as a result of prenatal drug exposure are likely to overwhelm the coping capacities of marginal parents, leading to increased incidence of family dissolution via child abuse, spousal abuse, and parental substance abuse.

Continuing substance abuse in parents results in a series of inter-related effects on childhood and adolescent psychopathology presenting for consultation. Over the course of the past decade an increasing number of children are being reared by grandparents, other family members, or foster or adoptive parents because of parental substance abuse. Many of these children are grieving in complex ways over the loss of a highly ambivalent relationship with parents. Those that remain in their families of origin are exposed to episodic and inconsistent parenting,multiple and unstable adult relationships, models of illegal or criminal behavior and substance abuse, family violence and sexual abuse, and risk of parental death. These children frequently present with early onset substance abuse, delinquency, depression, school failure, or non-compliance with medical care (Sirles et al, 1989). Adolescents from this group exhibit substance dependence, gang affiliations, violent behavior, self-destructive sexual activity, recurrent victimization, prolonged absence from home and school, suicide attempts, delinquency, and profound hopelessness about the future, preventing any positive investment in productive pursuits (Lewis et all, 1989). The consultant is faced with the task of providing this population with both appropriate and feasible long-term interventions, which may be mutually exclusive.

The greatly increased number of children living in poverty during the past decade has significantly amplified the impact of decreases in publicly funded mental health services, which will be addressed subsequently. Access to care is further impeded by competition for limited family resources, including transportation, parental time and emotional energy, and by alienation and disaffection from institutions of health care. Despite the intent of the Medicaid program, private sector mental health services remain beyond the reach of most poor families. Poverty limits the ability of parents to remove their children from physically and socially toxic and dangerous environments, so that multiple traumatization becomes increasingly frequent in clinical presentations. Limited access to community cultural and educational resources restricts opportunities to ameliorate pathogenic influences, so that children presenting for consultation have many fewer internal and external models of coping and creative positive adaptation. As a result the ability of the consultant to design and implement strategic interventions is compromised. Nowhere is this seen as dramatically as in children from homeless families.

A significant source of poverty in children which continued to increase over the past ten years is family separation and divorce. More than 25% of children in divorced families experience a substantial fall in economic status (Wallerstein and Corbin, 1991). Children of divorce are much more likely to present for psychiatric consultation in both in-patient and out-patient settings. Consultants are frequently faced with extremely complex family constellations in which previous tensions are inflamed by stresses of medical illness, battles over consent and custody erupt, and mutual blaming by divorced parents create a mine field. Psychiatric consultants whose work is based on systems theory often fare best in interfacing between these destructive families and medical personnel. A consequence of the increasing incidence of divorce is the involvement of psychiatric consultants in custody evaluations, in allegations of parental physical and sexual abuse of very young children, and in treatment of the psychopathological consequences of divorce.

Children and adolescents traumatized by violence have become increasingly prevalent during the 1980s (Pynoos and Nader, 1989). Exposure to large amounts of violence on television has become nearly universal, with well-documented effects on personality functioning and ego controls. Children and adolescents in inner city environments have both been direct witnesses of assaults and experienced the loss of friends and family members through violence. Perceived loss of safety and high levels of anxiety frequently result in identification with models of violence and enhance probability of gang affiliation. These identifications often interfere with thorough diagnostic assessment and preclude the formation of treatment alliances.

The spectrum of HIV-related illnesses affecting children and adolescents merits increasing attention. In addition to required consultation skills addressing chronic illness, death, dying, and loss, families with multiple affected members, either by intra-familial transmission or exogenous sources (hemophilia families) pose novel challenges. Codes of silence and secrecy in families as well as negative attitudes from the social environment further complicate consultation. Assisting in the optimal development of infants and children with AIDS, whether or not they are being raised by biological parents, has become a frequent request of child psychiatric consultants (Krener, 1991).

Over the past decade new challenges for the consultant have been presented by the influx of immigrants from non-Western cultures with highly structured traditional belief systems. Areas of the country impacted by Southeast Asian immigration have experienced the interface between diverse cultural and sub-cultural practices and the health care system (Nguyen and Williams, 1989). Consultants require basic knowledge of relevant cultures as well as the ability to work through conflicts with the aid of "cultural brokers" and ethnic community leaders. Child psychiatric consultants are asked to assess patients from recurrently traumatized and stressed families with widely divergent expectations of behavior and of sensory experiences (Kinzie et al, 1989). Families from each culture have distinct and unfamiliar patterns of family control and decision making, often leading to confusion in the negotiating process.

Other new patient populations for the child psychiatric consultant stem from advances in pediatric health care: long-term cancer survivors, adolescents and young adults with cystic fibrosis, transplant donors and recipients, and developmentally compromised survivors of extremely low birth weight. Each of these groups presents unique issues, but they have in common a history of prolonged intensive medical intervention, long-term uncertainties about outcome, family separations and profound alterations in the self-image of patients and family members. Families find themselves terrified and confused and at times narcissistically gratified to be at the forefront of new technology. They are often overwhelmed and disorganized by becoming newsworthy, or as a result of efforts to raise funds for medical care which frequently exceed the life-time earnings of parents. Psychiatric consultants in these arenas frequently make use of liaison work not only to benefit the milieu of specialized units, but also to keep abreast of treatment innovations, technical language, and treatment philosophies (Fritz, 1990).

Effects of Changes in Funding and Service Delivery Models

Changing patterns of reimbursement for medical and psychiatric services over the past decade have had an important effect on patterns of care in the public and private sectors. Institutional changes in case management, benefit regulation, ownership of hospitals, self-contained health care systems, and the virtual disappearance of a two-party model of treatment (Rafferty, 1991) have affected psychiatric consultation-liaison psychiatry with children and adolescents much more profoundly than has the impact of research or changes in clinical populations during this period. As in other areas of psychiatry, child psychiatrist's roles have been predominantly reactive rather than initiating. Many consultants have experienced the rapid pace of change with dismay and loss of sense of personal power.

In the early 1980s one of the first casualties of the changing health care environment was the continuity of relationship between the child, family, and primary care physician. As plans, groups, and organizations developed, flourished, and sometimes died, families discovered that cherished long-term relationships were severed, often unexpectedly and involuntarily. Child psychiatrists, as sub-specialists, were frequently exempted from the first round of organizational shifts, but stable coordinated-care relationships were disrupted and consultations were often precipitated by the family's loss of accustomed support. Over the past five years, the same organizational trends in private sector health care have expanded to include the subspecialist consultants, resulting in a second disruption of consultative relationships and of ongoing psychotherapy.

In the mid-1980s the explosive growth of for-profit corporate chain MacHospitals, with pre-printed treatment plan menus and large advertizing budgets, took advantage of generous funding of inpatient psychiatric and chemical dependency benefits for adolescents. Aggressive marketing and fast-track admission procedures resulted in increased rates of admission, diversions (often appropriate) of adolescents from the juvenile justice system, and the medicalization of family conflict. In response to the rapid cost escalation which ensued, managed care developed as a countervailing force, limiting admissions and decreasing lengths of stay. Lack of flexibility for funding of a full range of treatment alternatives (partial hospitalization, day treatment, residential treatment, placement in psychiatric and psychological level group homes, intensive out-patient treatment) paradoxically contributed to increasing length of hospital stays, and shifting of resources from out-patient to in-patient services. Recruitment by the for-profit hospital chains added to the discrepancy between needs and resources through the movement of child psychiatrists away from academic and public settings.

There have been positive consequences of the development of the for-profit hospital networks for child and adolescent psychiatry. Standards of care improved in some areas of the country. Public awareness of mental health issues and possibilities of treatment were increased. Well-funded educational programs have benefitted the mental health community and contributed to enhanced communication between child psychiatrists and other mental health professionals. Communication among professionals in widely separated geographical areas has been stimulated. Several models of collaboration between academic centers and for-profit hospitals have contributed to the training of psychiatry residents and child psychiatry fellows.

Parallel developments during the past decade in community mental health systems, in self-contained health maintenance organizations, and in managed-care capitated or indemnity-based psychological and psychiatric services, have resulted in a remarkable convergence on models of short-term, crisis-oriented psychiatric treatment with increased reliance on group therapy, behavioral management and psychopharmacologic interventions in all three systems. In response to these pressures, subtle degradations of clinical data, such as accentuating extent of pathology, overstating degree of suicidality until day of discharge, and shifts among diagnostic possibilities to those most likely to be reimbursed began to occur. Positive changes, such as greater clarity and definition of problem areas and treatment plans, earlier consideration of discharge plans, and more rapid coordination of services also eventuated, although the influence of the JCAHO Consolidated Standards in this regard was considerable. Similar effects have also occurred in out-patient consultation settings, including questionable shifts in diagnoses, disrupted referral relationships, briefer treatments, and fourth-party clinical decision making. One of the major detriments resulting from these changes has been a growing sense of powerlessness and insecurity in patient families, precisely the problem for which consultation was sought in the first place. Positive effects have also been noted, including more frequent and more focussed communication between consultants and primary care physicians.

Psychiatric consultative services to community-based institutions (schools, juvenile halls, preschool programs, special educational programs, group residential treatment facilities) have followed a biphasic pattern over the past decade, initially being marked by rapid expansion in the types and quantity of services available, followed by decrease in services because of uncertain funding of psychiatrists and other mental health providers. Ordinarily service cutbacks in community consultation settings would lead to decreased access to services, related to inconvenience, difficulties in communication with consultants in centralized secondary or tertiary care centers, and ambivalence by patients and families. In the current fiscal climate, access is further limited by waiting lists and service limitations, which discourage all but the most desperate.

Effects of Shifts in Professional Roles

Many recent changes in the function of child psychiatric consultants have resulted from shifts in role definition within mental health professionals and the emergence of new disciplines. The rapid increase in numbers of non-psychiatrist therapists and the re-medicalization of child psychiatrists have served to move child psychiatrists more clearly into the role of diagnosticians, consultants, and experts in child psychopharmacology. This trend has been further reinforced by the slow growth rate in numbers of child psychiatrists and the decreasing proportion of direct treatment services provided by them. In many areas psychiatric services to children are implemented by general psychiatrists with limited child psychiatric training.

Over the past five years in-patient psychiatric settings have been strongly effected by the results of Capp vs. Rank litigation in California and corresponding legislation in other states confirming psychologists as attending clinicians. Because this development took place at a time of expanding in-patient care, this transition took place relatively peacefully. In out-patient practice there has been a movement towards the formation of tri-partite practice groups (psychiatrist, psychologist, social worker), once the hallmark of the child guidance clinic. Larger groups based on the same model have developed to provide contractual services, either on fee-for-service or capitated basis.

The decades-long tension between child psychiatry and pediatrics (Kanner, 1937; Eisenberg, 1967; Anders, 1977; Fritz and Bergman, 1985; Work, 1989) has given birth to new disciplines of medical child psychology, with emphasis on behavior management, non-pharmacologic pain control, cognitive therapies, biofeedback, and hypnosis, and to behavioral pediatrics, which has focussed on the assessment and treatment of developmental crises, temperamental mismatch between children and parents, disorders of feeding, sleep, and elimination, learning disabilities, failure-to-thrive infants and toddlers, and survivors of high-risk perinatal crises. In several centers successful models of interdisciplinary training, research, and clinical practice have emerged, which have also contributed to the education of general psychiatrists and pediatricians (Fritz and Bergman, 1984).

RESULTANT DIRECTIONS OF CHANGE IN PEDIATRIC CONSULTATION-LIAISON PSYCHIATRY

The subsequent sections of this review will integrate the results of the multi-faceted influences on consultation-liaison psychiatry during the past decade, describe current models of education, research, and practice, define critical problem areas, and abstract implications for future development.

Pediatric Hospital Settings

The changing nature of the pediatric hospital environment has placed greater and more diversified demands on the child psychiatry consultant. Along with long-standing problems of role definition and status within the hospital community (Lewis and Vitulano, 1988), the consultant has to further define his or her role with respect to other mental health professionals and provide a clear delineation of expertise. Decreased lengths of stay and pressures for expedited discharge increase the demand for prompt evaluation and definitive intervention, especially in the face of declining external resources for referral and follow-up. Greater sensitivity to the systems aspect of consultation, understanding of the dynamics of the work- and life-space of pediatricians and pediatric residents, comprehension of the home environment of patients and their families, and above all, clarity in communication about the clinical situation, the family, school, and social environment, are all essential for the development and maintenance of a successful consultative relationship. Models of clear communication (Hamburg, 1987) have been helpful in this regard, especially for residents and fellows in a teaching hospital. Honest assessment of the resistance of child psychiatrists to solving problems in the consultative relationship (Lewis and Vitulano, 1988) may lead to a reduction in the vast number of pediatric inpatients with psychiatric disorders who do not receive psychiatric services.

The most critical, and often most neglected, step in the consultative process in child psychiatry is the preparation of the family for the consultation. Although time consuming for both the pediatrician and the psychiatrist and easily by-passed in the rush to assess the clinical situation, the outcome of the consultative intervention is largely determined at this stage. Unlike the situation in adult psychiatric consultation where the decision to involve the family is a possible outcome of an initial consultation, in child psychiatry the prior involvement of the parents and the working through of their understanding of the child's illness and possible resistances to psychiatric consultation must precede contact with the pediatric patient. A model of careful preparation, including a family conference with the pediatrician and a joint meeting of the pediatrician, psychiatric consultant, and parents has been delineated by Hodas and Honig (1983). Following such a model greatly increases the probability that a consultation will ultimately result in positive clinical results rather than being restricted to a greater understanding of the problem by the professional team. When combined with timely feedback to the pediatrician about immediate and long-term recommendations and outcome of interventions, a positive feedback circuit develops between consultant and consultee.

Out of successful consultative relationships come the opportunities for informal or formal liaison functions, including shared attention to clinical process and system effects, mutual support, development of clinical investigations, enhancement of administrative and clinical support services, and sharing of educational and training responsibilities. Pediatricians are more likely to be convinced of the value of psychiatric consultation-liaison services by personal experience rather than research data. The demonstration of effectiveness of psychiatric services in pediatric inpatient settings in cost reduction, decreased length of stay, and better clinical outcome awaits future research (Shugart, 1991).

Pediatric Out-Patient Settings

While in-patient consultation-liaison efforts have often suffered from repetitiveness, fatigue, stagnation, and burn-out, out-patient services have frequently been overwhelmed by the rapid pace of change over the past decade, driven largely by revolutions in health care finance and service delivery. Capitated systems provide disincentives for psychiatric referral if there is no corresponding reduction in costs for diagnostic studies or decrease in utilization of primary care providers. An increasing proportion of consultations are generated by family request rather than pediatrician initiation. Referrals continue to be generated, of course, by unexplained complaints following extensive work-ups, physician frustration over unsolvable problems, "obvious" psychiatric symptoms, and pressure from schools.

Pediatricians continue to have very high thresholds for recognition of psychopathology, failing to identify 50-80% of behavioral and emotional problems (Costello et al, 1988a). Children with high frequency of illness and service utilization are much more likely to be identified as disturbed (Costello et al, 1988b), and to be referred for psychiatric consultation. Disruptions to the continuity of primary pediatric care occasioned by health care system changes have a bidirectional effect on referrals for consultation. "Less obvious" symptoms are less likely to be noted or seen as significant, but the primary care provider also has access to a much diminished data base from which to plan interventions should he or she wish to undertake them without referral.

In hospital out-patient settings, various models of shared care between child psychiatrists, child psychologists, behavioral pediatricians, and other subspecialists have continued to evolve. The least complex, but also the least time-demanding format includes easy mutual access to medical records and low barriers to inter-clinic referral. The next higher level of involvement entails the presence of psychiatric consultants in other subspecialty clinics (Eisenhauer and Woody, 1989). Joint clinics with co-equal administrative responsibility provide the highest level of collaboration, but are highly dependent on the mutual respect and personal relationships of the subspecialists (Sturge, 1989). There is evidence that child psychiatrists who have had previous pediatric training function more effectively in each of these consultation settings (Fritz and Bergman, 1984). Consultative work is obviously enhanced by the availability in these settings of translators, developmental specialists, educational specialists, and clinicians with expertise with sub-cultural groups.

Community Settings

With the regression in political and financial enthusiasm for community mental health, child psychiatrists find themselves less often involved in community settings. Nevertheless, consultant relationships with schools, juvenile justice facilities, group homes and residential treatment facilities, day care centers and social service agencies have continued to be a significant part of child psychiatry training and practice. Comprehensive consultation and treatment services in community settings are most often found in teaching programs. The model outside of residency and fellowship training is most commonly for child psychiatrists to provide medication consultations, and sometimes diagnostic evaluations, in these settings, while non-psychiatrists provide the majority of assessments, individual and group treatment, and consultation to staff. Currently, child psychiatrists are proportionately represented in forensic evaluations regarding child custody and abuse issues.

Integrated Models of Consultation

Sturge (1989) has proposed an analysis of child psychiatric consultation which is elegant in its heuristic simplicity. He suggests that referrals be designated as requests for a) an opinion or assessment; b) a consultation, with continued primary responsibility held by the pediatrician; c) joint work, with mutual responsibility and effective ongoing communication; d) parallel work, with independent functioning of each participant; e) handover of care and responsibility. He describes situations best suited to each model, but stresses that the clarification of the model used and the explicit specification of responsibilities among all parties involved is essential for success. He depicts, as do Hodas and Honig (1983), that in an ideal consultation, that the primary physician physically joins the family (literally sitting on their side of the room) at some point during the consultative process to stress that the consultation is to the "system" of patient, parents, and pediatrician.

Fritz (1990) has described an "expanded model" of child psychiatric consultation services currently operating in three medical center training institutions. He notes the enthusiastic response of participants in the system, which include an interdisciplinary team of child psychiatrists, child psychologists, neuropsychologist, and pediatric-psychiatric nurses. Referrals are triaged to appropriate team members and are seen in specialty clinics designated for specific problems, inpatient and outpatient mobile consultations, a outpatient general psychiatric clinic coordinated with other pediatric subspecialities, primary medical management by child psychiatrists of psychologically complicated cases, and an inpatient psychiatric unit. Although this model demands high levels of resource commitment, leadership, and a sophisticated tertiary care setting, Fritz has found that there are significant financial and training benefits in comparison with more traditional consultation-liaison services.

CONCLUSION

Several familiar conclusions emerge from this review: the research base in child psychiatry remains sorely inadequate; clinical resources are extremely insufficient to meet demonstrated need; funding is highly inadequate even when services are otherwise available; subpopulations with the greatest need, trauma, and disability often have the fewest resources available; consultants are required to possess an extraordinary range of skills to function effectively; successful consultation is as dependent on attention to communication as it is to knowledge of psychopathology; changes in illness patterns and medical technology tend to steer the direction of consultative activities; and that broader social and political issues must be addressed on a continuing basis. It appears that the most effective model of consultative practice requires leadership, organization, clarity, and initiative, rather than the more traditional reactive responsiveness and passivity of consultation-liaison services.

Psychiatric consultation-liaison services have for too long had the image of "preaching in the wilderness", bringing to non-psychiatrist physicians often unwelcome messages about unconscious process, psychodynamics, interpersonal and system factors in medical care, and the need for attention to feelings. Despite the fatigue of the messengers, the message has gotten through. Child psychiatrists are no longer isolated in their attention to factors other than pathophysiology. In collaboration with other child mental health and developmental specialists cost-effective assessments and interventions are possible. The medicalization of child psychiatry and maturing of the identity of child psychiatrists has made *apartheid* obsolete as a model of development. Collaborative clinical practice, training, and research are likely to be more productive.

REFERENCES

Ainsworth,M. et al, 1978, "Patterns of Attachment: A Psychological Study of the Strange Situation". Laurence Earlbaum, Hillsdale, NJ.

Anders, T., 1977, Child psychiatry and pediatrics: the state of the relationship, *Pediatrics*, 60:616-620.

Baker,L. Cantwell,D.,1991, The development of speech and language, *in* "Child and Adolescent Psychiatry" M. Lewis,ed., Williams and Wilkens, Baltimore.

Bowlby,J., 1969, "Attachment and Loss, Vol. 1, Attachment". Basic Books, New York.

Brant, R. and Tisza, V., 1977, The sexually misused child. *Am. J. Orthopsychiatry* 47:80-90.

Brazelton,T.B., 1973, "Neonatal Behavioral Assessment Scale". (Clinics in Developmental Medicine, no.50). JP Lippencott, Philadelphia.

Brown, A. and Finkelhor, D., 1986, Impact of child sexual abuse: a review of the research, *Psychological Bulletin*, 99:66-77.

Campbell, M. et al, 1989, Naltrexone in autistic children:An acute open dose range tolerance trial, *J. Am. Acad. Child Adolesc. Psychiatry* 28:200-206.

Carey,W.B.,1970, A simplified method for measuring infant temperament. *J. Pediatr.* 77:188-194.

Cohen, D. et al, 1980, Clonidine ameliorates Giles de la Tourette syndrome, *Arch. Gen. Psychiatry* 37:1350-1357.

Coppolillo, H.,1991, The use of play in psychodynamic psychotherapy, *in* "Child and Adolescent Psychiatry", M. Lewis, ed., Williams and Wilkins, Baltimore.

Costello, E. et al, 1988a, Psychopathology in pediatric primary care: the new hidden morbidity, *Pediatrics*, 82:415-424.

Costello, E. et al, 1988b, Service utilization and psychiatric diagnosis in pediatric primary care: the role of the gatekeeper, *Pediatrics*, 82:435-441.

Cramer-Azima, F., 1991, Group psychotherapy for children and adolescents, *in* "Child and Adolescent Psychiatry", M. Lewis, ed., Williams and Wilkins, Baltimore.

Eisenberg, L., 1967, The relationship between psychiatry and pediatrics:a disputatious view, *Pediatrics*, 39:645-647.

Eisenhauer, G. and Woody, R., 1989, Child neurology and child psychiatry: current and future interfaces, *Psychosomatics,* 30:332-336.

Flament, M. et al,1985, Clomipramine treatment of childhood obsessive-compulsive disroder: A double-blind controlled study, *Arch. Gen. Psychiatry* 42:977-983.

Fritz, G., 1990, Consultation-liaison in child psychiatry and the evolution of pediatric psychiatry, *Psychosomatics*, 31:85-90.

Fritz, G. and Bergman, A., 1984, Consultation-liaison training for child psychiatrists: results of a survey, *General Hospital Psychiatry*, 6:24-29.

Fritz, G. and Bergman, A., 1985, Child psychiatrists seen through pediatricians eyes: results of a national survey, *J. Am. Acad. Child Psychiatry,* 24:81-86.

Garfinkle, B. et al, 1983, Tricyclic antidepressant and methylphenidate treatment of attention deficit disorder in children, *J. Am. Acad. Child Psychiatry* 22:343-352.

Green, A., 1978a, Psychopathology of abused chldren. *J. Am. Acad. Child Psychiatry* 17:92-97.

Green, A., 1978b, Self-destructive behavior in battered children. *Am. J. Psychiatry* 135:579-582.

Green, A., 1978c, Psychiatric treatment of abused children, *J. Am. Acad. Child Psychiatry*, 17:356-371.

Green, W., 1991, Principles of psychoparmacotherapy and specific drug treatments, *in* "Child and Adolescent Psychiatry" M. Lewis,ed., Williams and Wilkins, Baltimore.

Greenspan, S., 1981, "Psychopathology and Adaptation in Infancy and Early Childhood". International Universities Press, New York.

Hamburg, B., 1987, Consultation-liaison psychiatry, *Bull. N.Y. Acad. Med.*, 63:376-384.

Hodas, G. and Honig, P., 1983, An approach to psychiatric referrals in pediatric patients, *Clinical Pediatrics,* 22:167-172.

Hunt, R. et al,1985, Clonidine benefits chldren with attention deficit disorder and hyperactivity: Report of a double-blind placebo-crossover therapeutic trial, *J. Am. Acad. Child Psychiatry* 24:617-629

Kanner, L., 1937, The development and present status of psychiatry in pediatrics, *J. Pediatr.*, 11:418-435.

Kinzie, J., 1989, A three-year follow-up of Cambodian young people traumatized as children, *J. Am. Acad. Child Adolesc. Psychiatry*, 28:501-504.

Krener, P., 1991, HIV-spectrum disease, *in* "Child and Adolescent Psychiatry", M. Lewis, ed., Williams and Wilkins, Baltimore.

Lewis, D. et al, 1989, Toward a theory of the genesis of violence: a follow-up study of delinquents, *J. Am. Acad. Child Adolesc. Psychiatry*, 28:431-436.

Lewis, M.,1991, Intensive individual psychodynamic psychotherapy: the therapeutic relationship and the technique of interpretation, *in* "Child and Adolescent Psychiatry", M. Lewis, ed., Williams and Wilkins, Baltimore.

Lewis, M. and Vitulano, L., 1988, Child and adolescent psychiatry consultation-liaison services in pediatrics: what messages are being conveyed, *J. Devel. Behav. Pediatrics*, 9:388-390.

McLeer, S. et al, 1988, Post-traumatic stress disorder in sexually abused children. *J. Am. Acad. Child Adolesc. Psychiatry* 27:650-654.

Meltzer, H. (ed.), 1987, " Psychopharmacology: The Third Generation of Progress", Raven Press, New York.

Minuchin, S. and Fishman, C., 1981, "Family Therapy Techniques", Harvard University Press, Cambridge.

Murphy, L., Moriarty, A., 1976, "Vulnerability, Coping, and Growth". Yale University Press, New Haven.

Murphy, L., 1981, Explorations in Child Personality, *in* A. Robins et al (eds.) "Further Explorations in Personality. International Universities Press, New York.

Nguyen, N. and Williams, H., 1989, Transition from East to West: Vietnamese adolescents and their parents, *J. Am. Acad. Child Adolesc. Psychiatry*, 28:505-515.

Pynoos, R. et al, 1987, Life threat and post-traumatic stress in school age chldren. *Arch Gen. Psychiatry* 44:1057-1063.

Pynoos, R., and Eth, S., 1986, Witness to violence: the child interview. *J. Am. Acad. Child Adolesc. Psychiatry* 25:306-319.

Pynoos, R. and Nader, K., 1989, Children's memory and proximity to violence, *J. Am. Acad. Child Adolesc. Psychiatry*, 28:236-241.

Rafferty, F., 1991, Effects of health delivery systems on child and adolescent mental health care, *in* "Child and Adolescent Psychiatry", M. Lewis, ed., Williams and Wilkins, Baltimore.

Reiss, D., 1981, "The Familiy's Construction of Reality", Harvard University Press, Cambridge.

Shugart, M., 1991, Child psychiatry consultations to pediatric inpatients: a literature review, *General Hospital Psychiatry*, 13:325-336.

Sirles, E. et al, 1989, Psychiatric status of intrafamilial child sexual abuse victims, *J. Am. Acad. Child Adolesc. Psychiatry*, 28:225-229.

Stanton, M. et al, 1982, " The Family Therapy of Drug Abuse and Addiction", Guilford Press, New York.

Sturge, J., 1989, Joint work in paediatics: a child psychiatry perspective, *Archives of Disease in Childhood*, 64:155-158.

Terr, L.,1979, Children of Chowchilla. *Psychoanal. Study Child* 34:547-623,1979.

Terr, L.,1981, "Forbidden Games": Post-traumatic child's play. *J. Am. Acad. Child Psychiatry* 20:740-759.

Terr, L.,1983, Chowchilla revisited. *Am. J. Psychiatry* 140:1543-1550.

Thomas, A. et al,1963, "Behavioral Individuality in Early Childhood". New York University Press, New York.

Tronick, E. (ed.), 1983, "The Development of Human Communication and the Joint Regulation of Behavior". University Park Press, Baltimore.

Vallerstein, J. and Corbin, S., 1991, The child and the vicissitudes of divorce. *in* "Child and Adolescent Psychiatry" M. Lewis,ed., Williams and Wilkins, Baltimore.

Vallerstein, J. and Kelly, J., 1980, "Surviving the Breakup", Basic Books, New York.

Vork, H., 1989, The "menace of psychiatry" revisted: the evolving relationship between pediatrics and child psychiatry, *Psychosomatics*, 30:86-93.

'ates, A., 1982, Children eroticized by incest, *Am. J. Psychiatry*, 139:482-485.

'ates, T.,1991, Theories of Cognitive Development, *in* "Child and Adolescent Psychiatry" M. Lewis,ed., Williams and Wilkens, Baltimore.

:agar, R. et al, 1989, Developmental and disruptive behavior disorders among delinquents, *J. Am. Acad. Child Adolesc. Psychiatry*, 28:437-440.

CONSULTATION-LIAISON 1980-90 - THE HAWAII EXPERIENCE

Jon Streltzer, M.D.

Professor of Psychiatry
Univeristy of Hawaii at Manoa
John A. Burns School of Medicine

For half a century liaison psychiatry has been promoted as the way to integrate psychiatry into the whole of medicine.[1] Liaison psychiatry could humanize medicine as well as increase its effectiveness and efficiency. Despite numerous citations documenting the effectiveness of liaison psychiatry,[2,3,4] resistance to the approach on the part of physicians, including psychiatrists, has hampered development and remains widespread.[5] Nevertheless, spurred by initiatives from the National Institute of Mental Health, liaison psychiatry made remarkable progress in the 1970's. By 1980 almost all psychiatric residency training programs included consultation-liaison (C-L) in their curriculum.

C-L PSYCHIATRY IN HAWAII: 1980

C-L psychiatry showed great promise in 1980 in Honolulu, Hawaii, just as it did in the rest of the country. Although the sole medical school in the state (University of Hawaii) had no university hospital, the school had progressed out of its infancy and had solid affiliations with the major community hospitals. C-L services were provided at four main teaching hospitals.

For example, a typical liaison was established with a large oncology service. An interdisciplinary team met weekly. Regular rounds were made with housestaff and attending oncologists. A psychiatric resident and senior medical students on elective were assigned to the service.

The most highly developed liaison activity, however, occurred with what may have been the largest hemodialysis and kidney transplant program in the country.[6] The program had over 300 patients. There were several types of dialysis units depending upon the patient's ability to do self care. There was an extensive home dialysis program. Satellite facilities were present on several Hawaiian islands. Patients came from all over the Pacific, covering a geographic area larger than the continental United States. The patients represented a wide range of ethnic and cultural groups reflecting the population of Hawaii and the Pacific islands.

Consultation-Liaison Psychiatry: 1990 and Beyond
Edited by H. Leigh, Plenum Press, New York, 1994

This end-stage renal disease program engaged 10% of my time to develop psychiatric liaison services. I was able to hire a full time psychiatric nurse clinical specialist and take on a psychology graduate student. Two full time social workers completed the liaison team. In addition to providing consultation on request from physicians or nurses, liaison activities permeated all aspects of the program. All new patients were evaluated and assisted in their adjustment to maintenance dialysis. Protocols were developed for all treatment units to manage common events that could psychologically affect patients. For example, special care was given for patients who were transferred from one unit to another in order to facilitate adjustment to the new unit and to cope with the loss of the old, familiar unit. Procedures were in place to manage the effect of a patient death on staff as well as on other patients. All couples learning home dialysis were evaluated and predictions made as to their success with this modality.[7] The teaching nurses were helped to tailor their approaches according to the communication style of their patients. Cultural issues were commonly addressed in this context.[8,9] Special programs were developed for teenage dialysis patients. A men's group and a women's group were conducted focusing on sexual issues. Of course, regular meetings were held with the various nursing units and communication with physicians was continuous through ongoing participation in rounds. Thus, liaison activites were highly developed. Preventive and educational measures permeated the program, and, indeed, the liaison team influenced the structure of the program to create the most positive psychological milieu. Research was well-integrated into the C-L activities and a number of publications resulted.[10-15]

C-L PSYCHIATRY IN HAWAII: 1990

By 1990, however, C-L activities had diminished greatly. Financing issues caused cutbacks in the renal dialysis and transplant program and liaison activities ceased to the point that even psychiatric consultation rarely occurred. The oncology interdisciplinary team lost its funding and the character of oncology services changed. During the 1980's I was appointed training director of the psychiatry residency program and, while I continued to be responsible for resident rotations in C-L psychiatry, I had much less time available to spend on liaison activities. Increased C-L activity did occur when patients with AIDS became identified and there was a new demand for psychiatric consultation. A full-time psychiatrist was hired as part of an AIDS education grant. Services did not develop, however, and the position disappeared.

Other developments have shown more promise. The main teaching hospital has a large outpatient clinic facility designed to serve the indigent. This facility was taken over administratively by the University. This led to the development of new liaison services. A part-time liaison psychiatrist provides services to an HIV clinic and a primary care clinic. Psychiatric residents attend these and other outpatient clinics. A weekly teaching conference involves medical and psychiatric residents and other psychiatric faculty.

NATIONAL TRENDS

Has the Hawaii experience been reflective of national trends? The literature seems to reveal that this is indeed so. Despite the movement toward subspecialty status for C-L psychiatry, the enthusiasm of 1980 has been replaced by a more sober perspective of the opportunities for liaison psychiatry. For example, one recent paper entitled "A very modest proposal for 1990's C/L psychiatry"[16] called for a diminishment of expectations for what C-L psychiatry could accomplish. A remarkably prophetic article by Lipowski in 1979[2] described the great advances of liaison psychiatry of the 1970's, but warned of the great potential for subsequent decline. Lipowski noted that liaison psychiatry had already been through a previous cycle of rapid growth and high expectation followed by a long period of neglect and stagnation.

In order to determine what the literature has actually reflected about changes in consultation-liaison psychiatry from 1980 to 1990, I investigated the extent to which several pertinent topics were being published in selected journals. Articles (not including letters to the editor) focusing on the process of consultation or liaison were counted by searching the subject indexes of three C-L journals (International Journal of Psychiatry in Medicine, General Hospital Psychiatry, and Psychosomatics), and two prominent general psychiatry journals (American Journal of Psychiatry and Archives of General Psychiatry) for the years 1979-81 and 1989-91. Table 1 shows that C-L articles in the general psychiatry journals were quite infrequent in the 1980 period and they became rare in the current period.

Table 1

Articles in General Psychiatry Journals

Topic	1979-1981	1989-1991
C-L	12	4

Table 2 confirms that even within C-L journals, a similar downward trend occurred. Articles focusing on cancer or dialysis were also enumerated and a notable decline in the dialysis articles is present.

Table 2

Articles in C-L Related Journals

Topic	1979-1981	1989-1991
C-L	61	41
Cancer	25	20
Dialysis	17	6

For two C-L journals (International Journal of Psychiatry in Medicine and General Hospital Psychiatry), each article was reviewed and categorized into various subjects. Table 3 demonstrates the current interest in AIDS which was not known to exist in the 1980 era. Depression as a focus has been greatly increased. Articles related to surgery and OB/Gyn have increased substantially while internal medicine (including cardiology) has remained the same. Pain has increased somewhat while eating disorders have dramatically dropped.

Table 3
Articles in C-L Related Journals

Topic	1979-1981	1989-1991
AIDS	0	15
Depression	5	21
Surg/OB/Gyn	6	28
Pain	3	9
Internal Med	17	18
Eating Disorders	15	2

CHANGES IN CONSULTATION ISSUES

Consistent with the trend in literature, in Hawaii consultation activities with surgery have tended to eclipse relationships with medicine. Consultation requests from medicine are more likely to be patients for whom the primary problem may be psychiatric. Consultations from surgery frequently involve patients for whom psychiatric help is desired to further benefit patient care during surgical management. Surgeons appear more amenable to consultation recommendations. Surgeons are more likely to allow the psychiatrists to write orders in the chart. Issues of territoriality do not appear to be a significant concern between surgeons and psychiatrists. Internists, on the other hand, are more likely to feel that they understand the patient's psychology and that their views on psychopharmacology and management of sleep, pain, adjustment to illness, and sometimes even depression are more appropriate than the psychiatric consultant's views. This is in contrast to the older literature which tends to suggest that psychiatry relates much better to internal medicine than surgery.[7]

Many consults, particularly surgical, involve pain management. In contrast to 1980 and before, however, few are now associated with the undertreatment of pain.[8,9] Patient-controlled analgesia[20] has replaced Demerol 50-75 mg every 3-4 hours as the standard post-operative pain order. Surgeons now seem comfortable giving large doses of narcotics. Problems sometimes arise with overtreatment of pain. "Chronic pain" patients, who frequently have either a somatoform pain disorder or a drug dependence problem are able to find physicians who readily prescribe narcotics and benzodiazepines for extended periods. Helping these patients can provide much of the satisfaction in C-L psychiatry.[21]

In recent years the requirements for internal medicine residency training programs have placed new emphasis on the need to provide psychiatric training to their residents. In response the Department of Medicine assigned first year residents one month of psychiatry training. Partly because of lack of faculty resources, the C-L service was unable to accommodate a large number of residents, so a rotation focusing on inpatient and emergency psychiatry was developed. After three years, the medicine residency is being restructured with a new training director and the psychiatry rotation has been dropped. Ultimately, however, such requirements may be necessary to enable C-L psychiatry to flourish with medicine.

New developments in medical education are likely to have a significant impact on liaison activities in Hawaii. The medical school has moved to a radically new way of educating medical students - problem based learning.[22] Courses and lectures have been eliminated. Students learn in small groups. To a great extent, they determine their own learning agenda. The emphasis is on learning how to learn rather than passively receiving large amounts of information. A patient care focus permeates all learning activities, and there is no pure basic science. A biopsychosocial approach is explicit in the problem based learning format. For example, a problem case for a beginning medical student has to do with a woman with breast cancer. The case is designed so that a great deal of anatomy and biochemistry must be learned to understand the case, but the case also incorporates issues involving doctor/patient relationship, emotional response to illness, and family dynamics. Thus areas of concern to C-L psychiatrists are an integral part of the learning of medical students from the beginning.

Grants from the Robert Wood Johnson and Kellogg Foundations are influencing the clinical training of medical students in the same direction. Most of psychiatry is now to be learned in a primary care setting as is much of other specialties of medicine . Issues relevant to C-L psychiatry should readily become much more important than in the past.

In line with these changes, liaison activites are diminishing on inpatient services and expanding in the outpatient medical clinics. These current developments appear to offer new impetus and support for liaison activities. Whether these developments will permeate upward and influence medical and surgical residents and attendings remains to be seen.

REFERENCES

1. Z.J. Lipowski, Consultation-liaison psychiatry at century's end, *Psychosomatics 33*;128-33 (1992).

2. Z.J. Lipowski, Consultation-liaison psychiatry: past failures and new opportunities, *Gen Hosp Psychiatry,* 1: 3-9 (1979).

3. S.J. Levitan, D.S. Kornfeld, Clinical and cost benefits of liaison psychiatry, *Am J Psychiatry* 138: 790-793 (1981).

4. J.J. Strain, J.S. Lyons, J.S. Hammer, et al., Cost offset from a psychiatric consultation-liaison intervention with elderly hip fracture patients, *Am J Psychiatry* 148:144-1049 (1991).

5. M.H. Greenhill, The development of liaison programs, *in:* "Psychiatric Medicine," G. Usdin (ed), Brunner/Mazel, Inc., New York (1977).

6. J. Streltzer, A comprehensive model for providing psychosocial services to dialysis and transplant programs, *Dial Transplant* 13: 92-97 (1984.).

7. J. Streltzer, F. Finkelstein, H. Feigenbaum, et al., The Spouse's Role in Home Hemodialysis. *Archives of Gen Psych*, 33:55-58 (1976).

8. J. Streltzer, "Intercultural Marriages Under Stress: The Effect of Chronic Illness," *in*: Adjustment to Intercultural Marriage, W.S. Tseng, J.F. McDermott, T.W. Maretzki (eds), University Press of Hawaii, Honolulu (1977).

9. J. Streltzer, "Cultural Aspects of Adjustment to End-Stage Renal Disease," *in:* Psychonephrology II, N.B. Levy (ed), Plenum, New York (1983).

10. E.H. Yanagida and J. Streltzer, Limitations of psychological tests in a dialysis population,
Psychosom Med 41:557-567 (1979).

11. E.H. Yanagida, J. Streltzer, and A. Siemsen, Denial in dialysis patients: relationship to compliance and other variables,
Psychosom Med 43:271-280 (1981).

12. J. Streltzer, Sexual functioning in relation to overall psychological adjustment in kidney patients.
Dial Transplant, 10:753-756 (1981).

13. J. Streltzer, Coping with transplant failure: grief vs. denial,
Int J Psychiat Med, 13:97-106 (1983-84).

14. J. Streltzer, Diagnostic and treatment considerations in depressed dialysis patients,
Clin. Exper. Dialysis and Apheresis, 7:257-274 (1983).

15. J. Streltzer, R. Markoff, and B. Yano, Maintenance hemodialysis in patients with severe pre-existing psychiatric disorders,
J Nerv Ment Dis, 164: 414-418 (1977).

16. M.F. Weiner, J. Sadler, B.J. Fenton, et al. A very modest proposal for 1990's C/L psychiatry,
Gen Hosp Psychiatry 11: 231-234 (1989).

17. J.S. Golden, The Surgeon and the psychiatrist: special problems in psychiatric liaison, *in:* "Consultation-Liaison Psychiatry," Robert O. Pasnau, Grune & Stratton, Inc. (eds), New York (1975).

18. J. Streltzer and T.C. Wade, The influence of cultural group on the undertreatment of postoperative pain,
Psychosom Med 43: 397-403 (1981).

19. R.M. Marks and E.J. Sachar, Undertreatment of medical inpatients with narcotic analgesics,
Ann Intern Med 78: 173-181 (1973).

20. X. Sun, T. Quinn, and C. Weisman, Patterns of sedation and analgesia in the postoperative ICU patient,
Chest 101: 1625-32 (1992).

21. J. Streltzer, Treatment of iatrogenic drug dependence in the general hospital,
Gen Hosp Psychiatry, 2: 262-266 (1980).

22. A. Anderson, A conversion to problem-based learning in 15 months, *in*: "The Challenge of Problem-Based Learning," D. Boud and G. Feletti (eds), St. Martins Press, New York (1991).

CONSULTATION - LIAISON FUNDING: ISSUES FOR SERVICE AND TRAINING

James J. Strain, M.D.,[1] George Fulop, M.D.,[1]
and Jeffrey S. Hammer, M.D.[2]

[1]Division of Behavioral Medicine
and Consultation Psychiatry
Mount Sinai School of Medicine
One Gustave L. Levy Place
New York, NY 10029

[2]Brentwood Veterans Affairs Medical Center
UCLA, Los Angeles, California

INTRODUCTION

Methods to pay for both service and training for Consultation-Liaison Psychiatry (C-L), have confronted many obstacles since its inception as a recognized domain in psychiatry in the thirties (1-4). In fact, initial support for the first four university programs came from the Rockefeller Foundation that was intent on establishing psychiatric services within medical schools and teaching hospitals (5). With the development of more acute psychiatric inpatient units in the general hospital, the need for mental health service delivery to nonpsychiatric medical/surgical patients became even more apparent, and fostered the ascendency of the hospital wide psychiatric consultation services (6).

The frequency of psychiatric morbidity in the medical setting is significant. The funding for treating and teaching staff to manage medical and psychiatric comorbidity (PC) has been problematic and remains an obstacle for adequate health care delivery. In fact, fifty four percent of individuals with mental health problems were seen exclusively in the general health ambulatory care setting (7). By 1984 the Epidemiological Catchment Area five site survey by NIMH found that 62% of such individuals were now seen only in medical care settings (8).

The Hospital Cost Utilization Project demonstrated in 1985 that only .2% and .8% of patients were referred to psychiatry in rural non-academic and academic hospitals, respectively (9). Therefore, very few patients with mental illness in the medical setting, and the general hospital are being identified with these disorders, and of those who are, very few are being referred to psychiatry.

Consultation-Liaison Psychiatry: 1990 and Beyond
Edited by H. Leigh, Plenum Press, New York, 1994

Furthermore, Fulop, Strain, Hammer, and Lyons working in two hospitals - Mount Sinai (New York City) and Northwestern (Chicago) reported in 1987 that patients with PC remained in the acute care hospital almost twice as long as those with medical disorders alone (10). And, when the patients were 65 years of age or older, they remained even longer, if they had both medical and psychiatric symptoms. These authors also showed which medical illnesses were more likely to have longer length of hospital stay (LOS), e.g., toxic metabololic morbidities, neoplastic diseases, etc. In addition, they described which psychiatric diagnoses were associated with the longest hospital stay: dementia, affective disorders. Therefore, it was possible to target those medical illnesses which had significant amounts of psychiatric illness, and how this impacted and was associated with prolonged LOS and **increased** use of hospital resources.

Lyons, Hammer, Strain, and Fulop also demonstrated that the sooner the patient with PC was evaluated by psychiatry after admission to the hospital, the sooner they were likely to go home (11). That is, the earlier in the hospitalization the patient was visited by the psychiatrist - the shorter the lag time - the more likely the patient was to leave the hospital earlier. This is known as the "timing variable," or the timing phenomenon: the timing of the consultation is critical to the amount of hospital resources utilized.

Two other historical events are important to enumerate with regard to understanding the background on the funding of C-L psychiatry services. In the early 1970s stimulated by the increasing awareness of the frequency of psychiatric morbidity in the general health sector, the National Institutes of Mental Health (NIMH) Psychiatric Education Branch - under the direction of James Eaton - launched a pivotal support program for the funding of training for psychiatrists and physicians from other disciplines in the mental health care in the general medical setting (12). For the first time substantial funding could be competitively secured through training grant applications that supported faculty and trainees in the assessment and methodology of caring for the psychological needs of the medically ill. Unfortunately, by the 80s these training grants had been phased out.

The concept of cost offset research focusing on the benefits of providing mental health care to those in the general health setting with regard to not only mental health benefits, e.g., the reduction of psychiatric morbidity, but also the financial savings accruing from the reduction in medical costs after subtracting for the costs of the psychiatric intervention, launched a new genre of studies in the mid-seventies (13,14). Third party payers, e.g., New York State Employees Health Insurance Coverage, were also more aware and willing to fund payment for mental health care as a result of these health outcome studies undertaken by Mumford and Schlesinger (15).

NIMH COST OFFSET INITIATIVES

In the 1980s the American Psychiatric Association component on Consultation Psychiatry and primary care established a task force to examine the effectiveness of psychiatric interventions in the medical setting and the cost offset of such interventions. Shortly thereafter, recognizing a dearth in health service delivery research efforts in the C-L field, the NIMH established a series of technical workshops to promote grant submission for this effort. The conceptual framework behind this endeavor was that data describing the improved identification and management of psychiatric morbidity in the medical setting would not only enhance the patient's well being, but provide third party payers with the evidence that an investment in mental health care also enhanced physical status and cost offset effects. Concept proposals were invited and two workshops were held with experts at NIMH to assist in the the development of these complex proposals, which would examine not only the mind, but the body. The other feature of this work was that the general hospital consultation psychiatrist was to "team" up with another specialist: economist, methodologist, primary care specialist, etc. As a result of this initiative ten NIMH grants were awarded to study the phenomena of PC (Table 1).

TABLE 1. NIMH FUNDED STUDIES

1)	Wells:	Medical outcomes study
2)	Levenson:	Psychiatric consultation guided by screening
3)	Katon:	Randomized trial of psychiatric consultation with distressed high utilizers
4)	Katon:	Identification and treatment of depression in the primary care
5)	Smith:	Psychiatric consultation in somatization disorder: a randomized controlled study
6)	Smith:	Effectiveness of short term group therapy for somatization disorder patients
7)	Barsky:	Definition and course of hypochondriasis patients
8)	Barsky:	Associated features and treatment outcome with hypochondriasis patients
9)	Fulop:	Prospective study of psychiatric morbidity in the elderly admitted to an acute care general hospital.
10)	Strain:	Cost offset from a psychiatric liaison intervention with elderly hip fracture patients.

Wells working at the Rand Corporation reported in JAMA that the funtional disability for patients with major depressive disorders was equivalent to that found with diabetes, hypertension, arthritis, cardiac disease, and cancer (16,17): that the functional costs of depressive psychiatric morbidity was of the same magnitude as five of the most common and costly physical disorders in this country (16,17).

Levenson, at the Medical College of Virginia, hypothesized that psychiatric consultation would reduce health care utilization during and after medical hospitalization (18). His method employed a randomized controlled clinical trial of psychiatric consultation. After meeting inclusion criteria, 1541 patients were screened for depression, anxiety, confusion, and pain over a 21 month period. The 741 patients with "high" pathology or pain were divided into baseline and controls (N=232), contemporaneous controls (N=253), and an experimental consultation group (N=256). Levenson's outcome measures included LOS, hospital costs, post hospital psychiatric status, rehospitalization rates, and outpatient medical care use.

This study observed that the consultation patients were seen an average of one time by the psychiatrist, had heterogeneous medical diagnoses/services, and were of heterogeneous ages. Sixty three percent of the consult patients had an organic mental syndrome. After adjusting for disease severity using Disease Staging Clinical Criteria (19), no effect on psychiatric morbidity, hospital use, or post hospital medical care utilization was observed (e.g., depression or anxiety scores, support for completing activities of daily living, emergency room care, physician visits, medications, rehospitalizations, procedures, or the costs or charges for these services). However, concordance by the consultee, to enact the psychiatric recommendations were: recording psychiatric diagnoses in the discharge summary - 47.5%; drug recommendations - 52.4%; and diagnostic procedures - 32.8%.

There are several possible explanations as to why no positive impact was observed from the psychiatric intervention: 1) on the average a single visit by the psychiatrist; 2) heterogeneity of the patients' medical diagnoses and procedures; 3) the lack of concordance by the consultee in following the recommendations of the psychiatrist; 4) a relatively short LOS to begin with; and 5) black and poor patient populations where support networks and economic access were marginal.

Therefore, there may not have been a sufficient psychiatric intervention in a targeted group where it was known an intervention would make a difference - a mental illnesses that could be ameliorated within the parameters of one visit in an acute general hospital setting. The typical inpatient consultation service may be "hitting the ceiling" where the intervention can't make a difference. For example, in many delivery settings the LOS of the mother and newborn is 48 hours or less. It would not be anticipated that a psychiatric consultation intervention would shorten LOS when it was already so attenuated.

Katon et al performed a randomized trial consisting of a psychiatric consultation with distressed high utilizers of medical services (20). This study employed the Diagnostic Instrument Schedule (DIS) on every patient. A 1/2 hour interview of the patient with his/her primary care physician (PCP) was conducted with the conjoined development of a treatment plan for the psychiatric morbidity - depression. Therefore, primary care physicians were provided a conjoined consultation, consultation note, treatment plan, and an article regarding treatment for this kind of patient.

There was no difference between the control and the intervention groups with regard to: change in psychiartric morbidity or in health services utilization. However, the intervention physicians wrote significantly **more** antidepressant prescriptions, and the rate of use of antidepressants remained significantly higher in the second six months period after the intervention. No differences in costs between the control and the intervention groups was observed in health care utilization over a one year followup period.

Several issues may have effected the results that Katon observed. First, the design required that the psychiatrists work through another physician and not do the treatment themselves: in effect the intervention was indirect. Second, there remained the possible need for psychotherapy plus psychopharmacology in this patient group. This would encompass the need for adjunctive interventions, e.g., family, group, rehabilitation, etc. as well as drug treatment. Third, there was only a single consultation to a patient's physician. The presence of psychiatric morbidity in the medically ill may have required a more complex and vigorous intervention. Third, generation studies are currently underway.

Smith et al. examined the effect of a consultation letter on the health outcomes of care provided to somatization patients in a random assignment prospective study (21,22). The patient's physician was advised that their patient met criteria for somatization disorder and treatment recommendations were provided. After a period of one year, a random cohort of the patients were placed in a group therapy program as well (23). One year following the intervention, experimental patients reported greater functional capacity than control patients. The intervention resulted in a $526 reduction in medical and a non-significant $71 increase in psychiatric charges.

Those patients receiving group therapy were observed to have even greater physical well being and reduced costs. In addition to reducing total health care costs by 39%, the consultation letter improved physical functioning in a group of chronically impaired somatizing patients. Group therapy plus a consultation letter resulted in significantly better physical and emotional health in a one-year period during and after group therapy sessions, with a greater improvement in health associated with more group sessions (23).

In another study conducted by Smith, physicians with patients who had 6-12 physical symptoms received consultation with a psychiatrist and recommendations for the treatment of their somatizing patients (23). The patients with this intervention showed significant improvement which remained stable during the year following the intervention. The psychiatric intervention reduced annual medical care charges by $94 (10.7%) reduction in annual cost of care for medical problems.

Fulop has conducted a randomized prospective study of all patients over 65 years of age admitted to the Mount Sinai Hospital during one year (24). Three measures were employed to ascertain psychiatric symptoms and morbidity: the Geriatric Depression Scale (GDS), the Mini Mental State Examination (MMSE) for cognitive dysfunction, the Structured Clinical Interview for the DSM-III-R (SCID) (which also allowed the assessment of anxiety and alcohol disorders). Preliminary data on 475 elderly inpatients revealed that the SCID syndrome/symptoms disorders were:

anxiety symptoms (6 or more)	42.0%
panic disorder	0.2%
bipolar disorder	0.0%
dysthymic disorder	2.3%
major depressive disorder	15.0%
psychotic symptoms	5.0%

GDS scores greater than 10 and MMS values of <24 were observed in 32% and 38%, respectively. The percent of patients with any psychiatric morbidity was 48%. Fulop learned that patients with cognitive impairment stayed 14 in comparison to 10 days (p=<.001) and those with depression 13 versus 10 days (p=<.001). In an earlier report, when the medical illnesses and procedures were examined, arrythmias and GI disturbances in the elderly had no differences in LOS with or without psychiatric morbidity while those undergoing operating room and gastrointestinal procedures did. Therefore, the former in contrast to the latter are examples of patient populations for whom a psychiatric intervention in the general hospital may impact on the LOS and the use of health services resources use and would be a more optimal target for psychiatric consultation intervention.

In fact, the general hospital may serve as a "de facto" (7) mental health center, especially for the elderly patient. The general hospital affords an excellent opportunity to identify, initiate treatment, and begin aftercare for the psychiatric morbidity of the medical/surgical patient. Finally, very few elderly patients - 6% - are referred to the consulting psychiatrist in the general hospital despite the frequent occurrence of psychiatric morbidity (25).

Strain, Hammer, Lyons, et al. building on the findings of Levitan and Kornfeld (26) examined: the consultation rate; identification of psychiatric morbidity; change in psychiatric morbidity following a psychiatric liaison screen intervention; LOS; direct hospital costs; the indirect and direct costs to the patient during hospitalization, e.g., special duty nursing; and, at 6 and 12 weeks after discharge (27). Briefly, all patients over 65 admitted for the acute surgical repair of a hip fracture to two hospitals in separate cities (Mount Sinai Hospital - New York City) and (Northwestern Memorial Hospital - Chicago) were evaluated in a control and experimental year. Northwestern also had a contemporaneous control. During the control year the standard psychiatric consultation was requested by the orthopedic consultee. During the intervention year all patients who consented to the study had mental status screening by the psychiatrist within 48 hours of admission. If they were found to have psychiatric morbidity they were treated by several modalities by the psychiatrist: counseling, psychotherapy, psychotropic medications, group, family, conferences with ward staff, and a weekly multidiscipline conference with all the ward staff: attending orthopedic surgeon, nurse, social worker, rehabilitation therapists, and liaison psychiatrist - ombudsman rounds (28). This intensive multifactorial and multidiscipline intervention was called the **PSYCHIATRIC LIAISON SCREEN INTERVENTION** in contrast to the traditional consultation intervention. The identical psychiatric liaison screen intervention was applied at both teaching hospitals by separate investigators.

Only 10% and 5% of patients were referred by the consultee for psychiatric consultations in the **TRADITIONAL CONSULTATION YEAR** at Mount Sinai and Northwestern, respectively. During the **liaison** screen year 79% and 69% of patients were evaluted as some patients refused to participate in the study.

1. Over 50% of the elderly hip fracture patients in the **liaison** year were observed to have serious psychiatric morbidity, usually cognitive deficits.

2. The patients in the intervention year, in contrast to the base line and the contemporaneous control at Northwestern, went home on the average two days earlier.

3. The patients in the liaison intervention group had significantly less cognitive impairment at discharge at Mount Sinai, and significantly less depression at Northwestern.

4. At six and twelve weeks post discharge the liaison intervention group had fewer rehospitalizations and fewer rehabilitation days than the traditional consultation patients.

5. One could predict at admission on the basis of the mental screening measures whether the patient would have a prolonged LOS.

6. The patients' two day earlier discharge resulted in a savings of $178,000.00 at Mount Sinai and $57,000.00 at Northwestern. The psychiatrist's costs at each hospital were $20,000.00 which could all be offset from national health insurance reimbursement (Medicare).

However, there are many confounds in psychiatric intervention studies in the medical setting including this one which must be taken into account before the investigator is certain that he/she has a finding (29):

1. Effects can be transferred from the intervention ward to the control unit, and therefore the problem of contamination to the contemporaneous control ward in the same hospital.

2. Effects can come from the non psychiatric mental health care workers, e.g., social worker, nurse, etc.

3. The potential case mix may differ in the intervention and control year, e.g., seriousness of illness, socioeconomic status, educational level, age, employment, support/assistance at home, etc.

4. The difficulty in randomizing patients to a control or intervention ward in the acute care general hospital which must keep all of its beds full. The investigator does not have the freedom to admit to one versus the other kind of unit, e.g., a control or an intervention bed.

5. Although there is a need to study psychiatric interventions in different hospitals and in different communities with different funding systems, the institutional differences may account for the differences observed and not the intervention per se.

Psychiatric intervention studies are critically needed to demonstrate the demand for and the effectiveness of psychiatric care of the medically ill. These studies should focus on both psychiatric outcome, becoming less depressed, less anxious, less organic, less behaviorally disturbed, and at the same time address:

1. Does the psychiatric intervention improve mental status?

2. Does psychiatric care of the medically ill reduce the costs of overall medical care?

3. Is there a transfer of costs from the hospital to the ambulatory setting with earlier discharge?

4. Is the patient's functional status (physical status) equal to or better with earlier discharge?

This study has prompted five university hospitals to involve psychiatrists on their orthopedic units for assessment and treatment of the elderly hip fracture patient, and was the critical cost offset data required to support the funding of a consultation - liaison psychiatrist for this illness population. It will be essential for C-L psychiatrists to undertake health services and cost offset studies to demonstrate to hospital administrators, medical/surgical departments, and third party payers the significant advantage of supporting mental health services for the medically ill in the acute care hospital. The Forester, Kornfeld and Fleiss study in a radiology setting is another example (30).

However, the reduction of psychiatric morbidity in and of itself should be sufficient to warrant funding support for C-L training and staffing. It seems an unfair burden that a C-L intervention should also need to demonstrate, in addition, cost offset capability. For example, the reduction of cardiac symptoms with coronary artery bypass graft surgery (CABG) - pain, work and sexual dysfunction - has been demonstrated, but it has not been evaluated from the cost offset perspective - nor was it required to "pass that test" before it was financially supported by third party payors. Another example is that of social work services in the general hospital which are supported by Medicare Part A, and despite their acknowledged benefits, they have not been required to demonstrate cost offset effects from the interventions.

COST OFFSET FROM A HIGH RISK SCREENING SOCIAL SERVICE INTERVENTION

In order to provide psychosocial services to patients in a prompt manner, and to increase the sensitivity of identifying patients who need services, a pilot study was undertaken in a not for profit hospital to examine the benefits of a High Risk Survey program to screen medical/surgical inpatients for social risks (31). Patients were assessed at admission which generated referrals to the Psycho/Social Department of the hospital within 24 hours. Compared with the standard referral screening process in identifying patients at high social risk, the High Risk Survey referrals were able to shorten the time between admission and receiving the psychosocial intervention by 1.2 days, increased the sensitivity of identifying the need for referral by 35%, and shortened the average LOS by 6%.

The reduced LOS as a result of the high risk screening generated a savings of $1,096,802. If this pilot program had been implemented to the entire hospital population, rather than the 47% who participated in the study, the potential savings would have been 3.1 million dollars. This instructive high risk screening program offers an approach similar to the liaison screening intervention described above, and does not rely on the vagaries of the traditional referral consultation methods to the Psycho/Social Departments of the general hospital. Early detection - lag time - and intervention have been related to decreased hospital stay in a previous study (11). The frequency of PC, the need for screening, and the necessity for early intervention are recurring themes in the literature.

INNOVATIVE FUNDING PROPOSALS

A unique and important approach for obtaining fiscal support by "Screening Medicare Patients to Fund C-L Psychiatry" has been described by Koran and the Stanford group (4). Building on the concept of Fulop et al who identified medically ill cohorts in the general hospital who were at high risk for psychiatric comorbidity (10), Koran et al: 1) noted the most frequently encountered DRGs in their hospital, 2) identified those psychiatric complications or comorbidities (PC) which move the patient to a higher paying DRG, 3) calculated the increase in DRG value by including the psychiatric PC, 4) examined the Medicare patients admitted in the previous year, 5) established the value of finding one case, and 6) estimated the prevalence of all the PCs - noting the proportion of cases that will be screened and the sensitivity of the screening procedure.

This DRG screening methodology if implemented, could provide additional Medicare revenue for the hospital (4). The fiscal value of the screening is based upon enhanced DRG reimbursement from Medicare billings for additional service delivery which would in turn cover: 1) the costs of screening, and 2) the delivery of needed services. DRG cohort screening is an important "new" vehicle to not only identify patients with PCs and thereby, hopefully, attenuate psychiatric morbidity, but also to generate additional revenues from fee for services, currently not available for C-L divisions. However, Koran et al caution that the division of C-L "must be prepared to negotiate the distribution between the C-L service and the hospital of the incremental revenue generated by the screening program" (4). Strain et al. have discussed the Stanford model in their commentary: "A new tool for C-L funding: modified DRGs to reflect psychiatric comorbidity" (32).

This important study described above emphasizes the need to restructure the DRG system to take into account PC. To this end, C-L psychiatrists need to establish the frequency of PC and its contribution to the use of health services and their delivery and in which DRG groups.

With regard to cost offset from screening high risk patients for PC, one should also note that LOS may not be the best proxy for costs. In a study conducted at the Mount Sinai Medical Center, Fahs et al. discerned from a psychiatric intervention with elderly hip fracture patients admitted for acute surgical repair, that the most significant differences were noted in costs, but not in hospital charges or in the per diem rates, i.e., simple LOS times per diem calculations (33). By examining all the costs for room and board, laboratory studies, blood products, anesthesiology, etc. it was possible to observe a significant difference, whereas global charges and per diem per se did not significantly differentiate the screening and intervention group from the purely consultation control cohort.

CONSULTATION VERSUS LIAISON SCREEN INTERVENTIONS AND THEIR IMPACT ON FUNDING

An important parameter to enhance funding for C-L services as well as promote patient care in the general hospital is to adapt the liasion screen method for those patients at high risk for PC rather than await consultation which identifies a minimum of such patients. Non psychiatric physicians and nurses currently identify only a small percent of patients in the hospital with PC - less than 6% of the elderly - which means the majority are not cared for, they consume more hospital resources, and at the same time, a significant source of revenue has been overlooked for the C-L division (10). Of course such screening and treatment - when necessary - requires staffing, but billing for the screen/ intervention should provide an important source of revenue for this enterprise. For example, in the hip fracture study the psychiatric intervention and treatment of 142 patients during the intervention year required 282 patient visits, which under Medicare billing would have generated $20,000 - enough to purchase the time of the psychiatrist (who was paid for this study by the research grant).

The findings from the NIMH and other studies have major implications for hospital costs and should influence hospital administrators and departments of psychiatry as to the benefit of having C-L services available. In particular, liaison screen services for the elderly would be cost effective and superior to the conventional consultation methodology to treat PC in the general hospital. Such protocols for screening would: 1) have a high yield for PC in a vulnerable population, 2) allow early identification while in an acute care setting where adequate diagnosis and triage by experts could prevail, and 3) set in motion appropriate mental health aftercare in the ambulatory or nursing home environments.

FUNDING CONTRACTS WITH OTHER DEPARTMENTS

By the use of the liaison screen methodology and the development of the team approach to PC on acute medical and surgical wards, it is possible in many settings to establish a contract with a host department to have them reimburse for the psychiatric liaison services. At the Mount Sinai Hospital (NYC), it has been possible to establish contracts with the Departments of Nursing, Medicine, Transplantation, Otolarnyngology, Social Work Services, Rape Crisis, and Obstetrics and Gynecology. These liaison contracts prevail because liaison psychiatry, in contrast to consultation methods, screen all at risk patients, work with the medical and nursing team, assist in disposition of patients from the hospital, and arrange hospital aftercare for mental health needs. On many teams, e.g., the nursing and social service teams, the psychiatrist assists in reviewing and signing off mental health visits that can then be reimbursed by Medicaid to offset salaries of the host services. By this mutually important team - **LIAISON** - approach it is apparent to the host services, the benefits to their patients and their staffs. It also becomes apparent to the host services from careful patient record documentation of these collaborative mental health efforts of the cost offset accrued from the liaison contract, in contrast to the hit or miss functioning of the tradtional consultation referral methodology for which host services will **NOT** reimburse the divisions of C-L psychiatry. The MICRO-CARES optiscan C-L demonstration system generates reports for the host services as to the assessment, interventions and number of followup visits to their patients (34).

SURVEY OF FUNDING SOURCES FOR THE STAFFING OF C-L FELLOWSHIP TRAINING PROGRAMS

In an attempt to understand the funding of C-L services in teaching hospitals all institutions that listed the availability of a C-L fellowship in the Academy of Psychosomatic Medicine (1991) Guide to Fellowships were surveyed by a structured questionnaire by the authors. Of the 49 programs listed 47 responded to the mail/fax questionnaire. If the program had not answered within six weeks, there was weekly FAX followup until all programs which had fellows replied. Two institutions stated at the time of the study that they did not offer fellowship training despite the Academy listing. The survey examined the number and discipline of the C-L staff (Table 2), the source of funding (Table 3,4), and the number of optimal staffing for a 1000 bed acute care university teaching hospital (Table 5). The average number of full time equivalents (FTE) on the C-L services was 242 with an average annual budget of $324,000. The hospital and school contributed 71% to faculty, 74% to fellowship funding, and 84% to offset the secretarial salary. Almost all hospitals paid for a full-time secretary for the service.

TABLE 2. COMPOSITION OF C-L PSYCHIATRY SERVICE

Average Number of:	
Salaried full-time equivalent (FTE) MDs	2.4
Fellows	1.6
Secretaries	1.3
Nurses	0.8
Social workers	-

Average C-L Service budget: $324,664 (Range $40,000 - $550,000)

TABLE 3. FUNDING

Source	%
Grants	4.8
Department of Psychiatry	42.0
Hospital	29.0
Medical School	3.4
Other departments	6.3
Patient fees	13.3
Donations	1.0

TABLE 4. FUNDING SOURCES FOR SECRETARY

Source	%
Department of Psychiatry	42
Hospital	42
Patient fees	16

TABLE 5. OPTIMAL NUMBER OF STAFF

FTE MDs	3.2
Fellows	2.4
Secretaries	1.7
Nurses	1.5
Psychologists	1.1

FELLOWSHIP FUNDING BY FEE FOR SERVICE

A self funded position for a liaison fellowship on a hemodialysis unit was reported by the senior author (35). A model is presented for funding an authentic liaison training program, fully supported by consultation-generated revenue. This teaching and patient care program provided dissemination of psychological skills and knowledge to nonpsychiatric staff, training of the liaison fellow, and generation of sufficient revenue to offset its costs. A second fellowship funding model was established by the senior author by using a behavioral medicine ambulatory clinic concept (36). In this protocol the fellow could generate his fellowship stipend in 18 hours per week individually seeing patients and directing groups. Each patient had Medicaid coverage which permitted billing $74 per visit. At the same time the fellow taught biopsychosocial interviewing, assessment, and management in the medical clinics; participated in Divisional research projects; instructed medical students; and, attended a weekly fellow's workshop. Therefore, inpatient and ambulatory models are critical funding mechanisms for fellowship training when no funded departmental or hospital lines are available.

COMMENTARY

The research presented describe the need for mental health delivery services in the acute care general hospital for the medically/surgically ill, psychiatric intervention studies, and the current funding patterns for those programs that offer C-L fellowship training in the United States. It is apparent that two issues obtain: the frequent occurrence of psychiatric and medical comorbidity in the general hospital inpatient setting, and the fact that the majority of university medical centers offering fellowship training in C-L psychiatry fund staff (including secretaries) and fellowship positions. This would indicate a significant clinical base from which to launch a research effort that is so badly needed in this subspecialty of psychiatry. It also indicates the need to move from the consultation

- referral - model that exposes only the numerator of apparent and obvious mental/behavioral problems/disorders - and often late during hospitalization - to the liaison screen model which assesses all patients (the denominator) in an "at risk" cohort, e.g., elderly, hemodialysis, transplantation, for psychiatric and medical comorbidity at admission or early during hospitalization.

It is important to ask once again the question why does a medical intervention need to not only prove its effectiveness to ameliorate psychiatric morbidity in the medical setting, but that it must also be cost saving or have cost offset benefit as well? Is this demand put on the inpatient, outpatient, child, or other services within the traditional department of psychiatry? It may be an unfair demand to not only have to "prove" therapeutic effectiveness, but also to demonstrate cost offset. It is an unfortunate historical fact that C-L services were not "built" into the reimbursement schedule for inpatient services as were social work services and nursing; or that designated lines were not established in the same way they have been for patient advocates, clergy, and clinical nurse specialists. We think this is in part due to the difficulty of those in C-L to "speak" up for their efforts as have the other mental health professionals who are entering the general hospital setting with increasing momentum and funding.

It is in part due to the fact that many departments of psychiatry do not feel that medical and psychiatric comorbidity in the medical/surgical setting is their domain, or has high enough priority compared to their other pressing needs: major mental disorders, children, substance abuse, biological psychiatry, etc. Many departments of psychiatry feel that the consultation role can be filled by voluntary attendings who need to contribute professional time to maintain their appointments. It is in part also due to the continuation of the use of the consultation/ referral model that does not place psychiatry sufficiently central within other medical departments - to become liaison members of their faculty/attending/teaching/service teams - to argue for their fiscal support, or to jointly persuade the hospital administration to pay for psychiatric services among the medical/surgical inpatients, as social work, clinical nurse specialists and medical psychologists have so skillfully done as [liaison] members of medical/surgical teams. Succintly, consultation psychiatry is not sufficiently within medicine to request funding support, and the department of psychiatry may want to preserve any funds from hospital lines and medical school budgets for traditional psychiatry patients. Consequently, psychiatry itself becomes an obstacle to obtaining funds for CL.

Toward such an end three position papers were prepared to discuss the "Appraisal of Marketing Approaches for C-L Psychiatry" (37). This series of reports described: the "products" of C-L psychiaty, e.g., patient care, teaching (38); "segmenting and accessing the market" (39); the need to describe the consumers - administrators, other departments, and outside agencies - and the need to communicate with them in an understandable and provocative language (40). These essays offer important conceptual ideas and formulations for the marketing of C-L psychiatry. Although they may be criticized for the "commercialization" of a medical subspecialty, their statements point out the reality of contemporary medicine: the marketing concept is an attempt to sell, but it is also an effort to offer more adequate medical care and alleviate human suffering (37).

This chapter is based partly on work reported in General Hospital Psychiatry: A New Tool for Consultation-Liaison Funding: Modified DRGs to Reflect Psychiatric Comorbidity (14:119-123, 1992).

Acknowledgement: The authors wish to acknowledge the Green Fund and Ms. Mirjami Easton for their assistance in this work.

REFERENCES

1. F.G. Guggenheim: A market place model of consultation psychiatry in the general hospital. Am J Psychiatry 135:1380-1383 (1978).

2. M.F. Weiner, J. Sadler, B.J. Fenton, et al: A very modest proposal for 1990s C/L psychiatry. Gen Hosp Psychiatry 11:231-234 (1989).

3. J.J. Strain, L.H. Gise, G. Fulop: C-L Psychiatry: possibilities for the 1990s. Gen Hosp Psychiatry 11:235-240 (1989).

4. L. Koran: Screening Medicare patients to fund C-L psychiatry. Gen Hosp Psychiatry 14:00-00, 1992.

5. H.H. Greenhill: The development of liaison programs. In "Psychiatric Medicine," G. Usidin, ed., Brunner/Mazel, New York (1977).

6. Z.J. Lipowski: Consultation-liaison psychiatry: the first half century. Gen Hosp Psychiatry 8:305-315 (1986).

7. D.A. Regier, I.D. Goldberg, and C.A. Taube: The de facto US mental health services system: a public perspective. Arch Gen Psychiatry 35:685-693 (1978).

8. D.A. Regier, J.K. Myers, M. Kramer M, et al: The NIMH Epidemiologic Catchment Area (ECA) program: historical context, major objectives, and study population characteristics. Arch Gen Psychiatry 41:934-941 (1984).

9. J. Wallen, H.A. Pincus, H.H. Goldman, and S.E. Markus: Psychiatric consultation in short-term general hospitals. Arch Gen Psychiatry 44:163-168 (1987).

10. G. Fulop, J.J. Strain, J. Vita, et al: Impact of psychiatric comorbidity on length of stay for medical/surgical patients: A preliminary report. Am J Psychiatry 144:878-882 (1987).

11. J.S. Lyons, J.S. Hammer, J.J. Strain, and G. Fulop: The timing of psychiatric consultation in the general hospital and length of hospital stay. Gen Hosp Psychiatry 8:159-162 (1986).

12. J. Eaton: Personal communication.

13. E. Mumford, H.J. Schlesinger, and G.V. Glass: The effect of psychological intervention on recovery from surgery and heart attacks: an analysis of the literature. Am J Public Health 72:141-151 (1982).

14. E. Mumford, H.J. Schlesinger, G.C. Glass, et al: A new look at evidence about reduced cost of medical utilization following mental health treatment. Am J Psychiatry 141:1145-1158 (1984).

15. Personal communication.

16. K. Wells, J.M. Golding, and M.A. Burnham: Psychiatric disorder and limitations in physical functioning in a sample of the Los Angeles general population. Am J Psychiatry 145:712-717 (1988).

17. K.B. Wells, R. Hays, M.A. Burnam, et al: Detection of depressive disorders for patients receiving prepaid or fee-for-service care. JAMA 62:3298-3302 (1989).

18. J. Levenson: American Psychiatric Association Annual Meeting, Washington, DC, 1992.

19. J. Gonella, ed.: Disease Staging Clinical Criteria, Third Edition. Systemetrics, Santa Barbara, CA, (1990).

20. W. Katon, M. von Korff, E. Lin, et al: Distressed high utilizers of medical care. DSM-III-R diagnoses and treatment needs. Gen Hosp Psychiatry 12:355-362 (1990).

21. G.R. Smith Jr., R.A. Monson, D.C. Ray: Patients with multiple unexplained symptoms. Arch Intern Med 146:69-72 (1986).

22. G.R. Smith Jr., R.A. Monson, D.C. Ray: Psychiatric consultation in somatization disorder. A randomized controlled study. NEJM 314:1407-1413 (1986).

23. G.R. Smith: American Psychiatric Association Annual Meeting, Washington DC (1992).

24. G. Fulop, et al: American Psychiatric Association Annual Meeting, Washington DC (1992).

25. G. Fulop, J.J. Strain, E. Blank, and J. Ginsburg: Phases of late life development and referral to psychiatry. American Geriatric Association Annual Meeting, May 1987.

26. S.J. Levitan, D.S. Kornfeld: Clinical and cost benefits of liaison psychiatry. Am J Psychiatry 138:90-93 (1981).

27. J.J. Strain, J.S. Lyons, J.S. Hammer, et al: Cost offset from a psychiatric consultation-liaison intervention with elderly hip fracture patients. Am J Psychiatry 148(8):1044-1049 (1991).

28. J.J. Strain, D. Hamerman: Ombudsmen (medical-psychiatric) rounds. An approach to meeting patient-staff needs. Ann Intern Med 88:550-555 (1978).

29. M. Stein, A.H. Miller, and R.L. Trestman: Depression, the immune system and illness. Findings in search of meaning. Arch Gen Psychiatry 48:171-177 (1991).

30. B. Forester, D.S. Kornfeld, and J.L. Fleiss: Psychotherapy during radiotherapy: effects on emotional and physical distress. Am J Psychiatry 142:22-27 (1985).

31. J.S. Hammer, H.T.C. Lam, and J.J. Strain: The cost benefit and effectiveness of a social risk survey program at an acute care hospital (in press).

32. J.J. Strain, G. Fulop, and J.S. Hammer: A new tool for consultation-liaison funding: modified DRG's to reflect psychiatric comorbidity. Gen Hosp Psychiatry 14:119-123, 1992.

33. M. Fahs, J.J. Strain, J.S. Lyons, and J.S. Hammer: Economic methods in cost offset measurement. American Psychiatric Association Annual Meeting, May 1992, p 173.

34. J.S. Hammer, J.J. Strain, and M. Lyerly: An optical scan/ statistical package for clinical data management in C-L psychiatry. Gen Hosp Psychiatry 14:000-000 (1993).

35. J.J. Strain, B. Vollhardt, and S. Langer: A liaison fellowship in a hemodialysis unit: a self-funded position. Gen Hosp Psychiatry 3:10-15 (1981).

36. G. Rowan, J.J. Strain, and L.H. Gise: The liaison clinic: a model for liaison psychiatry funding, training and research. Gen Hosp Psychiatry 6:109-115 (1984).

37. J.J. Strain: An appraisal of marketing approaches for consultation/liaison psychiatry. Gen Hosp Psychiatry 9:368-371 (1987).

38. J.L. Houpt: Personal communication.

39. T.N. Wise: Segmenting and accessing the market in consultation-liaison psychiatry. Gen Hosp Psychiatry, Vol 9 (1987).

40. J.L. Holtz: Communicating an effective message. Gen Hosp Psychiatry, Vol 9 (1987).

COMPUTERIZATION AND CONSULTATION-LIAISON PSYCHIATRY IN THE 1990'S

Seth M. Powsner, M.D.

Department of Psychiatry
Yale University School of Medicine
New Haven, CT 06510

INTRODUCTION

Will this decade usher in effective, *psychiatric* computing? The past decade has certainly been the decade of *personal* computing. The increasing speed and decreasing cost of personal computers significantly improved our capacity to retrieve medical and patient information (Hale and DeL'aune, 1983; Hammer, Lyons and Strain, 1984). However, this wave of the information revolution has scarcely lapped the feet of most psychiatrists. For most psychiatrists, the last major change in information retrieval occurred when the Xerox copier became common in the work place. By reviewing the changes that accompanied the copier, we can anticipate the future as the personal computer becomes a more routine part of consultation-liaison psychiatry.

INFORMATION RETRIEVAL IN THE PAST

Three by five index cards were probably the most important pieces of equipment for rapid retrieval of medical information in 1980. The postal service delivered up to date medical information in the form of journal articles. A database of articles could be maintained with Steelcase filing cabinets and Pendaflex folders. But rapid, efficient access to the assembled medical information depended on three by five index cards.

In 1980, the maintenance of article files was important enough to be the subject of a lecture by Dr. Daniel Offer, the Chairman of Psychiatry at Michael Reese Hospital, Chicago, Illinois. Dr. Offer taught residents how to maintain a good collection of articles. He personally preferred the sequential filing method. Dr. Offer described carefully collecting important articles over the years and numbering each in sequence as he added the articles to the end of his files. He would then make up a number of index cards, one for each subject under which he might want to find the article in the future. Each card needed only note the subject matter and the sequential filing number. An

Consultation-Liaison Psychiatry: 1990 and Beyond
Edited by H. Leigh, Plenum Press, New York, 1994

impressive mass of information was then available simply by flipping through a set of three by five cards.

Three by five index cards are still in common use, for patient information as well as medical information. They allow rapid access to large article collections and they are still printed in the New England Journal of Medicine.

The most important piece of equipment for patient information retrieval in 1980 was the ball-point pen. The importance of the modern ball-point pen for medical record keeping is vastly underestimated. The same piece of equipment is used for notes and orders, data recording and signature verification, human readable markings and machine readable markings, plain paper and multi-part forms. The same ball-point pen works equally well with 8.5x11" chart paper as three by five index cards.

Dictaphones, IBM Selectric Typewriters, and microfilm all had some impact on the storage and retrieval of patient and medical information by 1980. They simplified making notes, or making notes legible, or making notes smaller. This sort of equipment did not change the basic nature of information storage and retrieval. Every step in the process of writing, reading, indexing, sorting, and filing, required human effort. Just having information implied that someone would read the text, make notes, index, and file it.

The introduction of the Xerox 914 Copier caused more of a change in medical information retrieval than anything since the invention of paper. Its introduction in the 1960's suddenly made it possible to copy information *without human effort.* Whole articles could be copied for future reference; no need to read them and write brief summaries in a notebook. Patient records could be copied. It was now possible to have a clinical database of sorts right in the office. Library and chart room leg work could be turned over to secretaries or students. No understanding of a particular subject was required to bring back a "Xerox" of an article or a chart.

The copier also facilitated the development of psychiatric rating scales. With a copier, any clinician or researcher could reproduce custom rating scales or reproduce forms to record histories, consultations, or even medical orders. No need to learn to make stencils or mimeo masters. Nowadays, when reviewing a medical or surgical chart, it is quite common to see sets of admission or pre-op or treatment protocol orders reproduced by a copier.

The name Xerox has become a verb in the English language; often we hear "Xerox me a copy." If it is true that language shapes thought, the machine has even affected our way of thinking. But this fundamental change has required decades. The 914 was introduced in the early 1960's. Only recently has every psychiatrist or trainee in a major department been given easy access to a copier the way they had easy access to a typewriter in 1960.

DEVELOPMENTAL PHASES OF A TECHNOLOGY

What were the developmental phases on the way to the ubiquitous office copier? First, there had to be a commercially available copier that really copied. The older thermal copiers accepted pieces of paper and produced sheets of substance that were useful, but hardly durable office documents. Second, people had to believe they could actually operate the copier. Some readers may remember the early TV advertisements showing a child making office copies; the follow-up advertisements showed a chimpanzee for anyone unconvinced by the first ad. Then came the long, third, "rising tide" phase of growing acceptance and application. The fourth phase, the assumption phase, in which came the assumption that a copier was a standard, required piece of office equipment, took place between 1980 and 1990.

For personal computers, the third, "rising tide" phase of their introduction into society was well underway by 1991, ten years after the introduction of the IBM PC. There are personal computers commercially available to do word processing, calculations, and graphics. There might be some argument about completion of the second developmental phase. Not all people believe that they can operate a computer. There are some psychiatrists who have had trouble, but most can learn. The frequently heard questions about *which* personal computer to buy are the hallmark of the third phase. The first phase of a technology is marked by the questions about *where* the item can be bought. The second phase is marked by questions of *whether* the item should be bought. The fourth and final phase is marked by a relative absence of questions since the item is assumed to be readily available in the office.

It was during the third phase of copiers that they became cheaper, smaller, and easier to operate. This is exactly what is happening with computers. What was less apparent, in the third phase, was that people began to experiment with copiers. One could copy the table of contents each month of a favorite journal. A small folder of such copies in the office permitted a quick check for recent articles. The task of fetching the article from the library could be delegated to someone else. It was possible to cancel a personal subscription and just copy the table of contents while browsing the library s subscription. A clinician might have first used a copier to make chart forms for insurance information. Later the form might be dropped in favor of actual copies of the patient s insurance card to be included in the chart.

Some copier experiments failed almost completely. Portable copiers, about three times the size of an electric razor and similarly shaped, have not proven useful to many consultants. Consultants do not need to copy four inch wide strips of chart pages often enough to warrant carrying such copiers around. Similarly, tiny, portable dictating machines have not found wide spread clinical use even though they seem ideal for quick notes. To be effective, the support staff has to transcribe and deliver a myriad of short notes dictated over the course of the day, or some support staff would have to pickup, transcribe, and return small cassettes each time a note is dictated. There is not much explicit discussion of experimentation in the rising tide phase. Such discussion would not go over well with administrators who control the purchase of new equipment. Equipment is purchased to accomplish a task. It is not openly purchased to reshape tasks.

In the current decade, the most interesting aspect of computers in consultation psychiatry will be the experiments with their application. When this phase is complete, the specific uses of computers in consultation psychiatry will be clear. This may not be of much comfort to those deciding how much to spend on computers today. For them, the results of some experiments are available and warrant review below.

EFFECTIVE APPLICATIONS OF COMPUTER TECHNOLOGY

Word processing for text and spreadsheets for basic business or statistical calculations are effective. No further experiments are necessary. They are so much better than previous alternatives that anyone who does either without a computer should seriously reconsider their current approach (Lieff, 1987; Powsner and Byck, 1991; Tanner, 1992).

The desktop computer is a definite improvement over index card files. Card files are easily set up on a desktop computer. Keyboarded entries are easier to read. The computer can take care of the tedious tasks of selecting, sorting, and printing once the information is on file. The computer may even take less space. On the other hand, the pocket computer is not a reliable replacement for pocketing three by five index cards.

Pocket sized keyboards and screens are problematic, and pen based pocket computers are not yet entirely reliable.

Desktop computers equipped with telephone modems allow on-line literature searches from the office. A typical search using the National Library of Medicine's *Grateful Med* software costs under $5. Literature searches are free in some medical libraries. The desktop computer's ability to access national on-line literature (card) files, combined with its ability to maintain smaller, personal bibliographic (card) files, can eliminate the need for article files. A convenient library (or office collection of journals) and a copier make it possible to assemble an entire, up to date bibliography for any subject right from one's desk (Haynes, McKibbon, et al., 1986; Bonham and Nelson, 1988).

Desktop computers are somewhat of an improvement over stand-alone word processors. Adding hard disk storage and free text indexing software offers an alternative to traditional filing systems. The average typewritten page occupies 3000 bytes of storage. This translates to about 300 pages per megabyte. A standard 40 megabyte hard disk costs $220 compared to $300 for a four-drawer filing cabinet. A 40 megabyte disk has the capacity to hold 12,000 single spaced, typed pages which is two dozen reams of paper.

The decreasing costs of personal computers make it entirely reasonable to search all the consultation reports transcribed for a consultation service. On the Psychiatric Consultation Service at Yale New Haven Hospital, all of the 2500 consult reports generated since 1987 (over 6 megabytes), can be searched on a desktop computer in about 30 seconds. They can be searched for anything expressed in the text (Perratore, 1991).

The advantage of text retrieval (free text database) becomes apparent when considering the medical events between 1980 and 1990. "AIDS" would not have been included in any list of important medical diagnoses back in 1980. The earliest citation indexed under "AIDS" by the National Library of Medicine is dated July 1982 and it was not indexed until 1983. In 1980, most consultants would not have coded their records for sexual preference and specifics of substance use, the significant other's sexual preference, or the significant other's drug use. This is exactly the kind of information required for quick review of consultations on patients likely to be infected with HIV. And much of this kind of information was probably noted in the text of the patient's history and social history.

If a consultant or consultation-liaison service had been able to store the full text of consult reports in a free text database back in 1980, a number of retrospective reviews could have been done five years later on HIV dementia. A search for the words "homosexual," "gay," or "intravenous drug abuse" and "confusion" or "disorientation" would immediately lead to cases of interest. There would be no need to read through hundreds or thousands of reports to code a new clinical research database.

By 1991, there were a number of commercially proven software packages available to search large collections of english text. There is no requirement that the information be in a particular format. There is no requirement that each new report be reviewed for indexing purposes. The software will simply keep track of all the words.

Two computer uses which are still considered experimental are electronic mail and pen-point computer input. Electronic mail or "email," message exchange computer to computer, works very well on a service where all the consultants will check their email regularly. However, the technology has not proven reliable enough for general use. Anyone who has tried to establish email contact with a colleague who uses different email software can attest to the difficulties. It is as if people writing with ball point pens could not write to people using typewriters and expect their letters to arrive. Once the technology is better established, the experiment will begin. The real question will be how well electronic mail compares with voice mail or the fax machine for inter-office communication. It will take a number of years of experience to answer this question.

Pen-point computers are the only serious contender to replace the three by five index card. Pen-point computers attempt to substitute for pen and paper. The computer supplies and stores the electronic ink. Handwriting recognition can be used to facilitate indexing, but saving the pen strokes guarantees rapid storage and retrieval of the same information used by clinicians today. The basic computer pen technology has been available for about twenty years. Recent developments in high capacity, low power semiconductor memory and developments in character recognition software have made tablet style computers a commercial possibility. However, the critical experiments in usage are just beginning (Linderholm et al., 1992; Baran, 1992).

EXPERIMENTATION

By recognizing the nature of technological change, specifically during the rising tide phase, the thoughtful psychiatrist can better identify effective computer applications as they emerge from amidst the many experimental ones. The hallmarks of a truly effective computer application are regular use in a number of different locations, moderate price, and understandable operation. The first two are characteristics of technology which has an established place in the market. The third is a characteristic of established purpose and reliability.

Some readers may undertake to computerize a task before it is established that computerization will be effective. This is an uncertain undertaking though sometimes reasonable. It is important to recognize that it could cost a lot more time or money than manually completing the original task. On the other hand it may be quite successful, or at least informative. Informed experimentation is key to this phase of computer technology.

IN CONCLUSION

Personal computers have caused some changes in consultation-liaison psychiatry between 1980 and 1990. The past and future impact of reliable, inexpensive computing is easier to understand if compared with the impact of reliable, inexpensive copiers. Both technologies have required many years to reach their current phase of development and application. Both technologies have matured through the phases of becoming commercially available as reliable pieces of equipment and becoming simple enough for most people to operate. Copiers have progressed through the long third, rising tide phase of growing acceptance and application; they are well into the fourth phase in which they are assumed to be standard, required pieces of office equipment. Personal computers are just finishing the second phase and entering the third phase. Consultation psychiatrists may benefit from efforts and experiments to apply computers in routine practice.

REFERENCES

Baran, N., 1992, The outlook for pen computing, Byte 17(9):159-164.

Bonham, M.D., Nelson, L.L., 1988, An evaluation of four end-user systems for searching MEDLINE, Bull. Med. Libr. Assoc. 76:22-31.

Hale, M. and DeL'aune R., 1983, Microcomputer use on a consultation/liaison service, Psychosomatics, 24(11):1103-1105.

Hammer, J.S., Lyons, J.S., Strain, J.J., 1984, Micro-cares: an information management system for psychosocial services in hospital settings, in: Proceedings of the Seventh Annual Symposium on Computer Applications in Medical Care, G.S. Cohen, ed. IEEE Computer Society Press, Los Angeles.

Haynes, R.B., McKibbon, K.A., et al. 1986, How to keep up with the medical literature: V access by personal computer to the medical literature, Annals of Int Med 105:810-824.

Lieff, J.D., 1987, Computer Applications in Psychiatry, American Psychiatric Press, Inc., Washington, D.C.

Linderholm, O., Apiki, S., Nadeau M., 1992, The PC get more personal, Byte 17(7):128-138.

Perratore, E., 1991, Document management software: a network under control, PC Magazine, 10(21):287-337.

Powsner, S.M., Byck, R., 1991, Implementing a computer system for psychiatric training, Academic Psychiatry 15(2):100-105.

Tanner, B.A., 1992, Automating reports with Microsoft Word, M.D. Computing 9(2):108.

A COMPUTERIZED DATABASE SYSTEM FOR PSYCHIATRIC AND CONSULTATION RECORDS

Hoyle Leigh, M.D.

Department of Psychiatry
University of California, San Francisco
Fresno VA Medical Center

ABSTRACT

We report the development of a clinical and educational computerized system for generating psychiatric records and consultation notes. Simultaneously, it generates the Patient Evaluation Grid (PEG) developed by Leigh, Feinstein, and Reiser -a bio-psycho-social inventory of the patient which serves an eduational as well as clinical function.

The PEG consists of the nine areas of investigation about patients formed by the intersection of the three dimensions of the patient (biological, personal, environmental) with three time contexts (current, recent, background). In addition, a PEG Management Form is displayed, with three dimensional diagnoses and management plans. The IBM program is menu-driven, and is directly inputted by the clinician in traditional format (Chief Complaint, Present Illness, etc).

The data base includes demographics, clinical and laboratory data, and administrative/financial data. The menus include programs for printing Narrative Summary, PEG, printed Consultation Note, Thank You note for the referring physician, billing, monthly report based on diagnosis or treatment, and customized research programs. This system has been used extensively at Yale University and at University of California, San Francisco, Fresno Division, in teaching medical students and residents as well as in clinical research.

INTRODUCTION

We proposed the Patient Evaluation Grid (PEG) as a tool to operationalize a bio-psycho-environmental model of the patient designed to provide comprehensive care for the patient (1-2). Since the publication of *The Patient: Biological, Psychological, and Social Dimensions of Medical Practice,* by Leigh and Reiser, the PEG has been adopted by a number of practitioners, and, particularly, by medical educators as a teaching tool to demonstrate the importance of the interaction among the three dimensions of the patient in understanding and managing patients (3-5).

Although the PEG in its original form was useful in teaching medical students, we were concerned that constructing the PEG involved the student's filling out an extra form. While the exercise itself was valuable, we felt that a method to generate the bio-psycho-environmental information without having to do additional writing would be more acceptable to those practitioners who were interested in understanding patients comprehensively, but whose limited available time precluded them from actually contructing the PEG.

As computers are becoming widely used in medicine in word processing and billing, there is a need to develop a computerized data base system that can be used clinically. We decided to develop a computerized data base for patients' clinical information, which would serve both traditional clinical needs as well as providing the comprehensive PEG information on patients. The program would be so designed that practitioners should need to input only one set of clinical data, but would acquire both traditional narrative data as well as the bio- psycho-environmental information displayed in the PEG format. We now describe such a program, the Leigh Patient Systems, (LPS) developed by the author.

THE LEIGH PATIENT SYSTEMS: A COMPREHENSIVE CLINICAL DATA BASE

The LPS is a MENU driven clinical data base system. LPS has two components: (1) Regular LPS Patient Database for outpatients, and (2) LPS for Psychiatric Consultation.

1. REGULAR LPS PATIENT DATABASE FOR OUTPATIENTS

Clinical Data and Traditional Narrative Summary

It is so designed that a clinician can input clinical data about patients directly into the computer instead of writing a narrative summary long-hand. After the patient's identifying information has been entered, the computer will prompt the clinician to enter clinical data in the order they are obtained. For example, Chief Complaint followed by Present Illness, duration, symptom severity, etc.

While considerable amount of text may be entered for present illness, and formulation, the amount of typing needed for the database is relatively small, as the menu-driven forms usually request one-word answers or quantifications. The amount of time required to complete a comprehensive LPS on a patient is approximately 10-30 min.

Generation of the Biopsychosocial Patient Evaluation Grid (PEG)

LPS automatically generates a PEG once the clinical data have been entered. Thus, the clinician inputs clinical data in the traditional format, and obtains a bio-psycho-environmental inventory concerning the patient. This function of LPS is especially useful in educating medical students and other trainees concerning the interaction of biological, psychological, and environmental factors in pathogenesis and patient management.

LPS also prints out the PEG-Management Form, in which diagnoses and problems in the biological, personal, and environmental dimensions as well as their proposed treatments are listed. PEG-Management Form draws the clinician's attention to the fact that treatment in one dimension of the patient may affect another dimension of the patient, and that patient management has to be comprehensive.

The PEG and PEG-Management Form are especially useful for the practicing clinician as a summary table for important aspects of the patient.

Automated Psychological Inventory

LPS can perform self-administered psychological questionnaires. Current version of LPS can administer and score the Marlowe-Crowne Social Desirability Inventory and the abbreviated version of the Taylor Manifest Anxiety Scale, and provide the clinician with a categorization of the coping style (i.e. repressor, true low anxious, true high anxious, defensive high anxious). As the "repression" dimension may have much bearing on the help-seeking and complaining behaviors (6)-i.e., the "repressors" may tend not to report high levels of distress in spite of lesions warranting distress, this automated inventory has been useful in our experience in identifying even low levels of complaints among repressors as being potentially significant.

Other self-administered questionnaires may be added to the LPS, such as the Hopkins symptom check list, and the Beck depression inventory.

Educational Uses

The automatic generation of the Patient Evaluation Grid (PEG) teaches the clinician and trainees the importance of biopsychosocial factors in pathogenesis and management. LPS also assists the educator and the trainee by listing the number of diagnoses of trainees's patients, the use of specific medications and other management modalities by trainees, as well as the number of patients each clinician has evaluated, is treating, or has terminated.

Another educational function of LPS is the direct interaction with the computer it provides for the trainees and the clinicians. Computer familiarity is thus achieved in the context of clinical work, which may further motivate the individual to learn more about computers and data bases for other applications as well.

Research

LPS utilizes the widely used and powerful relational database system, R:Base. Thus, a powerful research data base is created when LPS is utilized clinically. By using R:Base commands, each practitioner can create his/her own research queries of the LPS. For example, one can develop a program to compare the serum glucose levels of patients who are "repressors" vs those of patients who are truly "low anxious" as we have done at the Yale Behavioral Medicine Clinic (7). The data from LPS can be easily exported to statistical programs such as Systat.

Administrative Functions

LPS will provide an alphabetical listing of patients, a referral list, and a patient list by diagnosis. It will also print out bills (either for all patients, or for individual patient).

In addition to the menu options, one can easily develop other administrative applications, e.g., printing insurance forms.

Patients' demographic information may be inputted by the secretary, and may be accessible to selected nonclinical staff by the use of different levels of security codes.

2. LPS FOR PSYCHIATRIC CONSULTATION (LPS-CL)

Consultation-liaison (CL) psychiatry often suffers from the lack of standardized records because consultation notes are usually written on medical charts that do not form a part of the records kept in the psychiatric department. Such a lack of standardized records is often responsible for the difficulty that CL services encounter in claiming appropriate credit for the work done by their staff and in developing clinical research. There has been much interest during the past decade in using computerized data bases in consultation-liaison psychiatry (6). Existing computerized programs in CL psychiatry tend to be either too cumbersome, i.e., requiring the staff to fill out more than 15 pages of questionnaire and a secretary to input the voluminous material into the computer, or inadequate to meet the academic and research needs as the programs are not based on widely known powerful data bases.

The LPS for Psychiatric Consultation (LPS-CL) is a program specifically designed for Psychiatric Consultation Services. As the consultation psychiatrist has to evaluate, diagnose, and manage patients much more rapidly than in non-emergency outpatient settings, the LPS-CL utilizes briefer questionnaires, and the narrative summary is not as comprehensive or lengthy as is in the Regular LPS. Within LPS-CL there are two levels of comprehensiveness - i.e., the consultant may input either the "regular" consultation form or the "brief" consultation form.

A Consultation Summary is generated automatically by the LPS-CL. This feature provides an important advantage in consultation psychiatry --- *legible consultation notes.* The consultation summary uses a narrative format, but is less extensive and more focussed than the regular Narrative Summary generated by the Regular LPS.

LPS-CL is essentially similar to the Regular LPS described above except for the content of information requested. Data from LPS-CL are fully compatible with data from Regular LPS. LPS-CL automatically generates monthly and yearly summary of consultation statistics sorted by date received, in alphabetical order, according to consultant, and according to DSMIII-R diagnosis. It also provides periodic summaries for each resident of the number of diagnoses, psychotropic drugs and other management modalities recommended , etc.

3. SYSTEM REQUIREMENTS AND AVAILABILITY

Hardware

1. LPS requires an IBM-Compatible PC (Intel 386 Processor or better) with a hard disk and at least 640 K of Random Access Memory

2. A printer

Software

1. LPS is free-standing. It is based on R:BASE for DOS, that was compiled. To make changes or use the database as such, it is recommended that R:Base for DOS is also installed. Later versions of R:Base are OK, but the user may need to do a little editing to be able to use LPS.

Copyright

LPS is copyrighted by Hoyle Leigh, M.D.

Availability

Available directly from the author

An earlier version of LPS is also available to educational institutions through:
WISC-WARE
Academic Computing Center
University of Wisconsin-Madison
1210 West Dayton Street
Madison, Wisconsin 53706
(608) 262-8167

REFERENCES

1. Leigh H, Feinstein AR, Reiser MF: The patient evaluation grid: A systematic approach to comprehensive care
Gen Hosp Psychiatry 2:3-9, 1977

2. Leigh H, Reiser MF: *The Patient: Biological, Psychological, and Social Dimensions of Medical Practice, Third Edition*
Plenum Medical Publishing Co, New York, 1992

3. Leigh H: *Psychiatry in the Practice of Medicine*
Addison Wesley Publishing Co, Menlo Park, CA, 1984

4. Leigh H: A computerized system for psychiatric and consultation records. (Abstract) 1988 New Research Program and Abstracts
American Psychiatric Association 141st Annual Meeting
Montreal, Canada May 7-12, 1988 p 28

5. Leigh H: *Computers in Psychiatry*
Psychiatric Update Series, Volume 12, No. 3
Gene Usdin (Series Editor in Chief)
American College of Psychiatrists,
Medical Information Systems, Inc., Port Washington, NY, 1992

6. Linden W, Paulhus DL, Dobson KS: Effects of response styles on the report of psychological and somatic distress
J Clinical and Consulting Psychol 54:309-313, 1986

7. Jamner LD, Schwartz GE, Leigh H: The relationship between repressive and defensive coping styles and monocyte, eosinophile, and serum glucose levels: Support for the opioid peptide hypothesis of repression Psychosomatic Medicine 50:567-575, 1988

8. Hammer JS, Strain JJ, Hammond D, Lyons JS: Microcomputers in consultation psychiatry in the general hospital. Gen Hosp Psychiatry 7:119-124, 1985

DATABASING IN CLP PSYCHIATRY

Jeffrey S. Hammer, M.D.

UCLA/Veterans Affairs Medical Center West Los Angeles,
Los Angeles, CA

James J. Strain, M.D.

Mount Sinai School of Medicine, New York, NY

"DATABASING" FOR CONSULTATION - LIAISON PSYCHIATRY IN THE 1990's

THE PROBLEM

The epoch of the 1990's has proclaimed the need for documenting and recording information in nearly every category of endeavor: business, health care, teaching, government. This demand necessitates a move toward creating computerized database systems to collect, aggregate, and transform pertinent data into usable information. On all levels of health service delivery we need to understand not only what we are doing, but what we should not be doing. Never before has there been such an opportunity to document an enterprise and then re-examine what has been done, by whom, and for what indications.

The documentation of the delivery of health care lags behind many other industries where databasing is taken for granted and has reached a high level of proficiency on a daily basis: banking, securities, airlines, personnel search, marketing, payrolls, etc. There is an urgent need for clinical database management systems in order for us to understand and modify what is happening in the health care delivery system. Every clinical case should provide an opportunity to learn and contribute to a broad based denominator on the outcome of interventions. Such data can help in decision making by promoting service delivery changes on the basis of aggregate objective data over time as opposed to anecdotal or less objective case method approach. The resource investment required to achieve those outcomes should also be measured.

In the field of consultation-liaison psychiatry (CLP) the hand written consultation note remains the hall mark of the record keeping which is still extant. Although this note is often barely legible, it has not been structured to enforce the inclusion of essential variables, (e.g., employment status, living situation, stressors in the previous year), and does not mandate a recorded initial and closing diagnostic impressions, it continues as the primary documentation of the consultation process in the majority of teaching hospitals.

Consultation-Liaison Psychiatry: 1990 and Beyond
Edited by H. Leigh, Plenum Press, New York, 1994

It has been argued that only a narrative with personal biographical description and dynamic characterization of the individual is appropriate; to simply mark preselected variables is to dehumanize the interview and formulation process and make the record comparable to a description of the patients as if they were only particulate specifics like "vital signs."

Clearly, there must be some balance between the traditional hand written note and number coding (and crunching). In 1979 we described this dilemma and evolution: "The present version of the admission and termination forms for psychiatric consultation evolved from earlier attempts to record consultation data: these started with a handwritten 3" x 5" index card and progressed to an inventory of clinical, administrative and evaluation items (1)." The raison d'etre of this effort was to detail the clinical work load, ascertain administrative needs, evaluate the effectiveness of consultation programs, and codify consultation data for research purposes.

When this effort began in 1977 there were no recording forms designed specifically for data on non-psychiatric patients seen by a CLP Service. As the form was piloted, items were added, deleted, or reformulated in order to tap the desired information. Because of the response burden on the consultant it was necessary to compromise between inclusiveness and brevity. It was also envisioned that specific data from the consultant psychiatrist could be combined with information from the hospital database, so that variables available from this latter source would not have to be collected and recorded a second time on the CLP form. However, this concept had to be altered as data from the hospital computer was difficult and expensive to obtain and not available in a timely fashion, so that the form was reconceived to be self contained, (e.g., ethnicity, age, sex were collected directly to the form).

"To monitor case discussions that did not become formal consultations, an Informal Consultation Form was developed for use on units to which liaison fellows were assigned. A patient is registered if there are more than 5 minutes but less than 15 minutes of discussion, but no chart note is written and the patient is seen briefly, if at all (1). This issue of "subthreshold" consultations remains problematic and definitions as to what constitutes a recordable consultation, e.g., a "curb stone" consultation, have not been agreed upon. That is, the process component of CLP work remains an impasse in its definition and recording. Databasing of the process remains as problematic as databasing of the dynamics and formulation of the patient, and of the doctor-nurse-family-patient interaction. And, as it is understood that all of these hierarchical levels of information are important; it remains only a matter of time until we have the means to capture these important levels of knowledge to better understand the mind-body - self-other relationships in health and disease.

DEVELOPMENTAL LEVELS

With regard to the content of the database another dilemma is the need to contend with the developmental level of the patient. Hamburg thought she could adapt the adult CLP Form for use with children and youth at the Mount Sinai School of Medicine (2). After an enormous amount of effort she decided that actually three levels or databases were required: 1) under 5 years old; 2) latency; 3) post pubertal. The nature of the variables had to be in transition as was the developing child - preschool to school, family to peers, the achievement of milestones. The mental status assessment also had to be an evolutional instrument to be appropriate to the data that is obtained from the rapidly changing human organism. And, the source of the data needed to be altered from the caretaker exclusively to the patient him/herself.

Similarly, a database for the elderly will need to reflect the changes that confront them. The source of data may once again need to emanate from caretakers as elderly patients loose the capacity to speak for themselves, as their employment and social support system change, and when "the family" takes on a different generational structure. It has been stated that the DSM-III and DSM-III-R are not "medically ill or age fair," and less reliable and valid in such population or patient cohorts. Clearly, developmental algorithms will have to be constructed to take into account these life status changes, and need then to be reflected as variables in the database for that cohort.

DEGREE OF SPECIFICITY OF DIAGNOSES AND DRUGS

There is always the concern of the need for sufficient specificity and the need for ease in completion of the form by the consultant. It was the belief of the developers of MICRO-CARES that it was necessary to demarcate the specific Axis I, II, and III diagnoses so that the specific disorder could be addressed and examined. In contrast, in 1990, McKegney et al. (3) described an optically scanned consultation database which has data elements and an organization very similar to that published by Taintor, Gise, Spikes, and Strain, in 1979 (1), and the iterations that took place in the years that followed as described by Hammer, Lyons, and Strain (3-13) and Huyse, (14,15). It, however, does not provide the specific Axis I DSM-III-R categories, but rather codes "domains" of disorders. No code or identification numbers are recorded for either Axis I, II, or III diagnoses, limiting clinical research with this tool to specific state, trait or medical disorder entities. It is not possible, for example, to examine the frequency of major depression (296.XX), dysthymia (300.XX), adjustment disorder with depressed mood (309.00), or organic mood disorder (292.xx), all of which are commonly seen in the general hospital population. Furthermore, one could not separate out cancer of the prostate from other cancers, differentiate hypo and hyperthyroidism, or examine the diagnosis of hyperornithemia as described earlier. Although such a form may have the advantage of ease in its completion, it limits investigation, and makes certain evaluations impossible, and comprises the scientific rigor of CLP database research.

The McKegney approach does not permit the assessment of "initial" and "termination" impressions with regard to diagnostic considerations. Nor is there any method to assess the fate of the recommendations - were they carried out by the consultant, the consultee, or the other ward staff? Huyse et al. have demonstrated the importance of recording the outcome of recommendations and have built on the work of Leigh (16) and Popkin (17) to examine in detail psychosocial interventions and their implementation by the ward staff. Without such adherence-concordance data outcome studies are compromised by error measurement secondary to physician (consultee) noncompliance with psychiatric consultation recommendations. The issue of specificity must be answered by the user, but it is our concern that the database be at least as the rigorous as the medical record, which is the legal document for the hospital and the patient.

FLEXIBLE DATABASES

As described above there is a need for a flexible CLP database that can incorporate developmental issues, important new domains of data elements for a specific clinical situation, or investigations that require adding or substituting salient variables. It could be an entirely different database as was developed by Hamburg for children and youth or it could be adding a partial list - a "branch chain" to the core elements.

At times, clinicians may want to systematically collect a subset of variables for a particular period of time that would address a particular question. For example, the

Memorial Sloan Kettering Cancer Center psychiatry group suggested that a study of cancer patients should not only assiduously describe the Axis III state describing the tumor as specifically as possible, with regards to its ICD-9 codes, but also examine four critical variables not part of the core CLP database (18):

1. Tumor type: Blood - solid;
2. Nausea and vomiting;
3. Pain; and,
4. Suicidal thoughts, behaviors.

"Branch chains" would be helpful to examine the clinical situation of HIV infection, and Blumenfield and Wallack have proposed such a subset of variables (19). Since "branch chains" would permit a more complete description of patient population under consideration, it would be important to collect these data for a limited period of time as a complement to the core data set obtained on every patient for the clinical management database. However, to expeditiously carry out such a pursuit, a means to provide an easily produced flexible database would be essential. Most databases are structured and changes take time and can be costly.

INSTRUMENTS AND SCALES

Another form of "branch chain" would be standard instruments and scales, that have documented reliability and validity which the clinical investigator may wish to add to the CLP database for a specific time period and/or specific patient population. Although many instruments are problematic in the medical setting, since the majority of measures have been developed with the psychiatrically ill, and have not been field tested with the medically ill, such instruments would nevertheless buttress the clinical impressions of the consultant and augment the diagnostic assessment.

HOSPITAL DATA

Yet another example of a "branch chain" are the important data elements to be added for time limited studies available from the hospital computer, e.g., length of hospital stay (LOS), direct and indirect costs, anesthesia time, other consultations, units of blood, days in intensive care, surgical procedures, forms of insurance, etc. These "on-line" data can be helpful for certain kinds of clinical investigation as was shown by Lyons et al. (20), in the timing of consultation psychiatry and its effect on LOS and by, Fulop, et al, in their investigation of the impact of psychiatric comorbidity on LOS for medical/surgical patients (21). On the other hand the core database could be amended to collect some of these data elements if the hospital computer did not have them, or they were not readily available through such a source to the investigator. Methods to develop "branch chains" and CLP software to produce flexible databases will be described below. The need however, is for an approach which allows moving patient demographic, diagnostic and LOS data from the hospital mainframes and importing it electronically to database in the CLP microcomputer.

THREE LEVELS OF DATABASING

In the construction of a database it is important to keep three hierarchical levels in mind: 1) departmental; 2) divisional or section; and, 3) research. It would be useful for a department to decide on core elements which should be present in every database in every division, e.g., age, sex, date of admission, diagnoses, interventions, disposition. The department or even the institution than could peruse its entire patient cohort for age, sex, diagnoses, etc. to describe the population with whom it has been involved. This would also permit a department to draw databases from different divisions or sections without having duplication of data entry and data processing.

The second level revolves around the needs of a division or center and obviously must include variables pertinent to the population, problems, and process encountered in that setting. As said above, the child division would need different data elements from that of an adult CLP service. An inpatient service might need a different temporal coding of variables, e.g., the daily recording of medication changes, mental status alterations. An out patient department may want weekly, monthly or twice yearly summaries to accompany the process of ambulatory care. The CLP service for a minimum should include initial and then termination impressions to observe the evolution of the diagnostic profile during the hospitalization, and assure that those with rule out diagnoses remaining at discharge be assigned aftercare follow up. Therefore, there are **two** essential concerns for divisional or section databases: 1) which elements - variables; and, 2) what time reference for recording them.

A third level of integration is that dictated by special research projects that will draw on core and divisional data elements, but have their own specific data elements and timing needs for the research endeavor. For example, if one wanted to study those patients who move from the CLP service to the inpatient setting, it would be important to draw on both of the divisional datasets to complete the picture of the patient. What happens to CLP patients admitted to the inpatient service, and what was their profile while they were on medicine. Research protocols would rely heavily on "branch chains" and/or rating scales, but to be able to "pull" the data from the total contact with the patient before and after the commencement of the research protocol would be of great advantage.

Therefore, databases for the CLP setting should be integrated into the hierarchy of the departmental/ section/ and research needs to insure the compatibility of data elements and the most complete availability of information with the least amount of redundancy of data collection. The CLP service should shape its database to these other needs.

THE EVOLUTION OF THE MICRO-CARES SYSTEM

SOFTWARE AND HARDWARE

The 1977 version of the CLP database employed manually filled out forms, key punching, verification, an editing program that checked certain variables on the form for completeness and determined if they were "in range". However, error detection via computer was not as useful as supervisory interest in changing trainee behavior, although it directed where attention should be placed. The data was placed on a mainframe computer at a neighboring facility which generated print outs upon request, although the programming remained a problem, and there was considerable delay in receiving information. This approach permitted extensive retrospective analysis but did not allow for interactive report generation capability or immediate access to the data by the consultant or program director. No feed back or interaction with the data archive could be achieved on a daily ongoing basis.

The second evolutionary step for MICRO-CARES was at the Mount Sinai School of Medicine where the CLP database was moved from mainframe hardware to a minicomputer on site system - PDP-11 CLINFO (22). The CLINFO system with terminals throughout the medical center was a "user friendly" system which provides a statistical package that allows researchers and clinicians to maintain control over their own data: It did not require significant computer expertise or a programmer to access data, although it was not at a work station in the consultation office. It did have the additional feature of being an interactive system that accesses a mainframe computer for analyses of large numbers of cases with multiple variables. Furthermore, there were only a limited number of medical centers which had CLINFO so that the methods developed could not be exported to the majority of teaching hospitals and certainly not to the general hospital.

Although computers are of assistance in many areas of psychiatry, their pragmatic application to the general hospital and the consultation setting were compromised from the lack of a conceptual schema that would have utility in the university medical center as well as the community teaching hospital. In the former, one may find a variety of computer systems - mainframe, mini, micro, whereas in the latter, only the microcomputer maybe in place and affordable.

A principal asset of the microcomputer lies in its accessibility. As said earlier the great complexity and expense of mainframe computers combined with difficult to use programs and poor documentation tends to lock out the nonexpert user without the resources to hire a computer consultant. The computer consultant does not know CLP and the CLP psychiatrist does not know computers. Therefore, Hammer and his group at the Northwestern Memorial Hospital developed a stand-alone microcomputer system for on-line administrative requirements that provided essential day-to-day report writing for the establishment of census and billing, logs, medical chart notes, acknowledgement letters to the consultees, consultant's profiles of case loads, ad hoc reports, and cross tabulation summaries. These latter files permit the construction of subsets from the data as a whole for observations and hypotheses generation. Since the microcomputer is an interactive system, more complex statistical analysis was accomplished via associated mainframe machines, although the power of the microcomputer has increased so rapidly that many of the statistical manipulations of the data are now being performed on the microcomputer in the CLP office.

The initial MICRO-CARES (Clinical, Administrative, Research, Educational System) was designed around several highly popular software packages - dBase II and FMS-80 database management programs as well as the Wordstar-Mail merge word processing package. With the enhancement of computer power and the MS-DOS operating system the MICRO-CARES system was organized around a single integrated software application development package called METAFILE instead of the multiple, non-integrated programs used before. This METAFILE MICRO-CARES system has been well described in the literature (4,5).

The MICRO-CARES system is basically a clinical database management system. It is comparable to searching the medical record for information and its data should be as reliable as that found in the medical record. But in addition certain variables that might not be found in the medical record are systematically structured into the database form to help insure that data element is present when a review is undertaken. Too often the medical record does not have the variable the investigator might need, e.g., employment status, or previous mental health care. Many have misunderstood this important concept and feel that the database approach does not offer either reliable or valid data. It is not a research project with interrater reliability. It is a structured readily accessible medical record. With an instruction manual, a glossary defining each item, ongoing supervision and training, it should surpass the medial record in the quality of the data.

Several clinical situations have been examined: The problem of alcohol, the effects of the timing of psychiatric consultation in the general hospital, psychiatric emergencies, informed consent (24-25).

However, the system which was provided to several medical schools with an Upjohn Company educational grant was hampered by the length of the database, and the difficulty of manual entry of the data which took 10-15 minutes per case. To overcome these deficits based on use, in 1987 the MICRO-CARES database was considerably shortened, and an optical scan computer form was developed (Figure 1). It now required about 5 minutes to fill out each form, and 200-300 questionnaires per hour can be read by an optical scanner and directly inloaded to the computer in the consultation office. Optical scanning also enhances the accuracy of data entry.

FLEXIBLE DATABASE AND FORM GENERATION

Manual data entry was a "sore spot," which nearly extinguished user interest in MICRO-CARES. As said above in early 1987 with the use of National Computer Systems transoptic scanning devices, this problem was overcome. The four page scannable database form, however, had to be independently produced in volume quantities by an external vendor. The process involved three production phases: 1) "mock up designs," 2) production phase (which took about 4 weeks); and, 3) color and multiple page design, all of which contributed significantly to both cost and time. And once produced, the scannable database could not be modified without going through the same process all over again.

An approach close to ideal is one in which the user with his/her own hardware/software in their own offices could desk top publish optically scannable forms specifically tailored to their needs. This would allow for adding or dropping items. It would facilitate the development of CLP specific scales or instruments, which are "age, medical and psychiatrically comorbidity fair". For example, Edicott has proposed and Rapp and Vrana have confirmed, that with medically ill geriatric patients the substitution of non-vegetative symptoms, i.e., cognitive, for vegetative symptoms in the medically ill does not alter the detection of depressive disorders. It would be important to have the option to substitute the Endicott symptoms in a series of CLP settings to learn if they would be a more reliable approach to the diagnosis of depression in the medically ill. With a flexible form generator, such a questionnaire could be produced and used for a limited period of time. In such a manner a variety of variable alterations could occur at will and with little expense as the user is "unbound" from the static database form.

The sixth iteration of MICRO-CARES is the Medical Application Platform (MAP), and it contains the enhancements that permit new opportunities including desk top publishing which can replace commercially produced forms. Flexible optically scannable form generation is only a part of the process required for comprehensive data management. The entries in the specific locations on the scannable form which represent data elements, must go through a series of checks to insure their correctness. MICRO-CARES uses three mechanisms to insure the correctness of the data developed and entered within the context of the clinical situation: 1) The data from the form are printed for observation, i.e., Chart Note, that is placed in the medical record and can be verified against the other clinical data in that record., e.g., age, sex, medical diagnosis, data of admission, etc.

Reliability checks built into the software systems to determine if there are missing or double entered values within a specific range, and the systematic determination of "logic validation, " e.g., the year of the consultation in 1991 cannot be "2001." The computer program would "see" 2001 as out of range and not accept it. The data validation form printed for each case entered and returned to the consultant and supervisor for verification of ever item serves as another check. Finally mainframe data imported to the MAP is compared to similar data obtained by the consultant for criterion validation.

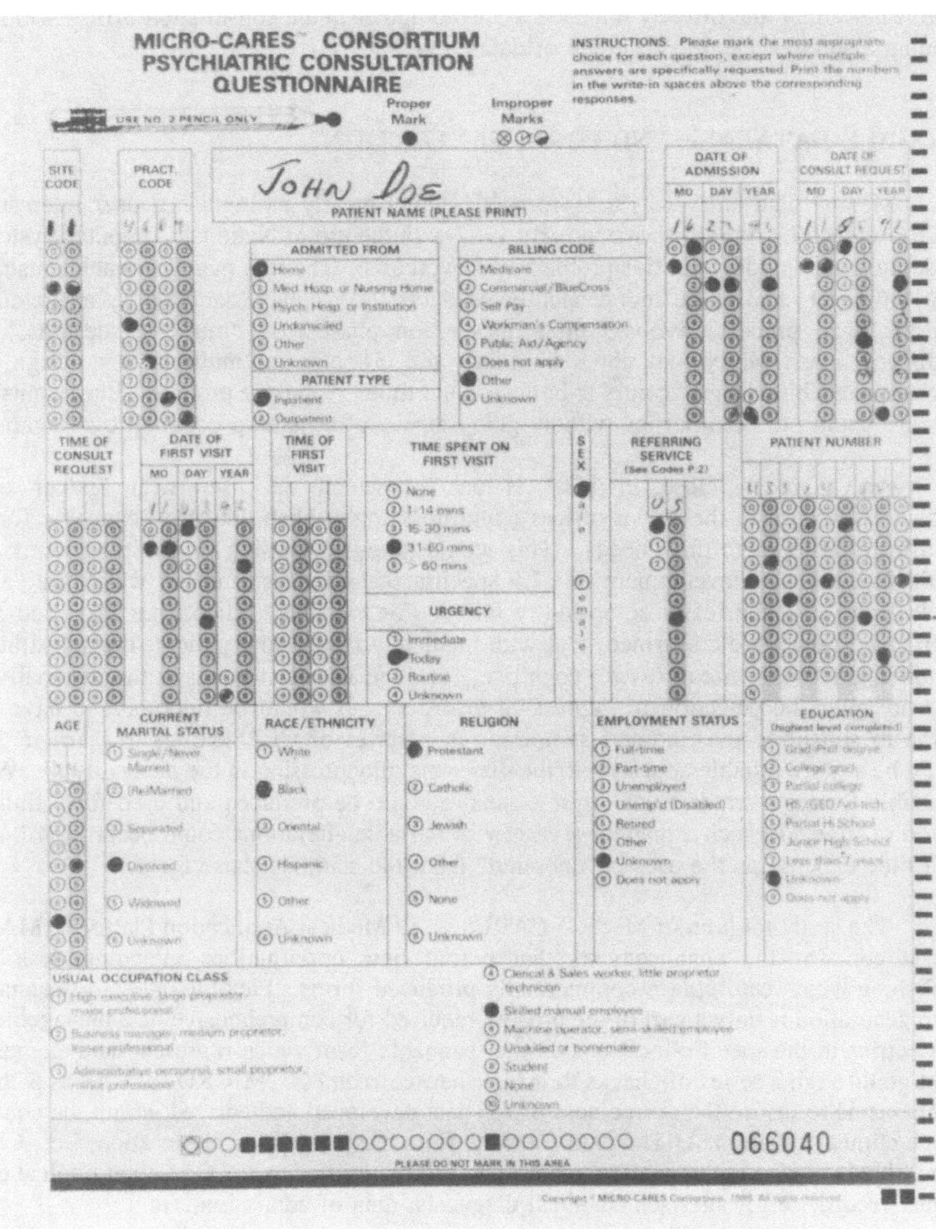

MICRO-CARES™ CONSORTIUM PSYCHIATRIC CONSULTATION QUESTIONNAIRE

USE NO. 2 PENCIL ONLY

Proper Mark

Improper Marks

INSTRUCTIONS. Please mark the most appropriate choice for each question, except where multiple answers are specifically requested. Print the numbers in the write-in spaces above the corresponding responses.

SITE CODE

PRACT. CODE

JOHN DOE

PATIENT NAME (PLEASE PRINT)

DATE OF ADMISSION: MO DAY YEAR

DATE OF CONSULT REQUEST: MO DAY YEAR

ADMITTED FROM

1. Home
2. Med. Hosp. or Nursing Home
3. Psych. Hosp. or Institution
4. Undomiciled
5. Other
6. Unknown

PATIENT TYPE

1. Inpatient
2. Outpatient

BILLING CODE

1. Medicare
2. Commercial/BlueCross
3. Self Pay
4. Workman's Compensation
5. Public Aid/Agency
6. Does not apply
7. Other
8. Unknown

TIME OF CONSULT REQUEST

DATE OF FIRST VISIT: MO DAY YEAR

TIME OF FIRST VISIT

TIME SPENT ON FIRST VISIT

1. None
2. 1-14 mins
3. 15-30 mins
4. 31-60 mins
5. > 60 mins

URGENCY

1. Immediate
2. Today
3. Routine
4. Unknown

SEX: Male / Female

REFERRING SERVICE (See Codes P.2)

PATIENT NUMBER

AGE

CURRENT MARITAL STATUS

1. Single/Never Married
2. (Re)Married
3. Separated
4. Divorced
5. Widowed
6. Unknown

RACE/ETHNICITY

1. White
2. Black
3. Oriental
4. Hispanic
5. Other
6. Unknown

RELIGION

1. Protestant
2. Catholic
3. Jewish
4. Other
5. None
6. Unknown

EMPLOYMENT STATUS

1. Full-time
2. Part-time
3. Unemployed
4. Unemp'd (Disabled)
5. Retired
6. Other
7. Unknown
8. Does not apply

EDUCATION (highest level completed)

1. Grad/Prof degree
2. College grad
3. Partial college
4. HS/GED/vo-tech
5. Partial Hi School
6. Junior High School
7. Less than 7 years
8. Unknown
9. Does not apply

USUAL OCCUPATION CLASS

1. High executive, large proprietor, major professional
2. Business manager, medium proprietor, lesser professional
3. Administrative personnel, small proprietor, minor professional
4. Clerical & Sales worker, little proprietor, technician
5. Skilled manual employee
6. Machine operator, semi-skilled employee
7. Unskilled or homemaker
8. Student
9. None
10. Unknown

066040

PLEASE DO NOT MARK IN THIS AREA

Figure 1.

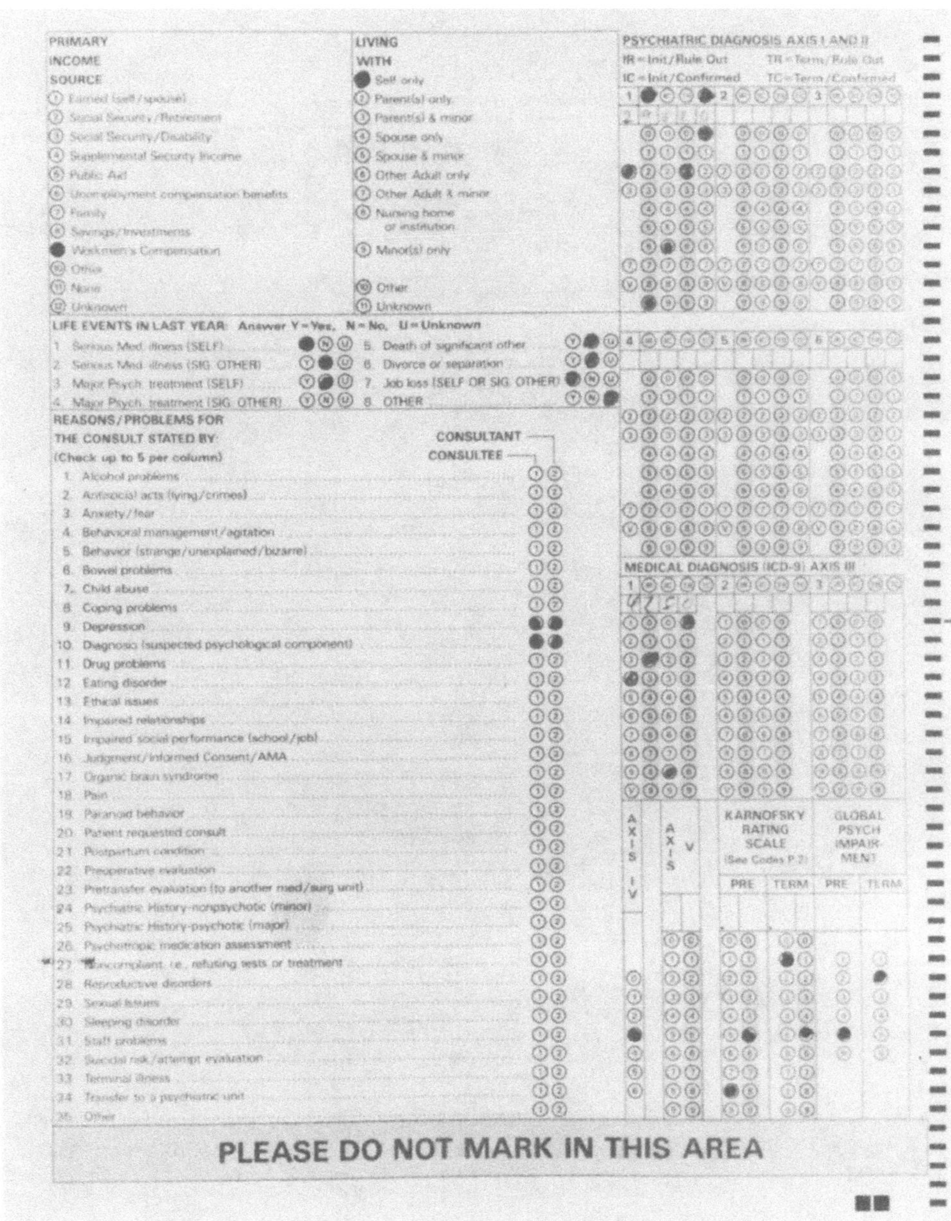

PRIMARY INCOME SOURCE
1. Earned (self/spouse)
2. Social Security/Retirement
3. Social Security/Disability
4. Supplemental Security Income
5. Public Aid
6. Unemployment compensation benefits
7. Family
8. Savings/Investments
9. Workmen's Compensation
10. Other
11. None
12. Unknown

LIVING WITH
1. Self only
2. Parent(s) only
3. Parent(s) & minor
4. Spouse only
5. Spouse & minor
6. Other Adult only
7. Other Adult & minor
8. Nursing home or institution
9. Minor(s) only
10. Other
11. Unknown

PSYCHIATRIC DIAGNOSIS AXIS I AND II
IR = Init/Rule Out   TR = Term/Rule Out
IC = Init/Confirmed   TC = Term/Confirmed

LIFE EVENTS IN LAST YEAR: Answer Y = Yes, N = No, U = Unknown
1. Serious Med. illness (SELF)
2. Serious Med. illness (SIG. OTHER)
3. Major Psych. treatment (SELF)
4. Major Psych. treatment (SIG. OTHER)
5. Death of significant other
6. Divorce or separation
7. Job loss (SELF OR SIG. OTHER)
8. OTHER

REASONS/PROBLEMS FOR THE CONSULT STATED BY:
(Check up to 5 per column)
CONSULTEE   CONSULTANT
1. Alcohol problems
2. Antisocial acts (lying/crimes)
3. Anxiety/fear
4. Behavioral management/agitation
5. Behavior (strange/unexplained/bizarre)
6. Bowel problems
7. Child abuse
8. Coping problems
9. Depression
10. Diagnosis (suspected psychological component)
11. Drug problems
12. Eating disorder
13. Ethical issues
14. Impaired relationships
15. Impaired social performance (school/job)
16. Judgment/Informed Consent/AMA
17. Organic brain syndrome
18. Pain
19. Paranoid behavior
20. Patient requested consult
21. Postpartum condition
22. Preoperative evaluation
23. Pretransfer evaluation (to another med/surg unit)
24. Psychiatric History-nonpsychotic (minor)
25. Psychiatric History-psychotic (major)
26. Psychotropic medication assessment
27. Noncompliant, i.e., refusing tests or treatment
28. Reproductive disorders
29. Sexual issues
30. Sleeping disorder
31. Staff problems
32. Suicidal risk/attempt evaluation
33. Terminal illness
34. Transfer to a psychiatric unit
35. Other

MEDICAL DIAGNOSIS (ICD-9) AXIS III

AXIS IV   AXIS V

KARNOFSKY RATING SCALE (See Codes P. 2)   GLOBAL PSYCH IMPAIRMENT
PRE   TERM   PRE   TERM

PLEASE DO NOT MARK IN THIS AREA

Figure 1 (continued).

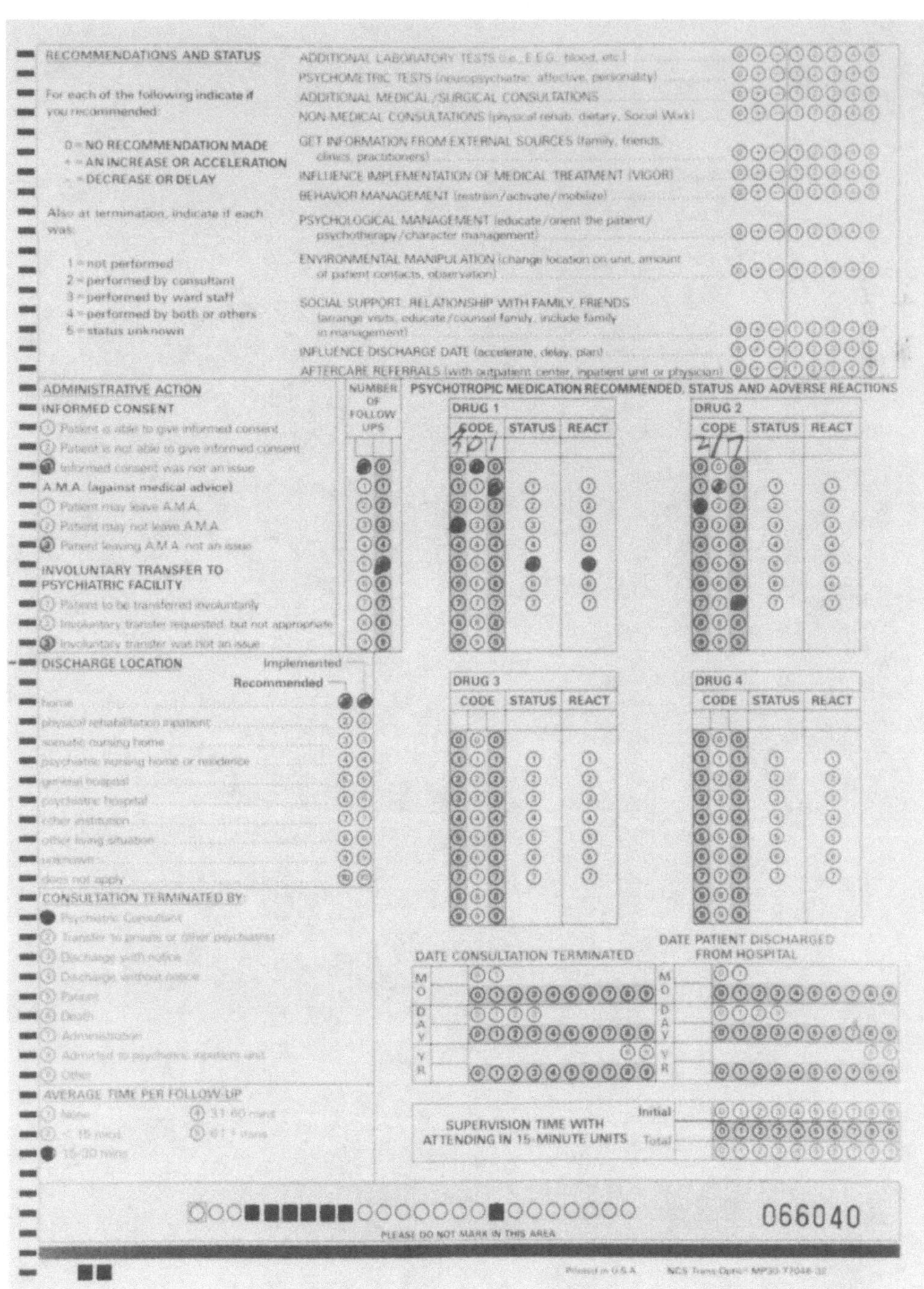

RECOMMENDATIONS AND STATUS

For each of the following indicate if you recommended:

0 = NO RECOMMENDATION MADE
+ = AN INCREASE OR ACCELERATION
− = DECREASE OR DELAY

Also at termination, indicate if each was:

1 = not performed
2 = performed by consultant
3 = performed by ward staff
4 = performed by both or others
5 = status unknown

ADDITIONAL LABORATORY TESTS (i.e., E.E.G., blood, etc.)
PSYCHOMETRIC TESTS (neuropsychiatric, affective, personality)
ADDITIONAL MEDICAL/SURGICAL CONSULTATIONS
NON-MEDICAL CONSULTATIONS (physical rehab, dietary, Social Work)
GET INFORMATION FROM EXTERNAL SOURCES (family, friends, clinics, practitioners)
INFLUENCE IMPLEMENTATION OF MEDICAL TREATMENT (VIGOR)
BEHAVIOR MANAGEMENT (restrain/activate/mobilize)
PSYCHOLOGICAL MANAGEMENT (educate/orient the patient/psychotherapy/character management)
ENVIRONMENTAL MANIPULATION (change location on unit, amount of patient contacts, observation)
SOCIAL SUPPORT. RELATIONSHIP WITH FAMILY, FRIENDS (arrange visits, educate/counsel family, include family in management)
INFLUENCE DISCHARGE DATE (accelerate, delay, plan)
AFTERCARE REFERRALS (with outpatient center, inpatient unit or physician)

ADMINISTRATIVE ACTION

INFORMED CONSENT
1 Patient is able to give informed consent
2 Patient is not able to give informed consent
3 Informed consent was not an issue

A.M.A. (against medical advice)
1 Patient may leave A.M.A.
2 Patient may not leave A.M.A.
3 Patient leaving A.M.A. not an issue

INVOLUNTARY TRANSFER TO PSYCHIATRIC FACILITY
1 Patient to be transferred involuntarily
2 Involuntary transfer requested, but not appropriate
3 Involuntary transfer was not an issue

NUMBER OF FOLLOW UPS

DISCHARGE LOCATION — Implemented — Recommended
home
physical rehabilitation inpatient
somatic nursing home
psychiatric nursing home or residence
general hospital
psychiatric hospital
other institution
other living situation
unknown
does not apply

CONSULTATION TERMINATED BY:
1 Psychiatric Consultant
2 Transfer to private or other psychiatrist
3 Discharge with notice
4 Discharge without notice
5 Patient
6 Death
7 Administration
8 Admitted to psychiatric inpatient unit
9 Other

AVERAGE TIME PER FOLLOW-UP
1 None
2 < 15 mins
3 15-30 mins
4 31-60 mins
5 61 + mins

PSYCHOTROPIC MEDICATION RECOMMENDED, STATUS AND ADVERSE REACTIONS

DRUG 1: CODE 401 | STATUS | REACT
DRUG 2: CODE 217 | STATUS | REACT
DRUG 3: CODE | STATUS | REACT
DRUG 4: CODE | STATUS | REACT

DATE CONSULTATION TERMINATED (MO, DAY, YR)

DATE PATIENT DISCHARGED FROM HOSPITAL (MO, DAY, YR)

SUPERVISION TIME WITH ATTENDING IN 15-MINUTE UNITS — Initial — Total

PLEASE DO NOT MARK IN THIS AREA

066040

Printed in U.S.A. NCS Trans-Optic MP30-77046-32

Figure 1 (continued).

CODE TRANSLATIONS

REFERRING SERVICE									
Anesthesia	= 01	General Surg.	= 19	Neurology	= 08	Orthopedics	= 12	Preventive Med	= 02
Card/Thor Surg	= 22	Gynecology	= 09	Neurosurgery	= 20	Otolaryngol.	= 13	Psychiatry	= 17
Dentistry	= 04	Hospice	= 27	Obstetrics	= 10	Pathology	= 14	Radiology	= 18
Dermatology	= 03	Infect. Dis.	= 06	Oncology	= 26	Pediatrics	= 15	Renal Medicine	= 07
Emergency Room	= 21	Medicine	= 05	Opthalmol.	= 11	Physical Med	= 16	Urology	= 24
______________	= 28	______________	= 29			Plastic Surg.	= 23	OTHER	= 25

KARNOFSKY SCALE: ESTIMATE FUNCTIONING DURING THE ONE MONTH PRIOR TO ADMISSION AND AT TERMINATION EXAM

ABLE TO CARRY ON NOR-MALLY. NO SPECIAL CARE IS NECESSARY	99%	Normal, no complaints, no evidence of disease.
	90%	Normal activity. Minor signs/symptoms of disease.
	80%	Normal activity with effort. Some signs/symptoms of disease.
UNABLE TO WORK BUT ABLE TO LIVE AT HOME & CARE FOR MOST PERSONAL NEEDS	70%	Cares for self, but can't perform normal activity or work.
	60%	Cares for self, but needs occasional assistance.
	50%	Requires considerable assistance and frequent medical care.
UNABLE TO CARE FOR SELF. NEEDS INSTITUTIONAL OR HOSPITAL CARE. DISEASE IS RAPIDLY PROGRESSING.	40%	Moderately disabled; requires special care/assistance.
	30%	Sever disabled; possible hospitalization; death not imminent.
	20%	Very sick. Hospitalization necessary.
	10%	Moribund with a fatal process progressing rapidly.
	0%	Died or will die within the week.

PSYCHOTROPIC MEDICATION RECOMMENDED, STATUS, AND ADVERSE REACTIONS

New = Agent started after patient arrived in hospital.

Old = Agent patient was taking at time of entry to hospital.

STATUS		REACTIONS	
1	New/Recc and Taken	1	Somatic/Definite
2	New/Recc and Not Taken	2	Somatic/Suspected
3	New/Recc/Taken-Discontinued	3	Psych./Definite
4	New/Recc/Unknown	4	Psych./Suspected
5	Old/Taken	5	No Adverse Reaction
6	Old/Discontinued	6	Unknown
7	Old/Unknown	7	Does not apply

CODES	ANTIANXIETY MEDICATION	
101	Alprazolam	XANAX
102	Chlordiazepoxide hydrochloride	LIBRIUM
102	Chlordiazepoxide hydrochloride	LIBRITABS
103	Clorazepate dipotassium	TRANXENE-SD
103	Clorazepate dipotassium	TRANXENE
104	Diazepam	VALIUM
104	Diazepam	VALRELEASE
105	Halazepam	PAXIPAM
106	Hydroxyzine hydrochloride	ATARAX
106	Hydroxyzine hydrochloride	ATARAX 100
106	Hydroxyzine hydrochloride	VISTARIL INTRAMUSC.
107	Hydroxyzine pamoate	VISTARIL
108	Lorazepam	ATIVAN
109	Meprobamate	EQUANIL
110	Oxazepam	SERAX
111	Prazepam	CENTRAX
112	OTHER	

	ANTIDEPRESSANT MEDICATION	
201	Amitriptyline hydrochloride	ELAVIL
201	Amitriptyline hydrochloride	ENDEP
202	Amoxapine	ASENDIN
203	Chlordiazep. & amitript.hydroch.	LIMBITROL
204	Desipramine hydrochloride	NORPRAMIN
205	Doxepin hydrochloride	SINEQUAN
205	Doxepin hydrochloride	ADAPIN
206	Imipramine hydrochloride	TOFRANIL
207	Imipramine pamoate	TOFRANIL-PM
208	Isocarboxazid	MARPLAN
209	Maprotiline hydrochloride	LUDIOMIL
210	Nortriptyline hydrochloride	PAMELOR
211	Perphenaz. & amitript.hydroch.	TRIAVIL
211	Perphenaz. & amitript.hydroch.	ETRAFON
212	Phenelzine sulfate	NARDIL
213	Protryptyline hydrochloride	VIVACTIL
214	Tranylcypramine sulfate	PARNATE
215	Trazodone hydrochloride	DESYREL
216	Trimipramine maleate	SURMONTIL
217	Fluoxetine hydrochloride	PROZAC
218	OTHER	

CODES	ANTIMANIC MEDICATION	
301	Lithium carbonate	ESKALITH
301	Lithium carbonate	ESKALITH-CR
301	Lithium carbonate	LITHOBID
302	Lithium citrate	CIBALITH-S
303	OTHER	

	ANTIPSYCHOTIC MEDICATION	
401	Chlorpromazine hydrochloride	THORAZINE
402	Fluphenazine hydrochloride	PERMITIL
402	Fluphenazine hydrochloride	PROLIXIN
403	Haloperidol	HALDOL
404	Loxapine hydrochloride	LOXITANE IM
404	Loxapine hydrochloride	LOXITANE C
405	Loxapine succinate	LOXITANE
406	Perphenazine	TRILAFON
407	Prochlorperazine	COMPAZINE
408	Thioridazine	MELLARIL-S
409	Thioridazine hydrochloride	MELLARIL
410	Thiothixene	NAVANE
411	Trifluoperazine hydrochloride	STELAZINE
412	OTHER	

	SEDATIVES, HYPNOTICS, ANTICONVULSANTS	
501	Phenobarbital	PHENOBARBITAL
502	Phenobarbital sodium	PHENO. SODIUM
503	Ethchlorvynol	PLACIDYL
504	Flurazepam hydrochloride	DALMANE
505	Mephobarbital	MEBARAL
506	Methyprylon	NOLUDAR 300
506	Methyprylon	NOLUDAR
507	Pentobarbital	NEMBUTAL EXLIXIR
508	Pentobarbital sodium	NEMB.SODIUM CAPS
508	Pentobarbital sodium	NEMB.SOD.SUPPOS.
509	Secobarbital sodium	SECONAL SODIUM
510	Temazepam	RESTORIL
511	Triazolam	HALCION
512	Diphenylhydantoin	DILANTIN
513	Carbamazipine	TEGRETOL
514	OTHER	

To program for these in house form generation possibilities and the automatic internal audit would have been impossible in the previously reported versions of MICRO-CARES, but the new version incorporates the vehicles to automatically resolve the form, and the users' desired reliability checks by a newly advanced software language and mechanism - the Medical Application Platform (MAP) - program writer and form generator (Figure 2). The MAP using its own procedural language - METAVIEW - is able to: 1) resolve the data form generation at will; 2) create the internal data files necessary to accomplish the desired studies and clinical data management operations; 3) creates the microcomputer screens, including the internal/automatic data checks and validation procedures; 4) organizes the output data streams into reports and formats to use with the desired statistical packages, e.g., SAS, or for transport to the hospital/medical school mainframe for enhanced statistical management, and 5) import either batch obtained or real time obtained patient records from the hospital mainframe.

OBJECT ORIENTATION AND RELATIONAL CHARACTERISTICS

The MAP employs a newer language - METAVIEW - which is "object oriented" and allows for the relative ease of integration of data sets coming from the hospital mainframe and at the same time is close to "fully relational" in its capacity to store data, thus allowing automatic linkage between multiple files of the same patient. Previously with MICRO-CARES Version 5 and many of the software packages currently available for the PC to manage clinical data sets, the research could have only one file open at a time, e.g., "Open Table one," "Close Table One," and then "Open Table Two, etc. With the current MAP structure one can "open" many files simultaneously so that the user can have access to enormous data sets across multiple files. For example, one could have in the PC on line contemporaneously a clinical data set plus information from structured instruments: Hamilton Depression Rating Scale, Quality Assurance, Medical Status, Psychological Sympotomology, Social/Demographic Information, Patient Satisfaction Forms, Mental Status/Cognitive Scales, Biological Measures, laboratory results, etc. The METAVIEW language employed in the MAP allows multiple files with one to one, and one to many relationships to be opened and automatically accessible at the same time. Thus, the economy of handling multiple domains of data maintained in disparate files within the system is significantly enhanced for the clinician/researcher in his/her own office. This capacity is utilized to create subsets of information, which creates subsets across multiple files and exports these subsets to report writers, spread sheets, and statistical packages e.g., SAS. As stated previously conceptual framework of the MAP also includes the tools for the computer to generate its own screens, forms, programs, menus and data validation routines. These are generated after the user answers prompts about his/her needs regarding variables in Branch Chains. MICRO-CARES was a stand-alone computer application which we built specifically for the CLP setting, while the current MAP is a program generator specially tailored to the medical environment and can be used throughout the medical care system and for multiple areas of interest. The critical evolutionary step for this function was enclosed by a language which allowed multiple users simultaneous access to data and by hardware progression to the point where local area microcomputer networks are commonplace. An attempt to do this using a minicomputer was reported by the authors in 1985, but was abandoned because of expensive considerations.

COSTS

The costs of maintaining a clinical database in CLP fall into three domains. First is the cost of the hardware elements, such as the microcomputer, monitor, transoptic scanner and printer. As most are aware, hardware prices have come down significantly since the first iteration of MICRO-CARES, such that a suitable microcomputer currently

Mainframe
Data
Transfer
Infrared
Grid Pad
MAP
Facilities
Import Other
User Data
Sets
MAP
Merge
Validate
Subset
Export
Report
Graph
SAS
User Defined
Scanner Forms
Output
Manual
Data
Entry
Input

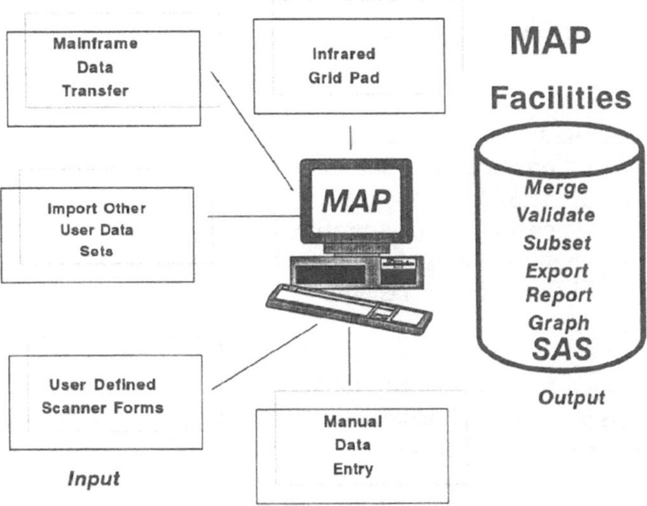

Figure 2.

costs approximately $2000, as apposed $6500 in 1983, a laser printer approximately $1300 as apposed to $5000 in 1984, and a transoptic scanner is available for about $3500. Of the 20 active sites using MICRO-CARES at this time, several have saved the cost of a scanner by sending forms to a sister site. The forms (plus floppy disks) are returned from the scanning to the local site, where the data on disk is imported into the microcomputer. The second element of cost is the software. The original cost of the MICRO-CARES software was $4500, but this has been reduced to $500 in the last year. The MAP software is currently a commercial product and currently costs $7500, including the desktop publishing elements. It is considered out of range for all but the wealthiest of institutions. However, the authors are currently working on a non-commercial version, which will be multi-user, and allow multiple Branch Chains on forms produced by the authors for approximately $500. Thus it is planned that in the near future that a workable multi-user version will be available for a total of approximately $2500 for hardware and software elements. The final element of costs is the ongoing maintenance and training required, which varies from site to site as does the time investment, both filling out forms and checking each one by the attending physician or supervisors. The "care and feeding" of the system to insure quality data input over time should not be underestimated.

EXTENSIONS IN THE USE OF THE DATABASE

PEDAGOGIC

With the current focus of the Joint Commission on Accreditation of Healthcare Organizations (JCAHO) on education (26), and the demand by graduate medical education training certification agencies for a complete listing of patient numbers and types patient outcome measures, the consultation data profile (CONDAT) becomes an important menu-driven report that highlights not only the specific patients seen, but displays the psychiatric interventions effected in a summary fashion. (Table I) (34). Drugs prescribed by each trainee can also be obtained.

The intervention section of this CONDAT demonstrates that this consultant did not interfere with or discourage any medical/surgical procedure - "zero decrease or delay;" recommended only one of 40 patients to have psychometric evaluations. It is apparent this consultant did little to decrease medical utilization or intervention by the consultee, ordered relatively few psychometric tests (N=5), or recommendations for behavioral management (N=6), environmental manipulations (N=8), social supports (N=9) or influenced discharge date (N=3). These are all areas for the supervisor to examine, to note if the psychiatric resident trainee is maximizing the use his therapeutic armamentarium with his consultation population. Such a display of interventions permits a supervisor to examine the kinds and frequency of interventions recommended by a consultant, compare them with the patient's diagnoses, and drug administration profile. In addition, the supervisor can check how many patients were discharged without notifying the psychiatric consultant and how often the prescribed recommendations were not followed, both indications of a possible breakdown in consultant-consultee relationships.

The database has be used to observe if a consultant is in the "defined" range for the average number of cases, usual numbers of follow-ups, absences of recommendations in certain expected domains, consultees' lack of compliance with their recommendations beyond the institutional norm, etc. Then the training director can discuss which trainees are the "outline" in prescribed areas based on expected performance from observations of the group as a whole - from the observed norms of the system in which the trainee operates. Such a method allows the clinician/researcher to continually examine the trainee's behavior against the group norm, against the trainee's own earlier performance, or against the performance of trainees at another institution.

TABLE I

CONDAT INTERVENTION SUMMARY

	NO RECOMMENDATIONS	INCREASE ACCELERATE	DECREASE OR DELAY
1. Laboratory tests	23	28	0
2. Psychometric tests	46	5	0
3. Medical/surgical consultation	42	9	0
4. Non-medical consultations	36	1	0
5. Get information from external sources	32	19	0
6. Influence implementation of medical treatment	40	5	0
7. Behavior management	45	6	0
8. Psychological management	32	19	0
9. Environmental manipulation	43	8	0
10. Social support (family friends)	41	9	1
11. Influence discharge date	44	3	4
12. Aftercare referrals	34	17	0

QUALITY ASSESSMENT AND IMPROVEMENT

In addition to regulatory pressure to document post graduate training, there is a similar requirement for medical departments and divisions to document improvement in the quality of their care (26).

Aided by computerized database systems, which include critical data/clinical elements, one can examine quality by using these elements as rate based indicators measured over time. Measuring and improving the quality and appropriateness of care through continuous monitoring and evaluation of clinical performance indicators is the hallmark of quality assessment and improvement programs today. Modern quality improvement models had their origin in structure, process and outcome as the domains or abstract construct for describing aspects of "quality of care" (27). The systematized computerization of a pre-agreed upon clinical database is a first and crucial step toward examine these constructs in the CLP setting. To date the computerization of a clinical database for the CLP setting has been fairly infrequent, and its use for Quality Assessment and Improvement activities almost is non existent.

Although process and outcome measures may overlap, consider the following. One could measure lag time between calling for a consultation and its actual initiation. If it were expected that a consultation should be answered within one hour, eight hours, or 48 hours, deviations or variations from expectations could be examined by consultant, by initiating ward or service by diagnosis, by reason for referral, etc. In examining all the cases - the denominator norms could be established for the group and those and those individuals who deviated significantly from those norms. Thus using a process variable - lag time answer to a consultation - one could describe in measurable terms, the quality of answering consultations by consultant. Individuals who performed better than expected could be used to teach the group about their practice patterns. The "average lag time" could be used as a benchmark in establishing the baseline for improvement efforts. It has been shown that lag time effects an outcome measure related to the efficiency i.e., LOS. (24,28). LOS in a hospital setting often is a measure of quality of care in that longer LOS leads to more frequent nosocomial infections and pulmonary embolis. The improvement in process outcome over time is the essence of current quality management efforts. Further, the variations in performance between individuals and for the aggregate may be used to construct focused evaluations/interventions to explain variation while reducing it. This leads to more predictable outcomes. These focused evaluation/interventions are a series of "yes or no" questions constructed as Branch Chains for concurrent use in specific clinical situations, i.e., hypertensive patients, who have bipolar disorder. They are not only data that is collected as, but act as "triggers, reminder, or teachers" to the practitioner who fills them out concurrently in this special clinical situation.

Numerous variables lend themselves to process/outcome examination: 1) who terminated the consultation, 2) number of follow-ups, 3) use of which drugs which diagnoses, 4) adverse drug side effects, 5) compliance with recommendations by the consultant, 6) amount of supervision for time spent in service delivery etc. In fact, the clinical database is a natural for many important outcomes in the consultation setting. The concept of an indicator - allows the establishment of norms from the denominator of any of these variables and then the performance of the decreet individuals (the numerator) as compared with these system developed norms. Outliers could be identified and subjected to further analysis for their appropriateness or not. If more medically ill patients on ACE inhibitors developed lithium toxicity over time, compared to other anti-hypertensive medications, both process and outcome could be improved by a dialogue between internist and psychiatric consultant which lead to a change in medication prescribing practices.

THE EUROPEAN CONSORTIUM

In addition to expanding the MICRO-CARES database, Huyse and colleagues have adopted the Optical Scan format to produce a similar database, which has been used in multiple European countries to derive a collaborative CLP registration and process dataset (29). Form production, scanning and data analysis are done at a single central site, with centrally based training and reliability requirements for more consistent multi-site studies. The process has been funded by common market governments. The increased rigor and reliability inherent of this centralized process is compared to that of the American group, is somewhat offset by the delay in providing reports to the local site with local sites not having an option to fully utilize their dataset for interactive pedagogic, administrative quality based endeavors. There is a planned merging of the strengths of both systems with a short form database developed by Smith, Huyse, Strain and Hammer anticipated in 1994 (30).

SUMMARY

This chapter explores the increasing need for CLP to utilize clinical database systems to permit ongoing service management, to detail and track pedagogic efforts, and to assess and improve the quality and appropriateness of care provided. Although MICRO-CARES and its 14 years of evolution is the primary focus, two other paradigms are discussed. The most recent iteration of MICRO-CARES with its ability to desktop publish and program optically scanned forms, import and export data to mainframe computers, and to provide multi-user departmental integration has flexibility advantages, but some cost disadvantages. Planned subsequent iteractions are described. These may have more universal application.

NOTE

This work has been supported in part by the Green Fund, New York City. Portions of this chapter have been previously presented in an article in General Hospital Psychiatry, May, 1993.

ACKNOWLEDGEMENT

The authors wish to acknowledge the assistance of Ms. Mirjami Easton and Mrs. Carolyn Brown-Turner in the preparation of this manuscript.

REFERENCES

1. Taintor Z, Gise LH, Spikes J, Strain J: Recording psychiatric consultations: A preliminary report. Gen. Hosp. Psychiatry, 20:139-149, 1979.

2. Hamburg, B: Personal communication.

3. McKegney FP, Schwartz CE, O'Down MA et al: Development of an optically scanned consultation-liaison database.
General Hospital Psychiatry 112:71-76, 1990.

4. Hammer JS, Lyons J, and Strain JJ: MICRO-CARES: An Information Management System for Psychosocial Services in Hospital Settings. *Proceedings SCAMC,* 8:234-237, 1984.

5. Hammer JS, Hammond D, Strain JJ, and Lyons J: Microcomputers and Consultation Psychiatry in the General Hospital.
General Hospital Psychiatry, 7:119-124, 1985.

6. Hammer JS, Lyons J, and Strain JJ: Evolution of a Stand-Alone Integrated Microcomputer Software System for Psychiatric Services.
Computers in Psychiatry/Psychology, Par I, 7:7-9, 1985.

7. Hammer JS, Lyons J, and Strain JJ. Core Structure and Application Design of a Stand-Alone, Integrated Microcomputer.
Computers in Psychiatry/Psychology, Part II, 7:8-10, 1985.

8. Hammer JS, Barrett TP, and Lyons J. Integration of Disparate Microcomputer Systems Using a Minicomputer as a Passive File Server in a Distributive Network.
Proceedings SCAMC,

9. Hammer JS, Lyons J, and Strain JJ. Extensions, Enhancements, and Computer Considerations of a Stand-Alone Microcomputer System for Psychiatry Services. MICRO-CARES.
Computers in Psychiatry/Psychology, Part IV, 16-20, 1986.

10. Strain JJ, Fulop G, Strain J, Hammer JS, and Taintor Z: An Approach to Psychiatric Teaching: The Evaluation of a Computer Enhanced Teaching Program.
Journal of Psychiatric Education, 10, #2, Summer 1986.

11. Lyons J, Hammer JS, and White RE: Computerization of Psychosocial Services in the General Hospital. Collaborative Information Management in the Human Service Department.
Computers in Human Services, 1986.

12. Hammer JS, Lyons J, and Strain JJ: Development of a Stand-Alone Microcomputer System for Consultation/Liaison Psychiatry Service.
Computers in Psychiatry/Psychology, Part III, 7:15-18, Winter 1986.

13. Hammer JS, Strain JJ, and Petraitis JM: Consortium Based Consultation/Liaison Research Commentary and Perspective.
International Journal of Psychiatry in Medicine, 17(3), 237-248, 1987.

14. Huyse F, Strain JJ, Hengeveld MW, Hammer JS, and Zwaan T: Interventions in Consultation/Liaison Psychiatry The Development of a Scheme and a Checklist of Operational Interventions.
General Hospital Psychiatry, 10,88-101, 1988.

15. Huyse F, Strain JJ, Hammer JS, Interventions in Consultation/Liaison Psychiatry. Part II: Concordance.
General Hospital Psychiatry,12:221 - 231, 1990.

16. Leigh H, Reiser M: A systematic approach to psychiatric consultation.
J. Psychosomatic Research 26:76, 1982.

17. Popkin MK, MacKenzie IB, Callies AL: Consultation liaison outcome evaluation system I consultant-consultee interaction.
Arch Gen Psychiatry 40:215-219, 1983.

18. Holland, J: Personal communication.

19. Blumenfeld, M, Wallack J: Personal communication.

20. Lyons J, Hammer JS, and Strain JJ: The Timing of Psychiatric Consultation in the General Hospital and Length of hospital Stay.
General Hospital Psychiatry, 8:159-162, 1986.

21. Fulop G, Strain JJ, Vita J, Lyons J, and Hammer JS: Impact of Psychiatric Comorbidity on Length of Hospital Stay for Medical/Surgical Patients: A Preliminary Report.
American Journal of Psychiatry, 144(7), 878-882, July, 1987.

22. Strain JJ, Norvell CM, Strain J, Mueenuddin T, Strain JW: A microcomputer approach to consultation-liaison data basing: Pedagog-Admin-Clinfo.
General Hospital Psychiatry 7:113-118, 1985.

23. Hammer JS, Lyons J, Strain JJ: MICRO-CARES: An information Management System for Psychosocial Services in Hospital Settings.
Proc. SMAMC, 8:234:237, 1984.

24. Lyons J, Hammer JS, Strain JJ, Fulop G: The timing of psychiatric consultation in the general hospital and length of hospital stay.
General Hospital Psychiatry 8:159-162, 1986.

25. Fulop G, Strain JJ: Psychiatric emergenicies in the general hospital.
General Hospital Psychiatry; 425-431, 1986.

26. Strain JJ, Tainto Z, Gise LH, Spikes J: Informed consent - mandating the consultation.
General Hospital Psychiatry 78:228-233, 1985.

27. Accreditation Manual for Hospitals Vol 1 - 1993, Chicago, Joint Commission Press.

28. Donabedian: Explorations in quality assessment and monitoring, vol I. In the Defination of Quality or Quality and Approaches to its Assessment. Ann Arbor, MI, Health Administration Press, 1980.

29. Ackerman AD, Lyons J, Hammer JS, Larsen DB: The Impact of Coexisting Depression and Timing of Psychiatric Consultation on Medical Patients Length of Stay.
Hospital & Community Psychiatry, 39:173-176, February 1988.

30. European Common Community - Research Grant Funding - 1990-1995, Brussels, Belgium.

31. Smith G, Huyse F, Strain J, Hammer J: Personal communication.

CONTRIBUTORS

Hoyle Leigh, M.D., Editor
Professor and Vice-Chairman
Department of Psychiatry
University of California, San Francisco
Director, Fresno Division
Chief of Psychiatry
Fresno VA Medical Center
2615 East Clinton Avenue
Fresno, CA 93703

Scott Ahles, M.D.
Associate Clinical Professor of Psychiatry
Fresno Division
University of California, San Francisco
Chief of Psychiatry
Valley Medical Center
445 South Cedar Ave
Fresno, CA 93703

Stuart J. Eisendrath, M.D.
Associate Professor of Clinical Psychiatry
Director, Psychiatric Consultation-Liaison Program
University of California, San Francisco
Langley Porter Psychiatric Institute
401 Parnassus Avenue Box F-0984
San Francisco, CA 94143-0984

Byron Eliashof, M.D.
Associate Clinical Professor of Psychiatry
University of Hawaii at Manoa
John A. Burns School of Medicine
Department of Psychiatry
1356 Lusitana Street
Honolulu, HI 96813

David Fox, M.D.
Associate Clinical Professor Psychiatry
Fresno Division
University of California, San Francisco
Director of Residency Training
Department of Developmental and Behavioral Pediatrics
Valley Children's Hospital
Fresno, CA 93703

George Fulop, M.D.
Assistant Professor of Psychiatry and Community Medicine
City University of New York
Mt. Sinai Hospital
One Gustav L. Levy Place
New York, NY 10029

Stephen R. Griffith, M.D.
Associate Clinical Professor of Psychiatry
Fresno Division
Department of Psychiatry
University of California, San Francisco
Medical Director
Chemical Dependence Treatment Program
Fresno Veterans Affairs Medical Center
2615 East Clinton Avenue
Fresno, CA 93703

Robert Hanowell, M.D.
Chief Resident
Fresno Division
University of California, San Francisco
2615 East Clinton Avenue
Fresno, CA 93703

Jeffrey S. Hammer, M.D.
Associate Professor of Clinical Psychiatry
University of California, Los Angeles
Director, Quality Management Service
West Los Angeles VA Medical Center
Los Angeles, CA 90073

Seth Powsner, M.D.
Associate Professor of Psychiatry
Department of Psychiatry
Yale School of Medicine
333 Cedar Street
New Haven, CT 06511

James Strain, M.D.
Professor of Psychiatry
Director, Division of Behavioral Medicine and Consultation Psychiatry
City University of New York
Mt. Sinai Hospital
One Gustav L. Levy Place
New York, NY 10029

Jon Streltzer, M.D.
Professor of Psychiatry
Director of Residency Training
University of Hawaii at Manoa
John A. Burns School of Medicine
Department of Psychiatry
1356 Lusitana Street
Honolulu, HI 96813

Lowell Tong, M.D.
Assistant Clinical Professor of Psychiatry
University of California, San Francisco
Director of Residency Training
San Francisco VA Medical Center
4150 Clement Street
San Francisco, CA 94121

Craig Van Dyke, M.D.
Professor and Chairman
Department of Psychiatry
University of California, San Francisco
401 Parnassus Rd.
San Francisco, CA 94143

INDEX

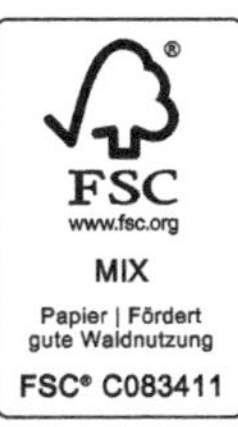

Zeitfracht Medien GmbH
Ferdinand-Jühlke-Straße 7
99095 Erfurt, Deutschland
produktsicherheit@kolibri360.de